The Formation of the Swiss Hospital System (1840–1960)

Pierre-Yves Donzé

The Formation of the Swiss Hospital System (1840–1960)

An Analysis of Surgeon-Modernisers in the Canton of Vaud

palgrave
macmillan

Pierre-Yves Donzé
Graduate School of Economics
Osaka University
Toyonaka, Japan

ISBN 978-981-19-3910-5 ISBN 978-981-19-3911-2 (eBook)
https://doi.org/10.1007/978-981-19-3911-2

This Palgrave Macmillan imprint is published by the registered company Springer Nature Singapore Pte Ltd.
The registered company address is: 152 Beach Road, #21-01/04 Gateway East, Singapore 189721, Singapore

Preface to the English Edition

This volume is the English edition of a book initially published in French under the title *L'ombre de César. Les chirurgiens et la construction du système hospitalier vaudois (1840–1960)*, by Editions BHMS. I offer my sincere gratitude to the publisher who has granted me the opportunity to produce an English edition. This book was based on a dissertation submitted in 2005 to the University of Neuchâtel, Switzerland, for the degree of Doctor of Philosophy. Research for the dissertation was conducted under the joint supervision of Professor Laurent Tissot (University of Neuchâtel) and Professor Vincent Barras (University of Lausanne). Nearly twenty years after the completion of this work, it is again a pleasure to express my deep gratitude to both for their guidance during my formative years as a historian.

Why publish an English version of this work today? My career has given me a unique opportunity to broaden my academic horizon. I have been carrying out research on the global dynamics of various industries, from watchmaking to luxury and fashion, food and medical devices. Moreover, I have had the chance to expand the scope of my interests and to analyse the formation and development of the healthcare business in Japan and globally. In recent years, I have benefited from friendly collaboration with several business historians and historians of medicine who have contributed to the renewal of my research interests. I would like to extend my warmest thanks to Paloma Fernández Pérez (University of Barcelona) with whom I share the desire to explore new dimensions of the history of healthcare industries to understand properly how this field has emerged and grown as a global business. My respectful acknowledgement goes to Akihito Suzuki (The University of Tokyo) who guided me through the twists and turns of Japanese historiography during my first years in this country. I wish also to thank Ken Sakai (Tohoku University, Sendai), Maki Umemura (Cardiff University), Ben Wubs (Erasmus University, Rotterdam) and Julia Yongue (Hosei University, Tokyo) for the fruitful discussions and exchanges on the business history of medicine. Finally, I offer my deep gratitude to Takafumi Kurosawa (Kyoto University) for all the academic and friendly debates we have had for so many years.

Beyond my personal career, the field of the business history of health and medicine has developed considerably during the last decade. Further to this, the shock of the COVID-19 pandemic and its deep impact on healthcare systems will undoubtedly attract attention to the historical foundations of health and medicine and the way they have developed over the years. Upon considering the book that I published in French in 2007 could contribute to a better understanding of these issues, I decided to prepare an English edition, addressed to a global audience. This book is not a mere translation of the original version. The introduction has been largely rewritten to include the contributions of new works published during the last twelve years. Moreover, details relating to Swiss local history and politics, which do not hold much meaning to the global audience, have been omitted. The English version is hence shorter than the original and more focused on the core arguments developed throughout the book: surgeon-modernisers became major actors in the formation of modern hospital medicine, and the hospital system is the appropriate scale to investigate this transformation.

Osaka, Japan
April 2022

Pierre-Yves Donzé

Contents

List of Figures

Chapter 4

Chapter 5

List of Tables

Chapter 5

CHAPTER 1

Introduction

Over the course of the twentieth century, the hospital has become one of the major and indispensable institutions of our contemporary societies. On an economic level, first of all, hospitals occupy a central place at the heart of public health, a sector that today represents more than 10% of GDP in most European countries (11.3% in Switzerland) and 16.8% in the United States.[1] Moreover, hospitals are often the main employers in their localities and operate with annual budgets that can exceed one billion francs.[2] The importance of today's hospital also has a social dimension, in that it has become a place of passage for the overwhelming majority of the population. Important stages of life, such as birth and death, now take place in hospitals. Finally, at the scientific level, the hospital appears to be the main place for the constitution and transmission of medical knowledge.

Compared to the largely marginal institution it was in the nineteenth century, intended primarily for a poor population, the hospital underwent a fundamental upheaval, not only in scale, during the first part of the twentieth century. This phenomenal growth leaves one wondering. What, indeed, may explain such a transformation? The classic and widely accepted interpretation—i.e., the development of medical knowledge, increases in the complexity of the techniques used and new scientific discoveries; in short, the march towards

[1] OECD figures for 2019, https://data.oecd.org/healthres/health-spending.htm (accessed 10 February 2022).

[2] In 2020, the Geneva University Hospitals, the largest hospital centre in Switzerland, employed more than 13,500 people, including more than 2500 doctors, and had an operating budget of more than two billion francs. Source: HUG website, https://www.hug.ch/faits-et-chiffres (accessed 10 February 2022).

P.-Y. Donzé, *The Formation of the Swiss Hospital System (1840–1960)*,
https://doi.org/10.1007/978-981-19-3911-2_1

a triumphant profession leading to larger and better-equipped hospitals—is insufficient, although it remains omnipresent in traditional historiography.[3] Medicine did not develop in a linear and constant manner. Nor did it have causal links with the hospital establishments in which it developed.

1 Influence of the Social History of Medicine

Since the 1970s, historians have endeavoured to bring the interplay of actors into new focus to show that the construction of hospital medicine not only responds to scientific imperatives, intrinsic to medical knowledge, but also to political, social and economic issues. The functions of the hospital in the city are indeed multiple and go beyond the singular framework of medical discoveries. For the most part, this new history of medicine has been structured around "medicalisation", a concept developed by Michel Foucault when he examined the reorganisation of hospitals that occurred at the end of the eighteenth century.[4] Thought of as the refocusing of these establishments on the care of the sick through the increasing intervention of doctors, medicalisation was then considered as a consequence of "the introduction of disciplinary mechanisms into the disordered space of the hospital".[5] This perspective has greatly inspired historians, particularly Anglo-Saxon ones,[6] who in turn have left their mark on research into the social history of medicine, such as that carried out by Othmar Keel on the transformation of hospitals into centres of medical practice and clinical education. Keel identifies hospital medicalisation as a decisive stage in the affirmation of the anatomical-clinical paradigm and defines it in this context as "the transformation [...] that takes place in various European countries in the eighteenth century of certain institutions of assistance or social regulation into therapeutic and medical-scientific institutions".[7] In Germany, Foucault's influence is also evident and historians make medicalisation an essential basis for social disciplining (*Soziale Disziplinierung*) in the nineteenth century. The strengthening of the sanitary police, the development of health insurance and the development of hospitals are generally interpreted as elements intended to ensure control over the working classes.[8]

[3] Jean Imbert (ed.), *Histoire des hôpitaux en France*, Toulouse: Privat, 1982.

[4] Michel Foucault, *Naissance de la clinique*, Paris: PUF, 1963.

[5] Michel Foucault, "L'incorporation de l'hôpital dans la technologie moderne", *Dits et écrits*, vol. 3, 1998, p. 517.

[6] Colin Jones and Roy Porter (eds), *Reassessing Foucault: Power, Medicine and the Body*, London/New York: Routledge, 1994.

[7] Othmar Keel, *The Advent of Modern Clinical Medicine in Europe, 1750–1815*, Geneva: Georg, 2001, pp. 29–30.

[8] Alfons Labisch and Reinhardt Spree, "Neuere Entwicklungen und aktuelle Trends in der Sozialgeschichte der Medizin in Deutschland - Rückschau und Ausblick", *Vierteljahrschrift für Sozial- und Wirtschaftsgeschichte*, 1997, pp. 171–210 and 305–321 and Francisca Loetz, *Von Kranken zum Patienten. "Medikalisierung" und medizinische Vergesellschaftung am Beispiel Badens 1750–1850*, Stuttgart: Franz Steiner Verlag, 1993.

However, the notion of medicalisation was diversified during the 1980s and 1990s, as in the work of the French historians Jacques Léonard, Jean-Pierre Goubert and Olivier Faure. For such authors, medicalisation is not only a process imposed by the ruling classes on the people, but the result of a real cultural revolution, in the sense that it is largely based on the internalisation by the population of new healthcare practices.[9] Today, medicalisation appears to be a polysemous concept whose use poses a number of problems. It is very rarely defined explicitly in the various studies and the term is used to define diverse realities, on a variable chronological scale. In general, medicalisation can be said to express an idea of process, moving from a state *before* to a state *after*, the latter being distinguished by a new situation in which medicine occupies a reinforced position. Several types of processes have been described by historians as medicalisation. For example, technical innovations (anaesthesia, antisepsis, bacteriology, genetics), the professionalisation of certain care functions (doctors, nurses, midwives), institutional reorganisations (such as the separation of the sick from the elderly in hospitals) or changes in the population's attitude (such as recourse to hospital care), have all transformed the practice of medicine and the consumption of healthcare. Faure highlights the deterministic nature that can result from the use of the term: "Identified as early as the Middle Ages by a greater presence of doctors, medicalisation would have developed unabated with clinical medicine, pastoral medicine and then the opening up to all of a hospital that had previously been reserved for the poor".[10] As he points out, the problem is that medicalisation is the bearer of a linear, deterministic, even teleological conception of the development of medicine over the last few centuries, with each innovation—and the new social uses it implies—being perceived as a step from the "less medicalised" to the "more medicalised".

2 Medicine as a Sociotechnical System

Research into the history of techniques, and more broadly into economic history, makes it possible to consider the construction of hospital medicine from a different angle. The notion of the "technical system" appears to be much more appropriate.[11] According to Bertrand Gille, technical systems are the result of a balance between various interacting techniques at a given time.[12] In this perspective, historical analysis highlights phases of equilibrium

[9] Jacques Léonard, *Les médecins de l'Ouest au XIXe siècle*, Paris: Champion, 1978; Jean-Pierre Goubert (ed.), *La médicalisation de la société française, 1770–1830*, Waterloo: Historial Reflections Press, 1982; Olivier Faure, *Genèse de l'hôpital moderne: les hospices civils de Lyon de 1802 à 1845*, Lyon: Presses universitaires de Lyon, 1982.

[10] Olivier Faure, "Vingt ans d'histoire de la santé", *Revue historique vaudoise*, 1995, p. 322.

[11] For a first approach to technical systems in economic history, see François Caron, *Les deux révolutions industrielles du 20e siècle*, Paris: Albin Michel, 1997.

[12] Bertrand Gille (ed.), *Histoire des techniques*, Paris: Gallimard, 1978.

and phases of readjustment of the system when a new technique appears or evolves. Moreover, the technical system is not autonomous but linked to other systems (economic, political and social), which have their own logic, and with which it is in constant interaction. However, Gille does not give a primary role to the actors: for him, the technical system results more from a cumulative process of all the techniques implemented at a given time than from a constructivist process resulting from the interplay of the actors.[13] It is thus quite conceivable and easy to apply Gille's model to medicine. The "medical-technical system" could thus be understood as the set of medical techniques existing at a given moment and grouping together machines and objects (e.g., operating tables, forceps, scalpels, stethoscopes), gestures gathered into bodies of doctrine (collected in books and taught in universities) and products (e.g., chloroform, catgut, cocaine, drugs). The appearance of a new technique, such as anaesthesia in the mid-nineteenth century, radiology in the 1890s or antibiotics in the 1940s, would then upset the balance of the medical-technical system, forcing it to readapt. Such an interpretation, even if it takes into account the interaction with other systems is, however, not sufficient. There is a great risk of giving too much importance to medical technology itself in explaining the construction of hospital medicine, and the use of Gille's concept only reinforces the evolutionary interpretation.

The notion of technical system conceptualised by Gille in the 1970s has greatly evolved, particularly thanks to the reflections of constructivist sociologists such as Thomas Hughes. The technical system, as the latter understands it, is not the mere accumulation of machines, tools, knowledge and technical gestures, but the interaction between these elements and modes of management, organisational models, financing policies and industrial interests. Technical systems are not autonomous products but are constructed and directed by actors.[14] Hughes thus uses the concept of a "sociotechnical system", i.e., a system that contains both technical and organisational elements.[15] The economic, political and social are not reduced to the environment, as is the case with Gille, but are considered as elements of the sociotechnical system. Applying the same perspective, François Caron highlights the problem of the transition from one sociotechnical system to another. He shows that certain dysfunctions or innovations, whether of a technical, political, economic or other nature, accelerate the instability inherent in any technical system and the search for a new equilibrium: industrial revolutions are thus seen as periods of profound upheaval which see the transition from one sociotechnical system to another.[16]

[13] Yves Cohen and Dominique Pestre (ed.), "Histoire des techniques", *Annales: Histoire, Sciences sociales*, 1998, pp. 735–738.

[14] Thomas P. Hughes, *Networks of Power: Electrification in Western Society, 1880–1930*, Baltimore: Johns Hopkins University Press, 1983.

[15] Ibidem, p. 465.

[16] François Caron, op. cit.

This way of understanding the history of technology and science has directly influenced the history of medicine. Several sociologists and historians have included medicine in their reflections on innovation and technical change. Following the work of researchers such as Thomas Hughes, Wiebe Bijker and Trevor Pinch in the 1980s,[17] some authors have taken an interest in the technical development of medicine and "there has grown a 'new school' which treats medical technology as another element in the social, political, and economic history of medicine, relating it to professionalisation, changing notions about disease, and the organisation of medical care".[18] Stuart Blume uses the example of medical imaging to show that the development of medical technology is the result of a social construction process.[19] In France, Bruno Latour's work on Pasteur and the construction of science in laboratories, which influenced a whole generation of historians of science,[20] should be highlighted.

Inspired by the work of Bijker and the sociologists of innovation, John Pickstone includes medicine within a broader context that he calls *Science, Technology and Medicine (STM)*, in reference to the acronym STS (Science, Technology and Society) used in the sociology of technology. He demonstrates that the evolution of medicine depends on the surrounding culture, on a society that is transforming and industrialising, and on changing intellectual training sites. The link between medicine and society allows a holistic history of the development of medicine.[21] Several authors close to Pickstone have studied particular aspects of the development of medicine from the STM perspective.[22]

In Switzerland, the social history of medical techniques is still underdeveloped and it is worth highlighting Thomas Schlich's excellent study on the development of osteosynthesis as the preferred method for treating fractures in the post-war period. By focusing on the social and economic dimension of this

[17] Wiebe Bijker, Thomas Hughes and Trevor Pinch (eds), *The Social Construction of Technological Systems. New Directions in the Sociology and History of Technology*, London/Cambridge: MIT Press, 1989 and Wiebe Bijker, *Of Bicycles, Bakelites and Bulbs: Toward a Theory of Sociotechnical Change*, London/Cambridge: MIT Press, 1995.

[18] Jennifer Stanton, "Making sense of technologies in medicine", *Social History of Medicine*, 1999, p. 438.

[19] Stuart S. Blume, *Insight and Industry. On the Dynamics of Technological Change in Medicine*, London/Cambridge: MIT Press, 1992.

[20] Bruno Latour and Steve Woolgar, *Laboratory Life: The Social Construction of Scientific Facts*, London: SAGE Publishing, 1979.

[21] John Pickstone, *Ways of Knowing: A New History of Science, Technology and Medicine*, Manchester: Manchester University Press, 2000.

[22] Roger Cooter, Mark Harrison and Steve Sturdy (eds), *Medicine and Modern Warfare*, Amsterdam: Rodopi, 1999; Jennifer Stanton (ed.), *Innovations in Health and Medicine: Diffusion and Resistance in the Twentieth Century*, London/New York: Routledge, 2002; Ilana Löwy (ed.), *Medicine and Change: Historical and Sociological Studies of Medical Innovation*, Paris/London: INSRM/John Libbey Ltd., 1993.

therapeutic innovation, he shows that the adoption of various technical discoveries by the medical world is, above all, the result of social power relations. In this case, osteosynthesis owes its existence to a group of young German-speaking surgeons who were socially downgraded—they were not involved in an academic career. They wanted to assert themselves in the surgical world and found alliances in the industrial world to impose their innovations.[23] In a similar way, Monika Dommann and Mariama Kaba have developed innovative work in recent years on the rise of radiology and the development of orthopaedics, respectively.[24]

However, this new field of research has still only rarely integrated the economic dimension into its reflections. The overwhelming majority of studies in the social history of medicine do not address the material framework in which innovations take place.

3 The Business History of Medicine and Hospitals

The application of analytical methods and concepts from the field of business history is still relatively rare. The few historians who have taken the step are mainly American and British.[25] The dramatic demographic growth and very strong urbanisation that the United States experienced at the end of the nineteenth century led to a profound restructuring of healthcare facilities, such as dispensaries and hospitals, to ensure the care of a constantly growing population. The change in scale that American hospitals underwent around 1900 implied a managerial and organisational reform that has not escaped the attention of historians.[26] The impact of Alfred Chandler's work on large American companies,[27] to which several historians of medicine (Thomas

[23] Thomas Schlich, *Surgery, Science and Industry: A Revolution in Fracture Care, 1950s–1990s*, Basingstoke: Palgrave Macmillan, 2002. A similar approach was followed by Takahiro Ueyama, "Capital, Profession and Medical Technology: The electro-therapeutic institutes and the Royal College of Physicians, 1888–1922", *Medical History*, 1997, pp. 150–181.

[24] Monika Dommann, *Durchsicht. Einsicht. Vorsicht. Eine Geschichte der Röntgenstrahlen, 1896–1963*, Zurich: Chronos, 2003 and Mariama Kaba, *Une histoire de l'orthopédie: L'Hôpital orthopédique de la Suisse romande dans le contexte international (18e-21e siècle)*, Lausanne: BHMS, 2018.

[25] Pierre-Yves Donzé and Paloma Fernández Pérez (eds), *The Business of Health: New Approaches to the Evolution of Health Systems in the World*, New York: Routledge, 2022.

[26] Charles Rosenberg, "Inward vision and outward glance: The shaping of the American hospital, 1880–1914", *Bulletin of the History of Medicine*, 1979, pp. 346–391.

[27] Essentially his book, *The Visible Hand: The Managerial Revolution in American Business*, Cambridge: Belknap Press, 1977.

Goebel,[28] Joel Howell, Barbara Bridgman Perkins,[29] Neil Larry Shumsky,[30] Paul Starr,[31] Steve Sturdy[32]) explicitly refer, should also be emphasised here. Sturdy states, for example, that it was not so much medical discoveries that influenced the development of medicine at the end of the nineteenth century but that "the most important changes in medical practice were to be found in the sphere of what might best be termed medical administration".[33] Taking the example of the city of Sheffield, he sees in the developments of medicine in the twentieth century a concern to rationalise an increasingly divided work on the industrial model in which the city was immersed. A similar approach was adopted by other British historians, such as Roger Cooter in his study of the organisation of orthopaedic surgery in the early twentieth century.[34] As for Shumsky, he argues that "the world of contemporary medicine is one of structure, bureaucracy, and organisation"[35] and explains the functioning of the San Francisco Municipal Clinic on the basis of Chandler's work. Finally, Bridgman Perkins demonstrated that the restructuring of American hospitals in the years 1900–1930 was based on organisational methods imported from the industrial sector that allowed the affirmation of medical specialities. The most convincing work on the role of administration and management in the transformation of hospital medicine remains, however, the classic and widely cited work by Joel Howell.[36] Using patient records from two American hospitals—New York Hospital and Pennsylvania Hospital in Philadelphia—from the years 1900–1925, he shows how medical technology asserts itself within hospitals and argues that hospital growth is as much about management as it is about technical aspects. The great merit of the book is indeed to show that the arrival of a new type of management makes it possible to think of the hospital in terms of growth. In the same spirit, Paul Starr links the development of hospitals, as well as the abandonment of their philanthropic nature, to the

[28] Thomas Goebel, "American medicine and the 'organizational synthesis': Chicago physicians and the business of medicine, 1900–1920", *Bulletin of the History of Medicine*, 1994, p. 640.

[29] Barbara Bridgman Perkins, "Shaping institution-based specialism: Early twentieth-century economic organization of medicine", *Social History of Medicine*, 1997, p. 420.

[30] Neil Larry Shumsky, "The municipal clinic of San Francisco: A study in medical structure", *Bulletin of the History of Medicine*, 1978, pp. 542–559.

[31] Paul Starr, *The Social Transformation of American Medicine: The Rise of a Sovereign Profession and the Making of a Vast Industry*, New York: Basic Books, 1982, p. 148.

[32] Steve Sturdy, "'The political economy of scientific medicine: Science, education and the transformation of medical practice in Sheffield, 1890–1922", *Medical History*, 1992, p. 130.

[33] Sturdy, op. cit., p. 128.

[34] Roger Cooter, *Surgery and Society in Peace and War: Orthopaedics and the Organisation of Modern Medicine, 1880–1948*, London: Macmillan, 1993.

[35] Neil Larry Shumsky, op. cit., p. 542.

[36] Joel Howell, *Technology in the Hospital: Transforming Patient Care in the Early Twentieth Century*, Baltimore/London: The Johns Hopkins University Press, 1995.

affirmation of the medical profession and declares that "surgery had [...] made hospital care profitable".[37] Several local or regional monographs have highlighted the detailed process of this organisational transformation.[38] According to the sociologists Marc Berg and Stefan Timmermans, the standardisation of the American hospital infrastructure at the beginning of the twentieth century was the first step in a movement that affected all medical practices in the 1980s and 1990s, and which saw the generalisation of "evidence-based medicine" built on standardised guidelines on a generally international scale.[39]

The actual financing of the hospital system has also been the subject of a significant body of work. Examples include the researches of Stephen Kunitz and Christy Ford Chapin on the American health insurance system,[40] and Steven Cherry, as well as Martin Gorsky and Sally Sheard, on hospital resources in Great Britain.[41] This type of study focusing on the problem of hospital financing has also been addressed since the 1990s outside the Anglo-Saxon sphere, with works such as those by the German historian Reinhard Spree on the development and financing of the German hospital system during the nineteenth century.[42] In Spain, the numerous publications of Margarita Vilar-Rodríguez and Jerònia Pons-Pons should be mentioned, as well as Pedro Pérez Castroviejo's innovative article on hospital management in the Basque Country in the years 1800–1936.[43] In the same vein, in France, Jean-Paul

[37] Paul Starr, op. cit., p. 157.

[38] David Rosner, *A Once Charitable Enterprise: Hospitals and Health Care in Brooklyn and New York, 1885–1915*, Cambridge: Cambridge University Press, 1982; Morris J. Vogel, "Managing medicine: Creating a profession of hospital administration in the United States, 1895–1915", in Granshaw Lindsay and Porter Roy (eds), *Hospitals in History*, London/New York: Routledge, 1989, pp. 243–260; Joan Lynaugh, *The Community Hospitals of Kansas City, Missouri, 1870–1915*, New York/London: Garland, 1989; James M. Wishart, "Class difference and the reformation of Ontario public hospitals, 1900–1935: 'Make every effort to satisfy the tastes of the well-to-do'", *Labour/Le Travail*, vol. 48, 2001, pp. 27–62.

[39] Marc Berg and Stefan Timmermans, *The Gold Standard: The Challenge of Evidence-Based Medicine and Standardization in Health Care*, Philadelphia: Temple University Press, 2003.

[40] Stephen Kunitz, "Efficiency and reform in the financing and organization of American medicine in the progressive era", *Bulletin of the History of Medicine*, 1981, pp. 497–515 and Christy Ford Chapin, *Ensuring America's Health: The Public Creation of the Corporate Health Care System*, Cambridge: Cambridge University Press, 2015.

[41] Steven Cherry, "Accountability, entitlement, and control issues and voluntary hospital funding c1860–1939", *Social History of Medicine*, 1996, pp. 215–233; Steven Cherry, "Before the National Health Service: Financing the voluntary hospitals, 1900–1939", *Economic History Review*, 1997, pp. 305–326; Martin Gorsky and Sally Sheard (eds), *Financing Medicine: The British Experience Since 1750*, New York: Routledge, 2006.

[42] Reinhardt Spree, "Krankenhausentwicklung und Sozialpolitik in Deutschland während des 19. Jahrhunderts", *Historisches Zeitschrift*, 1995, pp. 75–105 and Alfons Labisch and Reinhardt Spree (eds), *Krankenhaus-Report 19. Jahrhundert. Krankenhausträger, Krankenhausfinanzierung, Krankenhauspatienten*, Frankfurt: Campus Verlag, 2001.

[43] Margarita Vilar-Rodríguez and Jerònia Pons-Pons, "The historical creation of the hospital system in Spain: Private hospital sector strategies in relation to the development

Domin's recent work has shed light on the financial and political context of French hospital development in the nineteenth and twentieth centuries, renewing Maurice Garden's classic work on the Hospices Civils de Lyon.[44] Lastly, in Switzerland, a few rare publications address the issue of hospital financing and management from a historical perspective.[45]

Finally, the first attempts at an international comparison of hospital development have been made recently, often from an imperial and cultural history perspective, but also with the aim of highlighting different organisational and financial models.[46] In this context, the book *The Emergence of Modern Hospital Management and Organisation in the World 1880s–1930s*, published in 2021 by Paloma Fernández Pérez, stands out.[47] This work, based on rich original data and offering a truly global perspective, from Europe to Latin America, via the USSR and the United States, demonstrates how the adoption of new medical technologies and the transformation of hospital organisation are issues that affect all countries, regardless of the institutional framework. In most cases, Fernández Pérez highlights the obstacles, sometimes insurmountable, encountered by the pioneers of the new hospital medicine. Facing opposition from local authorities, philanthropists and other doctors, their modernising project was generally limited to a few hospitals before the Second World War.

4 The Interest of the Swiss Case

Through the lens of Fernández Pérez's book, the case of Switzerland offers the rare example of a successful early modernisation of the hospital system as a whole. It shows how a new generation of surgeons succeeded in transforming

of the public system", in Martin Gorsky, Margarita Vilar-Rodríguez and Jerònia Pons-Pons (eds), *The Political Economy of the Hospital in History*, Huddersfield: University of Huddersfield Press, 2020, pp. 17–59 and Pedro M. Pérez Castroviejo, "La formación del sistema hospitalario vasco: Administración y gestión económica, 1800–1936", *Transportes, Servicios y Telecomunicaciones*, 2002, pp. 73–97.

[44] Jean-Paul Domin, *Une histoire économique de l'hôpital (XIXe–XXe siècles)*, Paris: Comité d'histoire de la sécurité sociale, 2 vols, 2008 and 2013 and Maurice Garden, *Histoire économique d'une entreprise de santé: Le budget des Hospices civils de Lyon, 1800–1976*, Lyon: PUL, 1980.

[45] Vincent Barras and Marie-France Vouilloz Burnier, *De l'hospice au réseau santé. Santé publique et systèmes hospitaliers valaisans, XIXe–XXe siècles*, Sierre: Monographic, 2004; Thierry Christ, "De la bienfaisance privée à l'Etat social? Mise en place, financement et contrôle du réseau hospitalier et institutionnel (orphelinats, hospices) à Neuchâtel (1815–1914)", *Revue historique neuchâteloise*, 1997, pp. 23–51; Pierre-Yves Donzé, *L'hôpital bourgeois de Porrentruy*, Porrentruy: CEH, 2000; Pierre-Yves Donzé, *Bâtir, gérer, soigner. Histoire des établissements hospitaliers de Suisse romande*, Bibliothèque d'histoire de la médecine, Geneva: Georg, 2003.

[46] Mark Harrison, Margaret Jones and Helen Sweet (eds), *From Western Medicine to Global Medicine: The Hospital Beyond the West*, New Delhi: Orient Blackswan, 2009; Gorsky et al., op. cit.

[47] *Paloma Fernández Pérez, The Emergence of Modern Hospital Management and Organisation in the World 1880s–1930s*, Bradford: Emerald, 2021.

the hospital organisation in collaboration with the local authorities. The process was not without conflict: the surgeon-modernisers faced opposition from other doctors, who defended their own interests as general practitioners; from philanthropists, who wanted to retain control of the private hospitals they had founded, and; from traditional local elites, who fought against the rise of centralised investment in the university hospital. However, the negotiation between the various actors and the search for consensual solutions, under the aegis of the state, enabled Swiss hospital medicine to undergo a profound transformation in the first half of the twentieth century.

Of course, Switzerland is a federal state in which public health depends on the cantons, of which there were 22 during the period analysed in this book. The process of modernising hospital medicine was carried out in different ways in the different cantons. While generally succeeding in the urbanised regions that included medical faculties, the rural and Alpine cantons remained on the sidelines of this development until the second half of the twentieth century.[48] The case study chosen for this work is the canton of Vaud (see Fig. 1). It has several characteristics that make the analysis of the construction of its hospital system particularly relevant. First of all, of the five cantons with a medical faculty and a university hospital (Basel, Berne, Geneva, Vaud, Zurich), it is not limited to one city, like Basel or Geneva, but includes a vast hinterland,[49] which saw the establishment of various types of hospital establishments designed to care for a population that almost doubled between 1880 (235,349 inhabitants) and 1960 (429,512 inhabitants).[50] The relatively limited size of its territory (3200 km^2), nevertheless, makes it possible to examine in detail all the existing establishments within the system and not just the large ones. The role occupied by the secondary and peripheral hospitals, as well as the sometimes conflicting relations they have with other establishments, appear to be structuring elements of the hospital system. Moreover, the territory of Vaud did not evolve in a linear and homogeneous way during the period under consideration. The demographic growth and strong urbanisation that characterised these years called into question the territorial organisation of the canton. The relationships between the various hospitals were also affected by these structural changes. Finally, the canton of Vaud was governed throughout the period under consideration by the Radical-Democratic Party, which made the cantonal state an omnipresent and interventionist agent in the construction, and then the management, of the hospital system. The Vaud hospital system is therefore very diversified, with a public university hospital (Cantonal Hospital) and private specialised establishments (ophthalmology, orthopaedics and paediatrics) in the city of Lausanne, as well as about fifteen private general hospitals in the rest of the canton (local infirmaries/regional hospitals) and

[48] Donzé, *Bâtir...*, op. cit.

[49] Vaud is the fourth largest canton in terms of surface area, after Graubünden, Berne and Valais.

[50] *Annuaire statistique du canton de Vaud – 1985*, Lausanne: SCRIS, 1985.

private clinics for a wealthy clientele on the Lake Geneva Riviera. How will these various establishments react to the changes in the medical-technical system? Will they be the promoters or the obstacles?

To answer these questions, this book proposes an analysis that integrates the contributions of the social history of medical technology and the business history of hospitals in explaining the development of hospital medicine during the nineteenth and twentieth centuries. The concept of sociotechnical system elaborated by Thomas Hugues proves to be very useful to approach this phenomenon and to show that the profound reorganisation of hospitals at the end of the nineteenth century and in the first part of the twentieth century is similar to an industrial revolution, in the sense that François Caron understands it, i.e., the transition from one technical system to another. Several types of innovation, at once purely technical (new way of practising surgery), social (professionalisation of doctors) and economic (enlargement of the healthcare market), favoured the transition to a new "medical sociotechnical system", based on two main sub-systems: the hospital system and the medical-technical system (cf. Fig. 2).

By hospital system, I mean a set of institutional (public and private hospitals, clinics, medical faculties, nursing schools) and individual (doctors, patients, politicians, administrators) agents, interacting with each other and dependent on a common political, economic and social environment. The hospital system appears to be a structuring element of the medical market, with the bulk of the supply of care and infrastructure tending to be concentrated in this context from the end of the nineteenth century. It could then be organised according

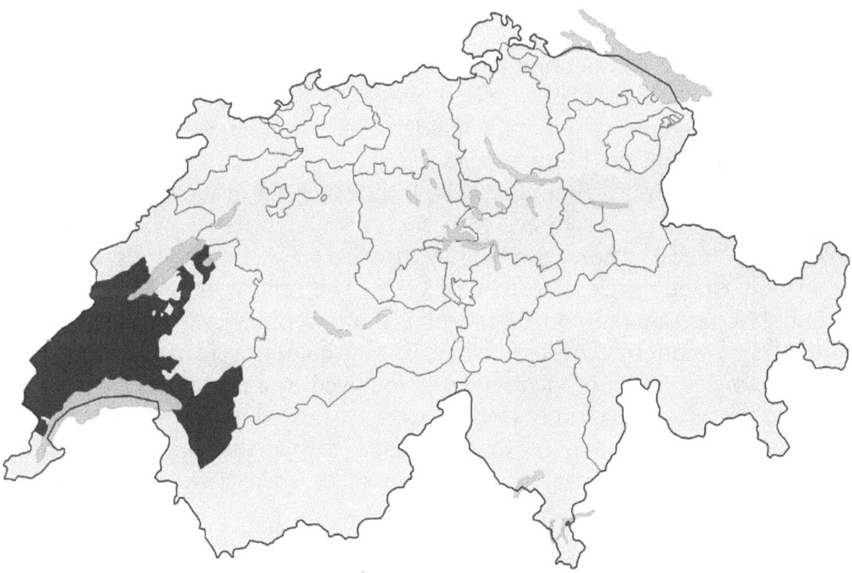

Fig. 1 The canton of Vaud (*Source* Wikimedia Commons)

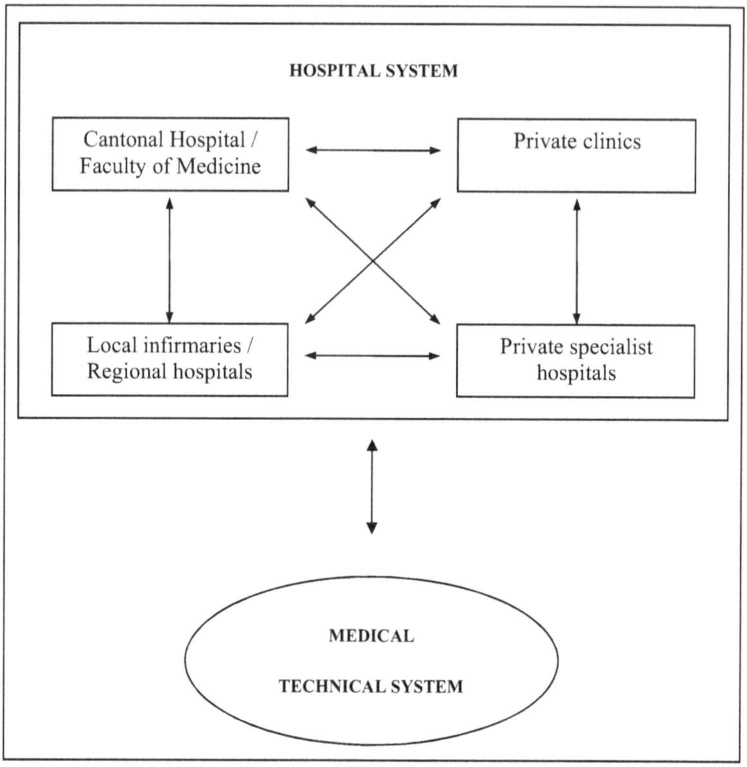

Fig. 2 The medical sociotechnical system in the canton of Vaud

to the principle of competition and the free market, or according to the principle of a regulated or even cartelised market, depending on the intervention of the various agents—the system builders dear to Hugues—and their power relationships within the hospital system.

As for the medical-technical system, I understand it in the sense of the way in which medicine is practised, with the various modes of work, machines, tools and technical gestures used in the act of caring; in other words, according to an understanding close to that of Gille. The upheavals that affected this technical system at the end of the nineteenth century and during the first part of the twentieth century resulted in a double movement of mechanisation and concentration of medical work, followed by a phase of the division of labour. This transformation of medical work was based on surgery, which itself underwent profound changes in the second half of the nineteenth century and around which hospitals were reorganised.[51] There was a standardisation

[51] Ulrich Tröhler, "Surgery (modern)", in W. F. Bynum and Roy Porter (eds), *Companion Encyclopedia of the History of Medicine*, London/New York: Routledge, vol. 2, 1993, pp. 984–1028.

of medical procedures and surgical equipment such as operating tables. The surgeon-operating room ensemble formed a real "healing machine" in which patients became interchangeable. This mechanisation allowed mass production, i.e., the treatment of an increasing number of cases. Hospitals thus became care production units and the practice of medicine tended to be concentrated there. From then on, the practice of medicine required access to a medico-technical infrastructure (operating theatres, laboratories, radiological facilities), which was concentrated in hospitals. This phase of mechanisation and concentration of medicine was followed in the interwar period by a phase of rationalisation, i.e., a strong division of labour—both vertical and horizontal—which gave the hospital the image of a multi-divisional enterprise and was mainly explained by the emergence of medical research and the affirmation of the professional specialisation of doctors. As Bridgman Perkins argues, these divisions of medical work have different functions that correspond to distinct moments in hospital development: "horizontal specialization allowed physicians to control their markets, and vertical specialization allowed them to control their work and their departments".[52]

This development of the medical sociotechnical system did not, however, take place smoothly and automatically: blockages and innovations were omnipresent. The development of the medical-technical system was closely linked to the development of the hospital system, and vice versa. System builders were involved at all levels. The question arises as to how the various agents reacted to the desire for change. Were doctors all in favour of transformations in the medical-technical system? What was their position with regard to the hospital? Similarly, did hospital administrators accept the transformation of medical techniques without question? How did they finance them? How did the population react to these changes? Did the state intervene in the hospital system? In what way and why? And, finally, what influence did these changes have on the relationships between the different hospitals within the hospital system? These various questions reflect multiple power relationships within the medical sociotechnical system. The transformation of hospital medicine can thus be imagined in various forms depending on the outcome of the conflicts and negotiations leading to a readjustment of the system.

The modernisation of hospital medicine in the canton of Vaud is first examined from the point of view of the medical-technical system and its creators: the surgeon-modernisers. This book confers a special place to surgery in the transformation of the hospital system during the years 1840–1960. The discipline of surgery appears as the main and initial vector of the transformation of the hospital system at this time. Surgeons were the ones who carried out the main innovations in the medical-technical system, which required the redeployment of hospital establishments. Their actions had a direct impact in terms of infrastructure that other fields of medicine would only experience in a second phase. The second chapter is, therefore, devoted to the study of

[52] Barbara Bridgman Perkins, op. cit., p. 424.

these surgeons and system builders, their professional training and the models that influenced it, as well as their careers in the various fields available to them or that they created for themselves. Special attention is given to the Cantonal Hospital of Lausanne and its surgical clinic, the canton's main hospital and the place where the vast majority of Vaud surgeons are trained. In writing a social history of medicine, the focus is on the actors of medical innovation, their interventions in the hospital system and the evolution of the medical-technical system. The following chapters focus on the reaction of hospitals to the readjustments of the medical-technical system, taking first the case of the Cantonal Hospital, then that of the regional hospitals.

The third chapter deals with the managerial and organisational aspects of the Cantonal Hospital. The transformation of medicine is not only the result of technical innovations. It requires a profound transformation of management methods and the arrival of a new generation of administrators. It necessitates the means to invest, to build the necessary infrastructure, as well as to learn about the healthcare market, to position oneself in it, especially in relation to private clinics and regional hospitals, and to create and respond to demand. The third chapter seeks to show, among other things, how a public university hospital manages to generate the financial resources necessary for its development and operation.

Alongside the Cantonal Hospital, the private charitable institutions (regional hospitals and specialised hospitals) play an important role in the hospital system, accounting for about half of the hospital capacity. The fourth chapter focuses on the intervention of surgeon-modernisers in these hospitals and on the consequences of their actions, in terms of management, organisation and financing. The aim is to show why and how small-scale charitable institutions are being transformed into modern, more highly capitalised enterprises that compete with other hospitals in the system.

Finally, the fifth chapter deals with the implementation of a cantonal hospital policy. The system-wide approach to hospital management highlights the process of reorganisation of the hospital system during the years 1945–1965 and considers this a response to a competitive system that did not satisfy its actors. This chapter continues the various themes discussed earlier, such as the division of labour at the university surgical clinic and the financing of the various establishments, which found a solution in the 1966 hospital plan. This new stage in the construction of the hospital system saw the arrival of public health planners, the new experts in hospital management who now organised health issues on a territorial rather than hospital level.

CHAPTER 2

Surgeons of the Canton of Vaud in the Nineteenth and Twentieth Centuries

1 Introduction

The work of surgeons underwent a profound change during the latter decades of the nineteenth century and early twentieth century. Techniques improved and diversified. Medical teams included a growing number of doctors, assistants, nurses and other helpers. Surgery also benefited from an increasingly complex infrastructure which soon made the hospital the centre of the healthcare system. The transformation of hospital medicine is not, however, a phenomenon that occurs automatically; it involves power issues, generating a whole series of conflicts that reveal the interactions between an academic discipline, medical practice and the organisation of hospital work.

This chapter discusses the evolution of the work of surgeons in the Canton of Vaud from the mid-nineteenth to the mid-twentieth century. It examines the considerable impact of César Roux, surgeon at the Cantonal Hospital of Lausanne (1887–1926) and the first professor of surgery at the Faculty of Medicine in Lausanne (1890–1926), who is considered to be one of the first representatives of the surgeon-modernisers in French-speaking Switzerland. Of course, surgeons of Roux's generation were not the first to develop new surgical techniques and equipment; for example, Mathias Mayor was the first head of the Surgical Department of the Cantonal Hospital (1806–1847) and designer of numerous surgical devices.[1] However, the innovations developed by surgeons in the first part of the nineteenth century, in Lausanne

[1] Jean-Charles Biaudet, "L'écharpe, le marteau et le tourniquet. Mathias Mayor, un chirurgien vaudois du début du XIXe siècle", in Guy Saudan (ed.), *L'Eveil médical vaudoise, 1750–1850. Tissot, Venel, Mayor*, Lausanne: UNIL, 1987, pp. 105–175.

P.-Y. Donzé, *The Formation of the Swiss Hospital System (1840–1960)*,
https://doi.org/10.1007/978-981-19-3911-2_2

as elsewhere in the Western world, were primarily aimed at the treatment of a particular ailment, isolated in the surgeon's daily practice. This was a completely artisanal conception of surgical work which did not exclude technical inventiveness but dealt with various patients in an individualised manner, according to the principle of singularity. Surgery was not practised in a centralised way in a particular place, nor in series. Things changed at the end of the nineteenth century with the arrival of a new generation of surgeons, generally trained at German schools. The innovations developed by Roux and his contemporaries concerned both the treatment of the condition itself and the organisation of the surgical work. Roux acquired new techniques from Theodor Kocher at the University of Berne and demonstrated a high degree of technical inventiveness, characteristic of the artisanal technical medical system. However, his expertise did not stop there. He gradually introduced new equipment (operating tables, sterilizers, X-ray equipment, etc.) which was concentrated in the hospital and enabled him to switch to a type of serial work organisation, similar to that used in industrial companies, particularly with the opening of a new university surgical clinic in 1914.

Some of Roux's students, once they left the University, moved outside Lausanne and obtained access to local infirmaries. These were small establishments of a philanthropic nature and with limited financial resources, whose primary aim was to help the working classes. From the 1900s onwards, these surgeon-modernisers, through the application of new surgeries, turned the local infirmaries into modernised hospitals which quickly entered into competition with the Cantonal Hospital. Arriving in the local infirmaries with a strong will to restructure and modernise, they embodied the salaried manager described by Alfred Chandler.[2] The spirit of managerial capitalism is very present in the hospitals. Surgeon-modernisers act as technical directors, dependent on a management committee and responsible for work organisation, technical innovation, flow management and care production. They are the promoters of the transformation of hospital medicine.

With the arrival of Pierre Decker at the head of the Surgical Department (1932), the second phase of the transformation of the medical-technical system began; that of the division of labour. This was confirmed under the professorship of Saegesser (1957). Research activities began to appear and led to the emergence of surgical specialties as well as a new mode of organisation based on the division of work, both horizontally and vertically. However, this new way of doing surgery required increased and centralised financial support at the Cantonal Hospital, whose Surgical Department clashed with the regional hospitals. Here, the medical service was directed by the surgeon-modernisers of the previous generation, draining a large proportion of the patients and public subsidies.

[2] Alfred D. Chandler, *The Visible Hand: The Managerial Revolution in American Business*, Cambridge: Belknap Press, 1977.

Surgery thus went through various phases during the period under consideration which had a direct impact on the development of the hospital system. The purpose of this chapter is to highlight the evolution of the technical medical system (work organisation, models, technical infrastructure, etc.) and thus the technical characteristics of hospital growth, the managerial and financial aspects of which will be addressed in the following chapters.

2 The Surgeons of the Canton of Vaud Through the Nineteenth Century (1800–1880): Surgery as a Craft

It is difficult to speak of *surgery* in the Canton of Vaud before the 1870s. Without a university to teach this branch of medicine independently, the distinction between doctors and surgeons remained vague. If we refer to the legal authorisation to practise medicine,[3] we can see that the overwhelming majority of practitioners called themselves *doctors* and *surgeons*. Moreover, the practice of medicine was essentially private so sources allowing the identification of possible specialisations in skills are almost non-existent. Finally, the local infirmaries founded by philanthropists in the 1840s and 1850s made no distinction between *medicine* and *surgery* until the very end of the nineteenth century (see Chapter 4). Under these conditions, the only place where a so-called *surgical* activity could be easily identified—that is to say, thought of as such—was the Cantonal Hospital, founded by the State of Vaud in 1806 through the purchase of the former Hospital of the City of Lausanne.

The first surgeon to work at the Cantonal Hospital, Mathias Mayor, is emblematic of the notion of surgery conceived as a craft. Neither the procedures used nor the working methods were clearly defined as a body of doctrine; for Mayor, "imagination makes the good surgeon".[4] He was a very inventive practitioner (e.g., using a constrictor with a rosary for the removal of tumours, treating fractures with the planchette, the so-called "Mayor sling", etc.) but his innovations did not aim to improve the organisation of surgical work. Mayor was a surgical craftsman in the sense that he treated each patient on a case-by-case basis, where each needed to be treated in the best possible way—which is where Mayor's inventive genius came into play. Mayor practised a lot at his home and not in hospitals, which reinforces the decentralised and artisanal organisation of his work.

[3] Official Directory of the Canton of Vaud (ODCV), various years.

[4] Jean-Charles Biaudet, op. cit., p. 107.

Table 1 Cantonal Hospital, heads of the Surgical Department, 1806–1926

Years of function	*Name*
1806–1847	Mathias Mayor (1775–1847)
1847–1863	Samuel Louis Larguier des Bancels (1806–1863)
1863–1866	Charles Pellis (1801–1877)
1866–1875	Louis Rouge (1833–1895)
1875–1887	Emile Dupont (1841–1901)
1883–1890	Victor Mercanton (1850–1910)
1887–1926	César Roux (1859–1934)

Surgery at the Cantonal Hospital Until the Mid-1870s

From 1806, the Cantonal Hospital of Lausanne was divided into two departments, one for internal medicine and the other for surgery. Until the mid-1870s, obtaining a hospital service was an important step in the career of doctors from the urban bourgeoisie, in the tradition of the Ancien Régime. As the hospital was still essentially a charitable and coercive institution, the title of *hospital doctor* had a strong symbolic and philanthropic connotation (Table 1).

In the continuity of the Ancien Régime, representatives of the local upper-middle-class mostly took up these posts. Mathias Mayor came from a well-to-do bourgeois family, linked to private bankers in Neuchâtel and Lausanne and strongly integrated into the medical world of the Enlightenment. He accumulated public offices and honours as deputy to the Grand Council (1808–1831), co-founder of the Société des sciences médicales (1829) and honorary professor at the Academy (1841).[5] Samuel Larguier des Bancels was the son of a judge and prefect of Nyon.[6] Similarly, Charles Pellis descended from a family of the old Vaud nobility. He was the son of the businessman and politician Marc-Antoine Pellis (1753–1809) and his brother was a professor of law at the Academy and a member of the Grand Council.[7]

The takeover of the hospital service by the old Lausanne families led to a reaction from other doctors who wanted to gain access to these prestigious posts. They attempted a coup de force in the Grand Council in 1842. A deputy asked for an increase in the number of doctors at the Cantonal Hospital but was refused by the Health Council, stating that the other doctors in Lausanne were seeking access to the Hospital "in order to create a name for themselves

[5] On the life of Mathias Mayor, see Jean-Charles Biaudet, op. cit.

[6] *Dictionnaire historique et biographique de la Suisse (DBHS)*, Neuchâtel: Attinger, 1917–1923, vol. 4, p. 455 and Olivier Robert and Franceso Panese, *Dictionnaire des professeurs de l'Université de Lausanne dès 1890*, Lausanne: UNIL, 2000, p. 722.

[7] He was Louis-Rodolphe Pellis (1791–1870), a lawyer, member of Parliament and professor of law. On the Pellis family, see *DHBS*, vol. 5, p. 241.

and a clientele".[8] Access to the hospital infrastructure as a working tool was not yet demanded by the medical profession. Doctors at the hospital did not owe their entire time to the institution. According to a regulation adopted in 1824, they had to make a daily visit to their departments and kept the rest of their time available for their private practice, which brought in the bulk of their income.[9] The hospital was not equipped with specific surgical equipment since the surgeon's office was held by a private practitioner who provided this service; Mayor used his own surgical instruments and Larguier did the same in the 1850s.[10]

Towards the middle of the nineteenth century, the hospital still occupied a secondary place in the professional practice of Lausanne surgeons. However, this conception of hospital medicine quickly came up against a growth in the number of hospitalisations (672 patients in 1830; 1259 in 1840; and 2206 in 1850) which required a stronger medical presence within the establishment. The State Council wished to remedy this deficiency by appointing an internal physician (1835)—a young doctor who had completed his studies, was appointed for a fixed period of time and would spend all his time in hospital service. The arrival of young interns made it possible to ensure a continuous hospital medical service without the chief physicians having to give up their private practice.

The Changes of the 1870s and 1880s

By the mid-1870s, a new generation of surgeons was emerging and influencing the institution. It was no longer social and family ties that allowed access to the position of hospital doctor; training became paramount. It should also be noted that the State intervened more strongly in hospital affairs during the 1870s, with the aim of improving the operation of the Cantonal Hospital and the care of patients. Dr. Emile Dupont, who graduated in 1865, was head physician of the Saint-Loup Hospital for several years (1866–1874) before being called to succeed Dr. Rouge in 1875.[11] Dr. Victor Mercanton, who was appointed alongside Dupont when the Surgical Department was split up in the new hospital (1883), came from the prestigious Lücke school where he had been an assistant in Strasbourg.[12] General practitioners who were proud of their title of "hospital doctor" faded away in favour of men for whom surgery was a particular branch of medicine, which was essentially practised in a hospital environment.

[8] Archives of the Canton of Vaud (ACV), K VIII B 38, letter from the Health Council to the Hospice Council, 27 December 1842.

[9] ACV, K VIII B 38, 1824.

[10] ACV, K VIII A 42/1, Hospice Council protocols, 4 January 1851.

[11] *Revue médicale de la Suisse romande (RMSR)*, 1901, p. 343.

[12] *RMSR*, 1910, pp. 737–738.

Dupont adopted the antiseptic method around 1875–1876.[13] Often retained in historiography as a decisive step in the advent of modern hospital surgery, this innovation was very controversial in the 1860s and 1870s, essentially for reasons of theoretical justification.[14] The germ theory of the Englishman Joseph Lister, the main designer of antisepsis, was discussed among British and European medical circles. It was not until the 1880s that it really became established, thanks in particular to the success of bacteriology, to which Lister linked his theory. In spite of the difficulties encountered on the theoretical level, from the end of the 1860s, many surgeons used all or part of Lister's antiseptic method for practical reasons: wounds healed better and more quickly.

The Canton of Vaud experienced similar debates between supporters and opponents of Lister, both on a theoretical and practical level, during the 1870s and 1880s. The *Revue médicale de la Suisse romande* is a good illustration of the many contradictory debates on this issue. As in Great Britain, antisepsis was essentially adopted by certain surgeons for practical reasons—it was an innovation that worked—but it came up against a problem of theoretical justification, reinforced by the sharp rise in treatment costs that it implied, and was denounced very early on by many hospital authorities, including those of the Cantonal Hospital of Lausanne.[15] Dupont himself had an aerialist conception of health which was not a priori favourable to the adoption of the Listerian method. In fact, in the presentation of his surgical service made in 1876, he underlined the apparent contradiction between the "exceptionally favourable hygienic circumstances"[16] in which part of his service was located, moved out of the city, in a place exposed to the sun and to the circulation of air, and the high incidence of erysipelas and pyaemia. Clean air and sunlight cannot cure postoperative infections, whereas Lister's method does cure many of them. He explained that practical considerations made him adopt antisepsis definitively: "these happy and unexpected results [...] I attribute to Lister's disinfecting method, which I now use exclusively and in the strictest manner".[17] He thus adopted flannel bandages instead of reusable cloth strips. On several occasions, this novelty was then invoked as the cause of the increase in the cost of medical material by the hospital administration (see Chapter 3). Dupont himself recognised that "all the necessary material is expensive, even very expensive. But it only takes a moment's reflection [...] to convince oneself that

[13] Dupont, "Le service de chirurgie de l'Hôpital Cantonal", *RMSR*, 1876, pp. 253–257 and 294–302.

[14] Michael Worboys, *Spreading Germs. Disease Theories and Medical Practice in Britain, 1865–1900*, Cambridge: Cambridge University Press, 2000.

[15] Ulrich Tröhler, "L'essor de la chirurgie", in Mirko D. Grmek (ed.), *Histoire de la pensée médicale en Occident*, vol. 3, Paris: Seuil, 1999, pp. 244–245.

[16] Dupont, "Le service de chirurgie...", op. cit., p. 254.

[17] Ibid., p. 255.

this reproach cannot constitute a serious argument".[18] In the longer term, the Listerian method could indeed be conceived as economical: "Without doubt, the bandage is expensive in itself, but the definite saving is in the fact that it heals more quickly, and consequently in a less considerable number of hospital days. Add to this the almost total disappearance of infectious complications of wounds, the possibility of performing more serious operations, such as, for example, the opening of joints, with complete immunity, the suppression, so to speak, of the action of the surrounding environment, and one will understand the ever-increasing favour with which Lister's disinfectant method is surrounded".[19] As early as 1875, Dupont received student nurses from the School of La Source to attend dressing sessions on patients where he probably taught them this new method.[20]

From this perspective, the hospital was no longer the only home for the poor that it had been since the Ancien Régime, but tended to become a place where the sick were treated. This institution thus became interesting for the medical profession, not only for honorific and symbolic reasons but also for professional training. This led young medical graduates to demand access to an internship. In 1879, seven medical students from the Canton of Vaud who had trained at the University of Basel requested that doctors who had graduated from all Swiss medical schools be accepted as interns, without having to pass the Vaud exams. They would like to have "the opportunity to do an internship in Lausanne, which would have many advantages for the Vaudois".[21]

In spite of these qualitative improvements, the number of hospitalisations in the Surgical Department remained extremely stable and reveals the saturation of its capacity. The number of patients in this department fluctuated around 900 per year. This problem was not new: the political authorities had been talking since the mid-1860s about constructing a new hospital outside the city to replace the buildings dating from the 1760s, which was completed in 1883. The opening of this 470-bed establishment was the occasion for a profound administrative and medical reorganisation (see Chapter 3). The surgery and medicine departments were split and remained so until the opening of the Faculty of Medicine in 1890. The second position of surgeon was given to Dr. Victor Mercanton. The Hospital now offered favourable conditions for the growth of hospitalisations: the number of patients in the Surgical Department increased from 1'036 in 1883 to 1'585 in 1890 and 2'345 in 1901.[22]

[18] Dupont, "Le service de chirurgie...", op. cit., p. 297.

[19] Ibid.

[20] ACV, K VIII B 61.

[21] ACV, K VIII B 18, collective letter to the Department of the Interior, 18 September 1879.

[22] Report of the State Council (RSC), Department of the Interior, 1883–1901. Figures for the Surgical Service are not known after 1901.

The arrival of César Roux to replace Dupont in 1887 was part of a dynamic of growth and modernisation of the Cantonal Hospital. A young and ambitious surgeon, he was a disciple of Theodor Kocher, determined to bring the new German surgery acquired at the University of Berne to the Canton of Vaud.

3 The Industrial Revolution in Surgery in the Canton of Vaud: César Roux and the German School (1880–1930)

César Roux was a true product of the new German surgery. After completing his medical studies at the University of Berne, he became an assistant to Theodor Kocher (1881–1883) and spent several months in 1881 visiting the clinics of some of the leading surgeons of the time, again in the German-speaking world. He visited Billroth in Vienna and Volkmann in Halle. On his return to Lausanne, he established himself as the main representative of the new German surgery.

The Model: Theodor Kocher and the German Surgical School

New surgical techniques were developed by surgeons in the German-speaking world during the second half of the nineteenth century.[23] Benefiting from both the mastery of favourable technical conditions—anaesthesia and antisepsis—and a working environment conducive to scientific research—the Humboldtian University—German surgeons carried out numerous innovations characterised by their invasive dimension, especially in abdominal and thoracic surgery. Whereas until then surgical practice was essentially reduced to the treatment of external pathologies, German surgeons turned it into a highly experimental discipline that aimed to open up the body in order to act directly on the organs.[24]

In addition to this technical dimension, it is important to emphasise an organisational characteristic which also played a role in the affirmation of the German model. The German hospital-university organisation, which favours proximity between medical faculties, university clinics and research laboratories, was conducive to the adoption of technical innovations in hospitals and to the concentration of medical work in hospital clinics. The hospital thus became an essential location for surgical practice and allowed the full affirmation of a new medical-technical system.

[23] Hans Killian, *Meister der Chirurgie und die Chirurgenschulen im gesamten deutschen Sprachraum*, Stuttgart: Georg Thieme Verlag, 1980, and Ulrich Tröhler, "The Rise of Surgery", op. cit.

[24] Ulrich Tröhler, "Surgery (modern)", in W. F. Bynum and Roy Porter (eds), *Companion Encyclopedia of the History of Medicine*, London/New York: Routledge, 1993, vol. 2, p. 992.

The German model has an undeniable attraction for Swiss doctors. In French-speaking Switzerland, one of the main promoters of this new surgery was a disciple of Billroth and Lücke, Theodor Kocher, professor of surgery at the Faculty of Medicine in Berne for 45 years (1872–1917) and winner of the Nobel Prize for Medicine (1909).[25]

The University of Berne was an essential training ground for young doctors in Western Switzerland. Among the 9800 students and the hundred or so assistants who were trained by Kocher during his career, several distinguished themselves in the implementation of this new surgery in modernised hospitals, both in the Canton of Vaud and elsewhere in French-speaking Switzerland. In the Canton of Vaud, the name of César Roux, who in turn became the master of a whole generation of surgeons, should be remembered, as well as those of his contemporaries who took positions in several local infirmaries throughout the Canton. Kocher's disciples also practised surgery in other Cantons, including Fribourg, Geneva and Neuchâtel. One of them was Dr. de Quervain, head of the surgery department of the La Chaux-de-Fonds Hospital (1897–1910) and consultant surgeon at the Le Locle Hospital in the Canton of Neuchâtel. He distinguished himself by his innovative spirit and developed numerous surgical devices, including an operating table which was produced by the Schaerer company in Berne and was a worldwide success. Later, Fritz de Quervain was appointed professor of surgery in Basel (1910) and then in Berne where he succeeded his master Kocher (1918).[26]

Kocher's influence and prestige in Swiss surgery is reflected in the founding of the Swiss Society of Surgery in 1913. At his initiative, 112 surgeons attended the founding meeting of the society at his University Surgical Clinic in Berne, electing Kocher as its president (1913–1916). He was succeeded by his students in the surgical chairs of Lausanne (César Roux, 1917–1918), Basel (Fritz de Quervain, 1919–1920) and Geneva (Ernst Kummer, 1921–1922). By participating in the foundation of this society, Roux asserted himself as a disciple of Kocher and the German school.

The Production of Surgical Equipment: A Product of the German School

Surgical practice became highly mechanised in the 1890s and 1900s with the adoption of new instruments, new operating tables and new types of sterilizers. The use of various mass-produced technical objects led to a standardisation of surgical practice, which in turn favoured the transition to mass surgery.[27]

[25] Ulrich Tröhler, *Der Nobelpreisträger Theodor Kocher, 1841–1917. Auf dem Weg zur physiologischen Chirurgie*, Basel: Birkhauser, 1984.

[26] Georges Terrier, "Le Dr Fritz de Quervain à la Chaux-de-Fonds (1894–1910)", *RMSR*, 1998, pp. 193–201.

[27] Thomas Schlich, *Surgery, Science and Industry. A Revolution in Fracture Care, 1950s–1990s*, Basingstoke: Palgrave Macmillan, 2002, pp. 46–64.

Schaerer AG is the leading Swiss manufacturer of surgical equipment, playing a decisive role in the mechanisation and standardisation of surgical activities.[28] Founded in Berne in 1893 by a mechanic, Moritz Schaerer, with the aim of manufacturing and marketing surgical and orthopaedic instruments. Schaerer soon began collaborating with a disciple of Kocher, Fritz de Quervain. Together, they developed a new type of operating table (eight patents registered between 1900 and 1942) made up of several autonomous and mobile trays which allowed the surgeon to give the patient's body the appropriate shape for the operation undertaken (see Fig. 1). In the words of its designer, this invention was intended to allow "the adaptation of new mechanical means to the new abdominal operating technique".[29]

The Schaerer company explained in a publication that "an operating table, in order to fulfil its purpose, must be adapted to all the requirements of modern surgery. Above all, it must be constructed in such a way that the patient can assume all the necessary positions and that changes can be made very quickly".[30] Thus, the originality of the de Quervain table is that it adapts the human body to a surgery whose various gestures are more and more decomposed. This veritable mechanisation of surgery is reflected in the explosion in the volume of teaching manuals in this branch: between the first edition of the very classic *Chirurgische Operationslehre* by Theodor Kocher (1892) and the fifth edition published in 1907, the number of pages increased from some 200 to nearly 1100.[31] As Thomas Schlich has shown in the case of osteosynthesis, the adoption by the medical profession of industrially produced and highly standardised material is an essential factor in the success and widespread dissemination of new medical methods.[32] The de Quervain table made it possible to adopt a working method in surgery based on interchangeability (of patients) and mass production (of care), as has been done for several decades in other economic sectors.

De Quervain presented his object at the first Congress of the International Society of Surgery, in Brussels in 1905, as well as in the prestigious *Zentralblatt für Chirurgie* the following year.[33] This table "built exclusively [...] in

[28] *Feuille officielle Suisse du commerce (FOSC)*, various years, Swiss patent database www.espacenet.ch (accessed July 2003) and the F 201 collection at the Schweizerische Wirtschaftsarchiv in Basel.

[29] Testimony of Quervain to the Société médicale neuchâteloise, 1939, unpublished and quoted in Ulrich Tröhler, "F. de Quervain, chirurgien pratique à La Chaux-de-Fonds (1895–1910): Un esprit physiopathologique à la conquête d'un terrain nouveau", *Gesnerus*, 1975, p. 202.

[30] *La construction*..., op. cit., p. 107.

[31] Ulrich Tröhler, "The Rise...", op. cit., p. 247.

[32] Thomas Schlich, op. cit.

[33] Fritz de Quervain, "Zur Operationstischfrage", in *Zentralblatt für Chirurgie*, 1906, pp. 321–323.

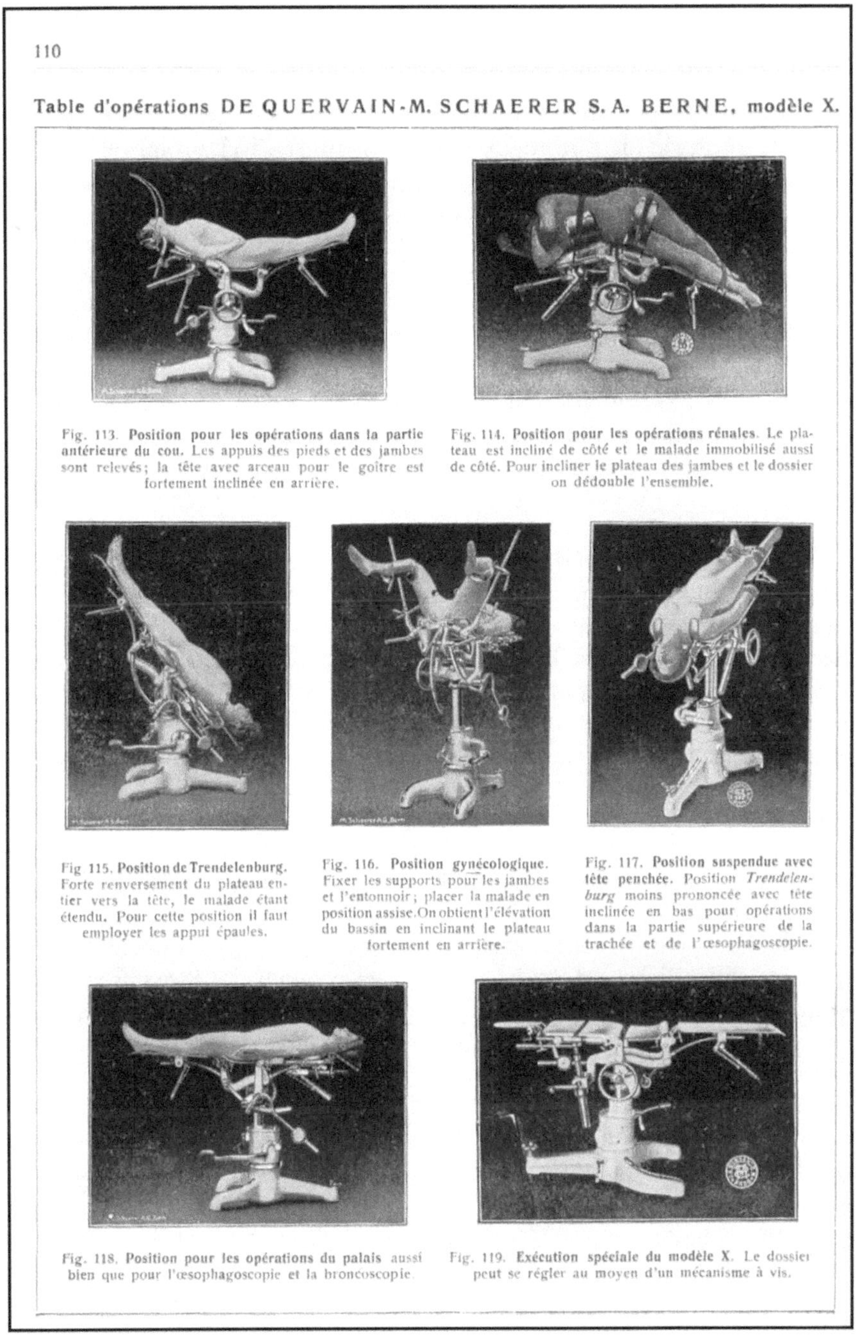

110

Table d'opérations DE QUERVAIN-M. SCHAERER S. A. BERNE, modèle X.

Fig. 113. **Position pour les opérations dans la partie antérieure du cou.** Les appuis des pieds et des jambes sont relevés; la tête avec arceau pour le goître est fortement inclinée en arrière.

Fig. 114. **Position pour les opérations rénales.** Le plateau est incliné de côté et le malade immobilisé aussi de côté. Pour incliner le plateau des jambes et le dossier on dédouble l'ensemble.

Fig 115. **Position de Trendelenburg.** Forte renversement du plateau entier vers la tête, le malade étant étendu. Pour cette position il faut employer les appui épaules.

Fig. 116. **Position gynécologique.** Fixer les supports pour les jambes et l'entonnoir; placer la malade en position assise. On obtient l'élévation du bassin en inclinant le plateau fortement en arrière.

Fig. 117. **Position suspendue avec tête penchée.** Position *Trendelenburg* moins prononcée avec tête inclinée en bas pour opérations dans la partie supérieure de la trachée et de l'œsophagoscopie.

Fig. 118. **Position pour les opérations du palais** aussi bien que pour l'œsophagoscopie et la broncoscopie.

Fig. 119. **Exécution spéciale du modèle X.** Le dossier peut se régler au moyen d'un mécanisme à vis.

Fig. 1 Quervain-Schaerer operating table, model X (*Source La construction des hôpitaux modernes et leurs installations. Ouvrage destiné à l'usage des médecins, architectes, ingénieurs, techniciens, personnel d'administration, étudiants et practiciens*, Berne, Maison Schaerer SA, 1930, p. 110)

identical series"[34] was a remarkable success; it was sold nearly six hundred times across the world in a few years, without counting the innumerable copies and forgeries of which it would have been the object.[35] Dr. de Quervain also built sterilisation installations at the beginning of his career, in La Chaux-de-Fonds. A former student of the bacteriologist Ernst Tavel, professor in Berne, who advocated the sterilisation of operating material, de Quervain developed at the end of the 1890s "autoclaves for hospital needs. The devices supplied by [Schaerer] were the first to be manufactured by him. They were devices with two atmospheres of overpressure, working with temperatures of 120 to 130 °C, while almost all his competitors were satisfied with autoclaves of the Schimmelbusch principle, with a maximum of half an atmosphere of overpressure".[36] Produced in series by Schaerer (nine patents registered between 1902 and 1939), these sterilisation installations were also commercial successes.

The mass production of surgical equipment was made possible by the intervention of external financiers who enabled the company to develop strongly. From the beginning of the 1900s, Schaerer sought to expand his workshop in the old town of Berne and move into an industrial stage of production to extend his market beyond the Berne medical network. In 1903, with the financial support of a local merchant, he transformed his company into a limited company. Branches and sales depots were opened in several European cities (Berlin, Brussels, Geneva, Lausanne and London). The international success of the company attracted interest and, in 1920, Schaerer was acquired by the German company INAG AG. The share capital of Schaerer was increased to five million francs in 1923, with the involvement of German businessmen from Credit Suisse. The German Siemens Group, to which INAG belongs, aimed to become the European leader in this sector between the two World Wars. Schaerer was a company in strong development and with broad ambitions when it intervened in the mechanisation and standardisation of surgery during the years 1890–1940.

In the Canton of Vaud, Roux and de Quervain played a considerable role in the commercial success of this company. In fact, two major Swiss producers of surgical equipment, the Bernese company Schaerer and the St. Gallen-based Hausmann, were fighting for the Vaud market in the 1900s. Being purely German-speaking, they did not seem to have any direct links with doctors in Vaud. It was, therefore, crucial for them to obtain the support of César Roux in Lausanne. The Hausmann company wrote to him in 1900 saying, "you have kindly promised [the Schaerer company] your protection [...] and that is why we take the liberty of asking you if, in this case, you would not also have some consideration for us. You will undoubtedly understand that we cannot

[34] *La construction des hôpitaux modernes et leurs installations. Ouvrage destiné à l'usage des médecins, architectes, ingénieurs, techniciens, personnel d'administration, étudiants et practiciens*, Berne, Maison Schaerer SA, 1930, p. 108.

[35] Terrier, "Le docteur Fritz de Quervain...", op. cit., p. 196.

[36] Testimony of Quervain quoted by Tröhler, "F. de Quervain...", op. cit., p. 202.

give up all our customers and that in spite of Mr. Schaerer, we will establish in Lausanne what [...] we did not do earlier".[37] In the end, Schaerer won in Lausanne with the opening of a branch in 1903. Schaerer's success in the Canton of Vaud was also due to the intervention of Quervain who, in 1897, acted as an expert of the equipment for the new Saint-Loup Hospital, which itself was to become a reference in French-speaking Switzerland. In the same way, the administrative authorities of the Montreux Hospital called on Roux in 1909 to supervise the organisation and equipment of their new surgical department.[38] Finally, Roux authorised Schaerer to include his name in the list of doctors quoted as references in their advertising catalogues published in the 1900s, among some fifteen medical personalities. On the strength of these successes, Schaerer became a key player in the development of hospitals between the two World Wars. In 1930, this company published a reference work on the subject, entitled *La construction des hôpitaux modernes et leurs installations. Ouvrage destiné à l'usage des médecins, architectes, ingénieurs, techniciens, personnel d'administration, étudiants et practiciens.*[39]

Roux in Lausanne: German Surgery and Radical-Democratic Networks

César Roux was the first doctor trained in the new German surgery to settle in the Canton of Vaud. However, there was no automatic link between the young doctor's professional training and his appointment to the Cantonal Hospital and then to the Faculty of Medicine. Roux had to establish himself in the medical profession as an innovative surgeon to benefit from the recognition of one's peers. But scientific and professional recognition is not everything; it was necessary to have political support.

Professional Recognition

Throughout his years as an assistant of Kocher, Roux expressed his desire to specialise in surgery. During the training trip to Germany and Austria he undertook in 1881, Roux spent most of his time in the clinics of the masters of surgery. He wrote to his fiancée that year: "I have learned above all a mass of practical and theoretical details that K[ocher] does not think to tell us. This does not mean that I appreciate V[olkman] better than K[ocher] but I am very happy to see them both. As for internal medicine, I cannot do much about it [...]. I can say that in short I sacrificed everything to surgery during my trip. Have I done well? The future will tell".[40] During his assistantship in Berne, Roux was already thinking about a career as a surgeon in the Canton of Vaud.

[37] ACV, César Roux Papers, letter from Hausmann to César Roux, 12 May 1900.

[38] Montreux Hospital, annual report, 1909.

[39] *La construction...*, op. cit.

[40] Letter from César Roux to Anna Bégoune, 31 May 1881, quoted in Jeanne-Marie Allier and Benjamin Baudraz, *Docteur César Roux. Lettres à Anna Bégoune et à quelques autres correspondants (1880–1933)*, Lausanne, Ed. d'en bas, 2003, pp. 128–129.

He wanted to be the first to develop the new surgery there and dreamed of a position as a surgeon at the Cantonal Hospital, the only place where he could put his acquired know-how to use. He wrote to his fiancée in 1881: "I can only go to L[ausanne] if I have the hospital".[41] A year later, in July 1882, he thought of giving up his position as an assistant and moving to the city of Lausanne, and consulted a former assistant of Kocher, Dr. Paul Niehans senior, who had recently been appointed surgeon at the Inselspital (Berne): "I told him of my project and of the fear of seeing a surgeon or surgeons set up before me, and spoke of the good opportunity, as my brothers call it. He didn't think for a minute and answered categorically that I had to present myself afterwards as a specialist, claiming that I had no right to do so now and that after another year I was sure to make a clientele quickly". "Even if there come half a dozen surgeons or so-called surgeons that will in no way prevent you from making your place in the sun with ease".[42] Roux thus extended his training time by a year.

When he moved to Lausanne in September 1883, he had the firm intention of taking up surgery. From December onwards, he helped the surgeons of the Cantonal Hospital, in particular with the extraction of goitres, a speciality acquired from Kocher.[43] In addition, Roux worked as a substitute surgeon during their vacations. He also operated on many occasions at home or in his private practice. Roux knew how to make himself known and did not hesitate to leave Lausanne on many occasions to carry out surgical operations in the surrounding countryside.[44] In the same way, some local infirmaries, such as the one in Montreux, called upon his services on several occasions.

Roux thus established himself among his colleagues in the Canton of Vaud as a doctor of the new generation who had embraced scientific modernism. Between 1883 and 1890, he presented about twenty papers at meetings of the local society of medicine (Société Vaudoise de Médecine, SVM) in which he revealed an innovative and modernist spirit that gave him a dominant position over the classical surgeons.[45] In 1883, as only a young doctor, he took the floor to denounce the obsolete character of certain operations performed by his colleagues. While Dr. de la Harpe presented a case of sciatic elongation with complications in November 1883, Roux declared that "the results of this operation are not very encouraging [...] and that it is now generally abandoned for these cases".[46] At the following session, in December 1883, he questioned the use of tin drains presented by Dr. Joël, to whom he declared that "the present tendency is rather to do without drains. A rigid drain is,

[41] Ibid., p. 146.

[42] Ibid., p. 204.

[43] Ibid., p. 224.

[44] According to letters written to his fiancée in 1883–1884. Allier and Baudraz, op. cit.

[45] See the minutes of the meetings of the Vaud Medical Society in the *RMSR*, 1883–1890.

[46] *RMSR*, 1884, p. 47.

moreover, not very rational; it can injure and oppose the coupling of the lips of a wound".[47] Moreover, Roux quoted operations performed by Volkmann or Kocher on numerous occasions, often to downplay the innovative nature of the cases presented by his colleagues or to justify the modernity of his own interventions. When his colleagues were surprised by the success of a certain surgical case, Roux replied that he "saw one by Volkmann and one by Kocher".[48] Similarly, when he presented an innovation—in this case, the injection of 5% phenic water against erysipelas in 1884—Roux placed it in the continuity of the work of the masters of surgery: "This observation thus confirms the experiences made at Kocher's clinic".[49] He also presented an economical method of catgut preparation (February 1884) and the use of dentists' milling machines in his surgical practice (November 1885); e.g., "for the twisting of vessels in surgical operations, and shows two models of forceps which can be adapted to the machine in question. [...] M. Roux shows again several models of circular saws for trepanning long bones, which can be adapted to the same machine".[50]

Finally, Roux also intervened in controversial issues. He defended the antiseptic method at a time when it was still being questioned by other doctors (December 1884). In addition, against the opinion of the majority of his colleagues, Roux defended a rapid surgical intervention in the case of femoral resection of tuberculosis patients (October 1885) or appendicitis (March 1889). His many operations enabled him to assert himself as a young surgeon of the new generation and a disciple of renowned surgeons with an innovative spirit. After becoming a professor of surgery (1890), he sent his assistant Perret in his place to present the last interesting cases he operated on at the Cantonal Hospital. Having reached the peak of his surgical career in the Canton of Vaud, Roux could afford not to present the results of his research to his colleagues of the SVM.

A student of the German surgical school, Roux had a particularly dominant image of his branch. In his inaugural lecture at the Faculty of Medicine (1890), he asserted that "the discovery of antisepsis has necessarily wiped out the experience acquired over several centuries; and the representatives most worthy of being listened to in the old school, seeing their reasoning sin by the base, will console themselves by giving the hand of the young to guide them anyway in the observation at the patient's bed".[51] This perspective was not limited to the surgeons of the older generations, but to the entire medical profession which saw itself subjected to the new surgery: "If it is true that one

[47] *RMSR*, 1884, p. 110.

[48] *RMSR*, 1886, p. 175.

[49] *RMSR*, 1885, p. 178.

[50] *RMSR*, 1886, pp. 111–112.

[51] *Discours et leçons prononcés à l'ouverture des cours du Ier semestre de l'Université de Lausanne*, Lausanne: Editions de l'Université, 1891, p. 160.

can be an excellent doctor without having a taste for surgery or the necessary skill in an operation, it is impossible to be a good surgeon without first being a good doctor".[52] This commanding position guided Roux's medical career.

Political Commitment: The Strength of Radical-Democratic Networks
In addition to professional recognition, Roux gained the indispensable support of the Radical-Democratic Party (RDP) in which the Roux family was actively involved. César's father, Benjamin Roux (1824–1876), was a local notable engaged in this party: a schoolteacher, he sat as a deputy in the Constituent Assembly, sat in the Grand Council in the ranks of this party for three years (1862–1865) and then held one of the three positions of Cantonal school inspector.[53] One of César's older brothers, Louis Roux, was a prominent figure in Lausanne politics.[54] He was a member of the Communal Council (1878–1882) and the Municipal Council, where he was director of schools (1882–1894). He was also a member of the board of directors of the bank Crédit foncier vaudois. These public offices enabled him to perform important functions in the hospital and university sectors, which undoubtedly contributed to the success of his younger brother. Louis Roux participated as a delegate of the municipality in the negotiations between the city of Lausanne and the Canton of Vaud which led to the creation of the University and the Faculty of Medicine (1890). He was also a member for more than ten years of the Health and Hospice Council, responsible for the Cantonal Hospital (1898–1908). Another brother, Félix Roux, had important connections in the field of public education even though he was not politically involved.[55] These two brothers were essential supports for César Roux. Their relations enabled them to offer him, in 1881–1882, the new position of surgeon created at the Cantonal Hospital.

César Roux himself joined the Radical-Democratic Party (RDP) on his arrival in Lausanne (1883). He held a seat as a municipal councillor during the years crucial for the future of his career (1885–1893 and 1898–1901). Among other things, he took part in the debate on the creation of the University and thus the Faculty of Medicine. Nevertheless, Roux's political career remained small; for example, he never held a seat in the Grand Council. However, Roux maintained networks that enabled him to be at the heart of political power in Vaud. He was part of the young modernising elite within the student society Helvetia, of which he was made an honorary member in 1885. This organisation brought together a number of lawyers, magistrates, university professors, engineers, pastors and doctors who were at the head of private companies and

[52] Ibid., pp. 160–161.

[53] Benjamin Baudraz, *Jean Roux du Villaret en Pragela réfugié à Bex en 1685 pour cause de religion. Son histoire et celle d'une partie de sa descendance au Pays de Vaud (1652–1900)*, Lausanne, 1995, pp. 162–179.

[54] Ibid., pp. 185–187.

[55] Ibid., pp. 187–189.

public or para-public institutions (University, Cantonal Bank, etc.) that were modernising the Canton of Vaud.[56] Finally, he was personally close to Louis Ruchonnet, leader of the Vaud RDP and federal councillor (1881–1893), acting as one of his doctors[57] and offering his son a position as an intern at the Cantonal Hospital in 1892.[58]

These political networks, coupled with his recognised professional skills, led to his appointment as professor of legal medicine at the Academy at the age of 27, six months after his move to Lausanne (1884). He was finally appointed doctor at the Surgical Department of the Cantonal Hospital (1887) and then professor of surgery at the Faculty of Medicine (1890).

Teaching Surgery in the Faculty of Medicine

Several historians have shown that the birth of medical specialties arose from the collective desire of doctors to be recognised for their knowledge and know-how specific to a type of disease or patient.[59] This repositioning in the field of medicine thus enabled doctors to emancipate themselves from certain supervisory bodies by creating a new social field whose hierarchy they controlled. The opening of new university chairs or the appointment of private professors in new fields of teaching were the result of conflicts and negotiations between young doctors and established professors, supported by the Faculty of Medicine, who accepted the making of an official new speciality to the detriment of their branch.

Surgery had a marked generalist character which the development of invasive methods in the second part of the nineteenth century only strengthened. The surgeon's reputation was thus based on his ability to undertake many types of operations. From this perspective, César Roux is a perfect example of a professor established in a vast field—surgery—who wished to keep control of it: he accepted the birth of specialties only on the condition that he remained their mentor. The medical specialities that succeeded in becoming independent of surgery were entrusted to close relatives (Demiéville) or loyal disciples (Perret, Vulliet). The case of gynaecology illustrates perfectly the problems encountered by doctors who did not come from the Roux network.

[56] *Helvetia: Livre d'or de la section vaudoise*, Lausanne, 1983.

[57] Félix Bonjour, *Louis Ruchonnet. Sa vie - son œuvre*, Lausanne, Imprimerie vaudoise, 1936, pp. 187 and 190.

[58] ACV, César Roux Papers, letter from Louis Ruchonnet to César Roux, 4 January 1892.

[59] Loris Premuda, "La naissance des spécialités", in Grmek, op. cit., pp. 253–269; George Rosen, "Changing attitudes of the medical profession to specialization", *Bulletin of the History of Medicine*, 1942, pp. 343–354; George Weisz, "The emergence of medical specialization in the nineteenth century", *Bulletin of the History of Medicine*, 2003, pp. 536–575; Lindsay Grandshaw, "Fame and fortune by means of bricks and mortar: the medical profession and specialist hospitals in Britain", in Roy Porter and Lindsay Grandshaw (eds), *Hospitals in History*, London/New York: Routledge, 1989, pp. 199–220.

Teaching Gynaecology

In the hospital built in 1883, gynaecology was attached to the Surgical Department while obstetrics was an independent department. This organisation was not called into question with the creation of the Faculty of Medicine in 1890, but the attachment of gynaecology to obstetrics, as well as the construction of a new maternity ward, were the subject of bitter negotiations for several decades. The foundation of the Faculty of Medicine was the occasion for Dr. Oscar Rapin, in charge of the maternity ward of the Cantonal Hospital since 1874 and professor of obstetrics since 1890, to claim for his department the gynaecology cases hospitalised for surgery, as well as the theoretical teaching of this branch and the construction of a new maternity ward.[60]

Unwilling to abandon the teaching of gynaecology, Roux, supported in this matter by prof. Kocher,[61] wrote to the Department of Public Instruction: "Having never seen special courses in gynaecology held, even in faculties where the professor of obstetrics forgets this one for that one, I have never had the idea of announcing a similar course - which is done only in Vienna and in some schools, during the holidays. I think, therefore, unless you decide otherwise, not to mention gynaecology, which will fit into the general teaching of surgery".[62] The State Council itself did not want to multiply the teaching, essentially for financial reasons.

This position aroused the anger of prof. Rapin, who wrote to the head of the Department of Public Education in 1891 and protested against the maintenance of gynaecology in the Department of Surgery: "The present organisation of disciplines places the Faculty of Lausanne in a situation of inferiority with respect to all the other Faculties in Switzerland. Here it has long been understood that the teaching of gynaecology is the indispensable complement to obstetrics. In Germany these branches are taught everywhere by the same professor, unless, in order to give more importance to these two branches, they are entrusted to two specialists, a midwife and a gynaecologist. [...] The way in which gynaecological teaching is distributed in Lausanne would be a step backwards, if it were definitive. It would correspond to the organisation that the Faculty of Berne had before 1869, when the special service of gynaecology was founded by prof. Breisky, 'accoucheur'. [...] The present organisation was sought to be justified by asking Professor Kocher in Berne for an advance notice. This choice sufficiently showed that one did

[60] ACV, K XIII 252 C, letter from Rapin to the Department of Public Instruction, 29 July 1890.

[61] ACV, K XIII 252 C, letter from Kocher to State Councilor Eugène Ruffy, 9 March 1889.

[62] ACV, K XIII 252 C, letter from Roux to the Department of Public Instruction, 6 August 1890.

not seek to clarify the question without bias; but simply to obtain the sanction of what one wished to establish".[63] Rapin also intervened at the Faculty Council and requested in 1892 the repatriation of gynaecology cases to the maternity ward for pedagogical reasons. He stated that, for his teaching, he needed this "gynaecological material which is currently at the disposal of the professor of surgery",[64] to which Roux replied that he had not wanted this situation but had inherited it when he arrived at the Cantonal Hospital. In order to calm the situation, Roux accepted in 1893 to put a small room in his Surgical Department at his colleague's disposal where he would be responsible for certain gynaecological cases. In spite of this half victory, Rapin was never able to teach gynaecology. He remained a professor only of obstetrics until his death in 1902.

The renewal of this chair was an opportunity to reorganise the branch of gynaecology and obstetrics. However, this teaching was not concentrated in the hands of a single professor. Guillaume Rossier, although a private doctor of gynaecology for more than 10 years, only obtained the position of professor of obstetrics and the direction of the maternity ward. As for the theoretical teaching of gynaecology, the Faculty decided to separate it from the surgical clinic and to give it to another private doctor of gynaecology, Maurice Muret. César Roux thus kept the gynaecological cases in his surgical clinic, only giving up the theoretical teaching which allowed him to concentrate on the practical aspects of his chair.

Roux's retirement made it possible to envisage a redistribution of tasks between the various professors of medicine (1926). The Faculty Council unanimously decided to transfer the entire teaching (theoretical and clinical) to the Maternity Hospital. A former intern and head of the clinic of prof. Rossier, Rodolphe Rochat, was entrusted with the teaching of gynaecology as a private doctor (1926), then as a professor (1929), as well as teaching obstetrics and acting as the director of the Maternity Hospital (gynaecology and obstetrics). After the death of his master (1929), he took over the whole with the help of two privatdozents. Rochat's arrival as the head of the chair of gynaecology and obstetrics corresponded exactly to the growth in the number of gynaecological cases treated at the Maternity Hospital following Roux's departure; their number doubled between 1927 (277 cases) and 1930 (561 cases), continuing to increase during the 1930s (679 cases in 1934).[65] With Rochat, the two branches in Lausanne were merged. His professional career during the 1920s appears to be a prelude to the union between gynaecology and obstetrics.[66] His attraction to the latter branch was confirmed as soon

[63] ACV, K XIII, 252 C, letter from Rapin to the head of the Department of Public Instruction, 14 February 1891.

[64] Archives of the University of Lausanne (AUNIL), minutes of the meetings of the Council of the Faculty of Medicine, 13 January 1892.

[65] ACV, K VIII D 62.

[66] Robert and Panese, op. cit., pp. 1088–1089.

as he obtained his medical degree (1920). Indeed, he held his first position as an intern at the Maternity Hospital with prof. Guillaume Rossier (1920–1922) before becoming head of the clinic (1923–1924). At the same time, Rochat completed internships in gynaecology, notably with prof. Faure in Paris (1921) and Bum in Berlin (1924). On the strength of these experiences, he opened his own gynaecological practice in Lausanne in 1924 and began an academic career. His reputation also rested on his management of the Montchoisi Clinic, intended for a wealthy clientele, which he founded in 1929 and where he became the obstetrician of the international gotha. Finally, Rochat became involved in national medical bodies to defend the merger of the two branches at a time when the boundaries between various medical specialties were becoming rigid. In 1930, he was appointed president of the Society of Gynecology and Obstetrics of French-speaking Switzerland. The autonomy of gynecology in relation to surgery and its union with obstetrics were materialised in the opening in 1937 of an annex to the maternity building, the Rossier Hospital, which housed the gynaecological clinic.

The Development of Orthopaedics

The empowerment of orthopaedics as a surgical branch is a perfect illustration of the issues involved in the emergence of surgical specialties outside the control of César Roux. Indeed, it took some twenty years of conflict and negotiation to achieve widespread acceptance of surgical methods in orthopaedics. However, unlike in Great Britain, for example, the orthopaedic surgeons in Vaud did not clash with other surgeons but with the older generation of orthopaedic doctors who wanted to maintain traditional methods of treatment.[67]

Until the beginning of the 1890s, orthopaedics in the Canton of Vaud were focused on treating congenital diseases, such as club feet, following on from the work undertaken by Venel at the end of the eighteenth century. Orthopaedic cases were mainly taken care of by a private institution, the Orthopaedic Hospice of French-speaking Switzerland (*Hospice orthopédique de la Suisse romande*), founded in 1876 in Lausanne by philanthropists from Geneva and Vaud.[68] This hospital was directed by a descendant of Venel, Henri Martin, who saw himself as both the guardian and the continuator of the family traditions and know-how.[69] This strong patrimonial dimension greatly explains the difficulties encountered by doctors, outside of this family, who were in favour of new ways of practising orthopaedics.

[67] Roger Cooter, "The meaning of fractures: orthopaedics and the reform of British hospitals in the inter-war period", *Medical History*, 1987, pp. 306–322.

[68] *Centième anniversaire de l'hôpital orthopédique de la Suisse romande*, Lausanne, Hospice orthopédique, 1976.

[69] Guy Saudan (ed.), *L'éveil médical vaudois, 1750–1850, Tissot - Venel - Mayor*, Lausanne, University, 1987, p. 95.

Originally, the Orthopaedic Hospice was an establishment "intended for children with deformities requiring orthopaedic treatment"[70] which did not admit adults. In such a context, the adoption of surgical methods for certain afflictions was not self-evident. The appointment in 1893 of a disciple of Kocher and Roux, Louis Perret, as assistant physician at the Orthopaedic Hospice very quickly brought to light the conflicts generated by the arrival of new ideas. In 1896, Perret obtained a position as a privatdozent of orthopaedics at the Faculty of Medicine, thanks to Roux's favourable notice, he sought to develop this specialty. Still under the orders of Dr. Martin, in 1898 he proposed to work voluntarily at the Hospice in exchange for the improvement of its medical equipment, which the committee of the establishment refused. The same year, supported by Roux, he proposed to the Faculty that they create a chair of orthopaedics: "Mr Perret offered the hospital service of the Orthopaedic Hospice for the students and asked that the Faculty organize the teaching of orthopaedics. Mr Roux thinks that the State should try to take an interest in the matter and to create an orthopaedic teaching in this establishment. He thinks that this would be the time to create this teaching".[71]

In 1899, Perret was appointed extraordinary professor and took on a former Roux intern, Placide Nicod, as his assistant. This intervention by the Faculty did not please the Hospice committee, which stated in 1900 that Perret "must refrain from doing surgery"[72] and put Nicod under the direct orders of Martin. At the same meeting, Martin asked that the maximum age of patients admitted (12 years) be more strictly observed. This restriction was a protectionist measure against the affirmation of surgical methods which rather take care of adult patients whose afflictions were not congenital but resulted from injuries and accidents. Finally, Perret was dismissed from the Orthopaedic Hospice in 1901 for having persisted in his surgical activities. He no longer had a hospital ward and lost his position as an extraordinary professor. From then on, orthopaedics was not taught at the University until 1913, when the Faculty Council agreed to grant a position as a privatdozent to Nicod, who remained in the service of the Orthopaedic Hospice.

Perhaps more conciliatory than his predecessor, Nicod did not assert himself a priori as a surgeon. He knew how to get into the good graces of the Hospice committee, which perceived him in 1902 as a "resolute supporter of Dr H. Martin's orthopaedic treatment".[73] However, the Hospice administrators were soon disillusioned, stating in 1905, "Mr. H. Martin explains that Mr. Nicod does surgery little by little, in the same way that Mr. Perret once tried to do it, while going, it is true, faster than Mr. Nicod does at present".[74]

[70] ACV, Orthopaedic Hospice Papers, regulation of 1 November 1876, art. 1.

[71] AUNIL, minutes of the meetings of the Council of the Faculty of Medicine, 2 July 1898.

[72] ACV, Orthopaedic Hospice Papers, Committee Minutes, 22 March 1900.

[73] Ibid., 9 October 1902.

[74] Ibid., 16 November 1905.

In the early 1910s, he developed a surgical method of treating tuberculosis which attracted several people disappointed with heliotherapy.[75] This led to the opposition of Dr. Edouard Martin, cousin of the founder of the Hospice, member of its committee and a renowned orthopaedic surgeon in Geneva, who "wished the hospice to remain orthopaedic, and that tubercular patients should not be too invasive, so that the establishment would not become too surgical [...]".[76] It seems that after this, Nicod made himself more discreet for a time. He would have performed operations out of sight, in the Bois-Cerf Clinic where he hospitalised his private clientele, as well as in the kitchen of the Orthopaedic Hospice after the death of Martin.[77]

In the end, Nicod was appointed as a privatdozent in 1913 and succeeded in imposing the need for surgical orthopaedics by around 1915. While he never mentioned surgical interventions in his annual reports, he alluded to them for the first time in 1915 when he wrote that "surgical interventions on muscles, tendons, bones and joints are often necessary and, in these cases, the operative act must be considered as a valuable adjunct or complement to the previous means [...]".[78] From this year onwards, references to surgical activity become more and more important. In addition, the question of a new hospital building, in which the Surgical Department would play a major role, was openly discussed during these years. As early as 1914, the Hospice committee approached the State to ask for support for its new building project, which the State Council accepted in 1916 (with the provision of a plot of land near the Cantonal Hospital). In return, the Orthopaedic Hospice submitted to the condition issued by the Faculty Council—and proposed by Roux—that "the professor of orthopaedics be appointed by the government and not by the Hospice committee".[79]

In addition to these conditions issued by the State, it is important to underline the arrival of two doctors who were committed to the new surgery within the Hospice committee: Jacques de Montmollin, chief physician of the Pourtalès Hospital in Neuchâtel (1903), and a former intern of César Roux, Gustave Delay (1918). Both promoted the acceptance of surgical methods in the treatment of orthopaedic conditions. Delay, in particular, played a determining role in the assertion of medical power within the Hospice. He noted, in 1920, that "conflicts between the administrative and medical management are very frequent in establishments such as ours. [...] He shows the origin of this antagonism, which has been increased recently by the development of orthopaedic science. He does not believe in the possibility of a

[75] Michel Gross, *Placide Nicod. Un pionnier de l'orthopédie moderne*, Yens-sur-Morges, Cabédita, 1993, p. 44.

[76] ACV, Orthopaedic Hospice Papers, Committee Minutes, 12 December 1912.

[77] According to Gross, *Placide Nicod...*, op. cit., p. 37.

[78] ACV, Orthopaedic Hospice Papers, Annual Report, 1915, p. 5.

[79] AUNIL, minutes of the meetings of the Council of the Faculty of Medicine, 18 November 1914.

two-headed management. The management must be medical, as was decided at the Cantonal hospital [...]".[80] Indeed, Nicod had to face the hostility of the bursar, who also functioned at times as a nurse and masseur and "who was Mr. Martin's right-hand man [and] remained in the old orthopaedic methods". The committee then followed Delay. In 1921, it appointed Nicod as director of the Hospice and subordinated the bursar to him, putting an end to the Martin period. The policy of appointing members of the Hospice committee between the two World Wars perfectly reflects this predominance of medical concerns; in the years 1926–1947, there were seven doctors and one nurse among the nine people who joined it. The opening of new buildings in 1927 embodies this turn from philanthropy to medicine. Located directly next to the Cantonal Hospital, they were designed to accommodate modern surgery, with the installation of an operating theatre equipped with high-tech equipment from the Schaerer company, an X-ray facility and a physiotherapy institute.[81]

After 1927, the development of surgical treatments allowed a new type of patient to be treated: the accident victim. The development of car traffic led to a sharp increase in the number of victims of road accidents; for the whole of Switzerland, this figure rose to 8539 in 1930 (including 412 deaths), 12,012 in 1950 (453 deaths) and 35,701 in 1960 (1303 deaths).[82] In the Canton of Vaud alone, traffic accidents affected 1050 people in 1950 and 4266 in 1960.[83] The increased mechanisation of the industrial and agricultural sectors only reinforced this trend. A real accident market was therefore created during the inter-war period and experienced a strong expansion in the 1950s, which largely benefited the affirmation and development of surgical methods in orthopaedics. The arrival of this new, generally adult, clientele resulted in a decrease in the proportion of children and adolescents hospitalised. The under-18s were still largely dominant until the end of the 1920s, when they represented nearly 85% of hospitalisations, but their proportion fell sharply during the 1930s, falling from 84% of patients in 1930 to 68% in 1939.[84]

It was in this context that orthopaedics was recognised by the Faculty of Medicine: Placide Nicod was appointed full professor in 1931. The adoption the following year of FMH titles to regulate the various medical specialties confirmed the surgical dimension of orthopaedics: according to the regulations adopted by the Swiss Medical Chamber in 1931, specialisation in this

[80] ACV, Orthopaedic Hospice Papers, Minutes of Executive Committee Meetings, 30 December 1920.

[81] Ibid., 20 March 1921.

[82] *Annuaire statistique de la Suisse*, 1930–1960. These figures were not published until 1929.

[83] Figures by Canton were not published in the 1930s.

[84] ACV, Orthopaedic Hospice Papers, annual reports, 1928–1939.

branch required an additional four years of study, two of which were spent in a Surgical Department.[85]

The Radiology Laboratory

The discovery of X-rays by Röntgen in 1895 was an important event for surgical practice and the development of hospitals, not only because X-rays soon became a safe and objective diagnostic tool, but also, and above all, because they helped to spread a certain idea of medicine among the public which was not without effect on the growth in demand for care.[86]

In the beginning, doctors did not yet know exactly what this discovery could be used for in their daily practice but they realised the importance of studying this new technology which allowed one to see inside the body. In 1897, the Health and Hospices Council considered the creation of a radiology service at the hospital and asked Roux to report on this issue.[87] The following year, this council decided to install radiology apparatus to carry out "medical research by the Röntgen ray process".[88] Even if he did not yet perfectly know how this technique worked, Roux already saw its potential usefulness and the first laboratory was installed in his surgery department. This decision led to a reaction from the dermatology professor Emile Dind, who obtained access to the installation for the entire Vaud medical corporation (1898).

The installation was minimal—no employee was especially attached to it—but it already allowed the taking of a few X-rays (118 in 1898 and 416 in 1901) and met with a certain amount of success: 2.2% of patients were X-rayed in 1898 and 7.7% in 1901. The hospital administration, which saw this as an opportunity to collect new revenue to develop the equipment, agreed to the doctors' requests and authorised the expansion of the laboratory. New equipment was purchased in 1904 and the laboratory was entrusted to a German chemist, Reiss. A second radiology laboratory for radiotherapy was opened in the same year in Prof. Dind's department, for the use of the entire medical profession.

Reiss left his post shortly afterwards and was replaced by a disciple of Roux, Frédéric Wullyamoz (1906–1916), who was particularly interested in radioscopy. He developed surgical instruments allowing the extraction of foreign bodies under radioscopic control—the subject of his thesis, directed by Roux and accepted in 1910. Another pupil of César Roux, his nephew Jacques Roux, completed a thesis on *The use of X-rays before appendectomy* (1913). The aim was clearly to study the usefulness of this innovation for surgical practice. Finally, Wullyamoz created a radioscopic operating table but this invention was quickly abandoned when the danger of the rays was recognised; he died in 1917.

[85] *Bulletin des médecins suisses*, 1935, p. 654.

[86] Howell, *Technology in the Hospital…*, op. cit.

[87] ACV, K VIII B 6, minutes of the Health and Hospice Council, 1897.

[88] Ibid., 2 March 1898.

This phase, the setting up and acceptance of radiology, was made all the easier by the fact that this service gradually became profitable for the Cantonal Hospital. The first fees for the use of the X-ray installation were paid, as early as 1904, by patients or external doctors for their clients. They soon became an important financial resource for the hospital (2.2% of the operating income in 1904 and 10.6% in 1910) and helped to make its growth possible (see Chapter 3).

The resignation of Wullyamoz in 1916 was the occasion to reform the organisation of radiology, in the context of the profound restructuring of the Cantonal Hospital during the inter-war period. The two laboratories of the establishment—the radiography laboratory of the Surgical Department and the radiotherapy laboratory of the dermatology department—were brought together under the technical and administrative direction of a single doctor. It was not one of Roux's students who was appointed to this position, but a former head of Prof. Dind's clinic, Roger Isenegger (1916–1921). When Isenegger resigned in 1921, radiology was a branch that had become independent of other medical specialties. The Faculty Council then turned to the leading specialist in radiology in French-speaking Switzerland, Alfred Rosselet. Holding doctorates in science (physics) and medicine, he had organised the radiology department of the Cantonal Hospital in Geneva (1917–1920) before joining Auguste Rollier's tuberculosis clinic in Leysin (1920–1922). With his arrival in Lausanne, radiology became an independent department of the Cantonal Hospital. The following year, he was entrusted with a course in radiology as a private lecturer (1923) and then as a professor (1926). He also became known as one of the initiators of the Anticancer Centre in French-speaking Switzerland (*Centre anticancéreux romand*), founded in Lausanne in 1924. Rosselet established himself as an equal to other professors of medicine.

The Surgical Policlinic

The teaching of the surgical policlinic—small ambulatory surgery—was very quickly separated from the Surgical Department and attached to the Cantonal University Policlinic, founded in 1892.[89] This organisation actually took over the activities of the Central Dispensary, a private philanthropic institution opened in 1887 by about twenty doctors. The departure of the surgical policlinic was completed without any apparent problem, as the University Polyclinic did not compete with the clinical services of the Cantonal Hospital. It essentially provided free outpatient care to the poor, rapidly diversified its services with the multiplication of types of treatment (ophthalmology 1904, tuberculosis 1906, ENT 1912, nerve diseases 1913, venereal diseases 1919, infants 1923, dentistry 1923) and was very successful with the public. There were more than 17,000 consultations in 1895 and more than 30,000 per year

[89] *Policlinique médicale universitaire, 100 ans, 1887–1987*, Lausanne, PMU, 1987, 66 pp. and Guy Saudan, "Dispensaire et policlinique à Lausanne: 100 ans de médecine et société", *RMSR*, 1989, pp. 267–277.

in the 1900s and 1910s.[90] Roux himself was personally in favour of an agreement between the Central Dispensary and the Faculty of Medicine. He wrote to this effect to the Department of Public Education in 1891, insisting on the fact that the ambulatory consultations of the Cantonal Hospital could not replace a Policlinic and that the latter was an essential element of a Faculty of Medicine.[91] In 1892, the University Polyclinic was entrusted to a close friend of César Roux, Paul Demiéville; a former student of Theodor Kocher, he was the father-in-law of one of Roux's daughters.

Empowerment of Non-clinical Chairs: Operative Medicine and Occupational Health

If a specialty was not linked to clinical teaching, its autonomy was much less problematic. Branches such as operative medicine (courses on cadavers) or occupational health were essentially theoretical. Their creation did not call into question any hospital services and allowed César Roux to abandon these secondary teachings in order to concentrate on more prestigious fields, such as the surgical clinic.

As far as operative medicine was concerned, Roux acted in two stages. First of all, in 1894, he asked the Department of Public Education for authorisation to hire a special assistant at his own expense.[92] Five years later, he intervened at the Faculty Council and asked to be relieved of the teaching of this theoretical branch (1899). He proposed that it be entrusted to Louis Perret, who was experiencing serious difficulties at the Orthopaedic Hospice. The Faculty accepted Roux's proposal and Perret held the chair until 1934.

As for the chair of occupational health, it was created in 1913 because of its inclusion in the federal medical examinations following the adoption of the law on accident insurance. Initially, the Faculty wished to appoint Henri Secrétan to this post, whose professional experience made him an excellent candidate. Established in Lausanne in 1885, he worked for several insurance companies and specialised in the care of injured people. He also wrote a book on the subject of work-related accidents.[93] But Secrétan declined the Faculty's offer and the latter turned to an internal solution. The Faculty Council asked for the nomination of a former chief of clinic of Roux, Henri Vulliet, who obtained the position.

[90] Saudan, "Dispensary", op. cit., p. 273.

[91] ACV, K XIII 252 C, letter from Roux to the head of the Department of Public Instruction, 30 November 1891.

[92] ACV, K XIII 252 C, letter from Roux to the Department of Public Instruction, 30 April 1894.

[93] Henri Secrétan, *L'assurance accidents, notes chirurgicales et professionnelles*, Genève: Eggimann & Cie, 1906.

Roux's Disciples

Roux's importance for a whole generation of doctors was due not only to his dominant position at the Cantonal Hospital of Lausanne but also to the fact that he was the first to teach surgery at the Faculty of Medicine and did so for 36 years (1890–1926). It is nevertheless difficult to determine who exactly were the disciples of prof. Roux. Indeed, if all the students enrolled at the Faculty of Medicine in Lausanne between 1890 and 1926 attended surgery courses, does this make them Roux's disciples? Similarly, it is difficult to assess the impact of a semester of internship in surgery on the future of a medical career and on the know-how acquired. To one degree or another, the hundreds of doctors who graduated from the University of Lausanne up to 1926 were all pupils of Roux, at least in the sense that they participated in the dissemination of a mythical image of their master.

However, in view of the development of hospital surgery, the number of disciples can be considered much smaller. Let us look at the doctors who actually worked alongside Roux in the Surgical Department of the Cantonal Hospital: the heads of clinics and the interns.[94]

Chiefs of Clinics

The position of chief of clinic was created by the Faculty of Medicine (1890) to be occupied by a doctor who acted as an intermediary between the professor and the subordinate body (interns, nuns, nurses). At the time of Roux, he also functioned as an assistant doctor: he directly assisted the master during operations and sometimes directed the intervention himself.[95] It was an important position that allowed him to acquire a wide experience in surgical matters. Twelve doctors succeeded one another, for an average period of three years.

Some of these heads of clinic did not go on to make a career in surgery—Maurice Campart, Louis Senn and Hermann Seiler established themselves as generalists in Lausanne, Geneva and Berne, respectively, but they were exceptions and Louis Senn attempted to return to the surgical scene by running to succeed Vulliet as chair of surgery (1932).[96]

Several of them played a decisive role in the dissemination of the new surgery and the development of hospitals in areas that had previously remained on the fringe. Gustave Clément, who returned to Fribourg in 1900, operated in his private clinic and held the post of surgeon in the two main Fribourg establishments, the Bourgeois Hospital and the Cantonal Hospital, also working as a consultant surgeon in various regional hospitals. As for Victor

[94] *Catalogue des étudiants de l'Université de Lausanne*, 1891–1922.

[95] Marina Borboën, *Etude des livres opératoires de l'Hôpital Cantonal de Lausanne de 1891 à 1930. Contexte et évolution de l'anesthésiologie*, University of Lausanne, unpublished doctoral thesis in medicine, 1996.

[96] AUNIL, minutes of the meetings of the Council of the Faculty of Medicine, 10 October 1932.

Table 2 Chiefs of the surgical clinic of the Cantonal Hospital, 1891–1923

Period of office	*Name*
1891–1893	Hermann Seiler
1893–1894	Maurice Campart
1894–1896	Henri Vulliet
1896–1899	Gustave Clément
1899–1901	Victor Vella
1901–1905	Louis Senn
1905–1908	Paul Campiche
1908–1910	Albert Reverdin
1910–1914	Jacques Roux
1914–1920	Léon Picot
1920–1923	Samuel Cuendet
1923–1925	Gustave Piotet

Vella, he settled in Ticino and took charge of the surgical services of the hospitals of Lugano and Mendrisio while operating at the Clinic of Moncucco. He was the first surgeon-moderniser to settle in this Canton and became an undisputed authority until his death in 1921.[97] Finally, two heads of clinics took charge of the modernisation of local infirmaries in the Canton of Vaud, Cuendet in Yverdon, and Piotet in Aubonne, Nyon and Rolle (Table 2).

Other heads of clinics went on to become academics and hold chairs of surgery. Henri Vulliet was appointed privatdozent shortly after his time as a chief of clinic (1898). In addition to his activities in hospitals—a surgeon at the Children's Hospice (1910–1926)—he worked as a professor of occupational health (1913–1926) and succeeded Roux on his retirement (1926). Albert Reverdin, on his return to Geneva, founded the Clinique Beaulieu with his cousin, the famous Geneva surgeon Jacques-Louis Reverdin (1919), and obtained a position as assistant surgeon at the Faculty of Medicine in the department of Prof. Kummer. Finally, Paul Campiche moved to the United States and became a professor at the San Francisco Medical School (1908).

Lastly, César Roux looked after his relatives. His nephew Jacques Roux and his son-in-law Léon Picot were appointed chief surgeons for exceptional periods of five years each, an experience that was all the more useful for the former as he later assisted César in his private clinic. As for Picot, he joined the group of surgeon-modernisers in the Canton of Vaud and took up a post at the Children's Hospice after the departure of Vulliet (1926–1957).

These few destinies highlight the importance of the position of chief of clinic in the construction of a surgical career. Surgery, as taught by Roux, was a generalist branch; there was no room for the emergence of surgical specialties.

[97] Virgilio Chiesa, *L'Ospedale civico di Lugano*, Bellinzona/Lugano, 1944, p. 111.

Table 3 Career of the interns of the surgical clinic of the Cantonal Hospital, 1891–1922

Professional career	*Number*	*As a % of*
Generalist or other than surgery	23	37.1
Surgeon-modernizer	16	25.8
Prof. at the Faculty of Lausanne in another field	3	4.8
Prof. of surgery outside Lausanne	5	8.1
Not identified	15	24.2
Total	62	100.0

Source *Catalogue des étudiants de l'Université de Lausanne*, 1891–1922
Note Names are not mentioned after 1922

Most knowledge was transmitted by the master. His closest disciples became renowned general surgeons and participated in the diffusion of the know-how acquired in Roux's Surgical Department.

Interns

The internship was a period that usually took place directly after graduation from medical school and could last from one to four or even five semesters. It is during this internship the young doctor acquired their practical training. He or she was present during operations, under the orders of Roux and the head of the clinic. Many doctors did a surgical internship even though they knew they were destined for a career as a general practitioner or as a specialist in another branch of medicine: if we add the professors of medicine who taught a branch other than surgery, they represent more than half of the interns. Several of these doctors who did not make a career in surgery were committed to the local infirmaries in their region of residence, for which they sometimes provided part of the internal medicine service (Henri Céresole in Morges, William Francken in Nyon, Félix Mercanton in Montreux, Charles Miéville in Vevey). They also proved to be promoters of the development of infirmaries, alongside the surgeons who modernised them. Even if they did not benefit directly from the modernisation of the hospital for their professional practice, it nevertheless contributed to the prestige of the medical profession as a whole (Table 3).

A quarter of Roux's interns had a surgical career, several in the local infirmaries of the Canton of Vaud which they reorganised and modernised: Samuel Cuendet and Ernest Demiéville in Yverdon, Henri Curchod in Saint-Loup, Walter Moehrlen in Orbe and Henri Vuilleumier in Bex. Others did the same outside the Canton of Vaud, such as the brothers Alfred and Victor Vella in Ticino, Alfred Germanier in Sion,[98] Albert Reverdin in Geneva, Fritz Dumont

[98] Vincent Barras and Marie-France Vouilloz Burnier, *De l'hospice au réseau santé. Santé publique et systèmes hospitaliers valaisans, XIXe-XXe siècles*, Sierre, Monographic, 2004, pp. 278–280.

in Berne and Félix Augsburger in Moutier. These men were of considerable importance in the development of the regional hospitals because they brought in the new surgery and played an essential role in their modernisation (see Chapter 4). Then, several interns became key figures in Lausanne's surgery between the two World Wars. They held various positions as privatdozent or professor at the Faculty (Decker, Paschoud, Vulliet) and competed for the renewal of their chairs. Finally, some made a career abroad, such as Jean Brossy, who settled in London in 1916 and was appointed a member of the Royal College of Surgeons of England in 1919, or Paul Campiche in San Francisco, André Crotti in Colombo (USA) and Paul Calame in Shanghai.

Vocational Training at the Roux School: Predominance of Practice and Rational Organisation of Work

César Roux had a completely utilitarian vision of surgery. His teaching had to be useful and applicable. With such a conception, he belonged to the radical-democratic rationalist elites who brought science and technology to the Academy, where he had been teaching since 1884 and which they transformed into a University (1890), the role of this school being to train the modernising leaders that the Canton of Vaud needed (engineers, doctors, magistrates, etc.).[99]

As soon as the Faculty of Medicine opened, Roux made sure that his students had an essentially practical training. In 1891, he asked the Faculty Council to require candidates for the professional examination to have previously completed a practical training period in a hospital.[100] Three years later, he requested the Faculty to intervene with the Federal Council to propose the exemption of interns from military service; according to Roux, it was necessary to "give more importance to the hospital internship and less to the barracks service, whereas it is the other way around at present. Young doctors are constantly forced to interrupt their internship to go and manoeuvre in [the] army".[101] Although he did not obtain the support of the federal authorities on this precise point—to which he returned in 1908—Roux was not alone in demanding practical training in hospitals for young doctors. Similar demands were made by other universities, in particular the University of Zurich, with the aim of harmonising medical studies in Switzerland and making them compatible with those in Germany. A six-month internship in a hospital was compulsory and, from 1909 onwards, a one-year internship was required. Due to the limited capacity of regional hospitals, most of the training took place in Lausanne, in the Surgical Department of the Cantonal Hospital.

[99] Laurent Tissot, *Politique, société et enseignement supérieur dans le Canton de Vaud. L'Université de Lausanne, 1890–1916*, Lausanne, Payot, 1996, p. 341.

[100] AUNIL, minutes of the meetings of the Council of the Faculty of Medicine, 14 July 1891.

[101] Ibid., 16 May 1894.

Under Roux, young doctors learned to work in a hierarchical, rationalised and mechanised framework. This type of work organisation was the result of a double influence on Roux: that of German surgery in his formative years and that of the technical culture that permeated the family environment. During his training period in Vienna with Prof. Billroth (1881), Roux said he was very impressed by the number of assistants and the organisation of the work. In a letter to his fiancée, he wrote, "there are eight assistants, only two of whom deal with the wound; the others literally play the role of nurses [...]".[102] The highly hierarchical organisation of the surgical clinics of the German school reflects a culture of order and obedience. But it must also be remembered that this was a time when limited and developing surgical knowledge allowed professors of surgery to have a theoretical and practical grip on all the work of their clinic. The training of surgeons was still very generalist and the absence of autonomous surgical specialities played in favour of a hierarchical organisation of work, although this was not an absolute rule.

The importance of technical culture in Roux's family circle must also be emphasised. His two older brothers, Félix and Louis, both had a career at the Lausanne Industrial School, one of the most important training centres for engineers in the Canton of Vaud,[103] while his sister Marie married Hermann Amstein, a professor of mathematics at the University. One of César Roux's daughters, Marie-Hélène, obtained a doctorate in physics.[104] The Roux family was thus immersed in a technical and scientific culture in which the rational organisation of large work units (private companies, public administrations, hospitals, etc.) was an omnipresent concern.

In his generalist conception of surgery, Roux was the head of the department and everyone owed him absolute obedience. So when, in 1914, Henri Paschoud, an ambitious young 27-year-old intern, asked to be appointed head of the clinic, Roux replied: "If you want to stay here, you must learn to obey and not to discuss".[105] The hierarchical nature of the surgical clinic can also be seen in the division of labour around the operating table. According to a British surgeon who visited the various university surgical clinics in Switzerland in 1910, "in every hospital the professor is the chief, his assistants being essentially subordinates".[106] He was particularly impressed by the organisation of the Surgical Department of the Cantonal Hospital in Lausanne: after operating on a patient in his auditorium in front of his students, Roux passed the patient's body to a back room to be stitched up and dressed by assistants and moved on to the next patient. This organisation allowed the professor to

[102] Allier and Baudraz, op. cit., p. 96.

[103] *L'Ecole industrielle Cantonale. Notice historique*, Lausanne, Payot, 1902, 234 pp. + appendices.

[104] Maxime Reymond, *César Roux*, Lausanne: L'écolier romand, 1935.

[105] According to a letter from Henri Paschoud to César Roux, 5 June 1931. ACV, César Roux Papers.

[106] H.S. Souttar, *Les Cliniques chirurgicales en Suisse*, 1923.

Table 4 Operations of the Surgical Department, physician in charge of the operation, 1891–1920

	1891	*1892*	*1893*	*1898*	*1899*	*1901*	*1903*	*1910*	*1919*	*1920*
Operations	945	930	1068	1178	1168	1336	1230	1027	1329	1313
Roux	599	601	627	624	596	601	554	452	292	355
Roux (in %)	64	64	59	53	51	45	45	44	22	27
Chief of clinic	–	–	–	259	257	–	–	–	558	394
Chief of clinic (in %)	–	–	–	22	22	–	–	–	42	30
Other	346	329	441	295	315	735	676	575	479	564
Other (%)	36	36	41	25	27	55	55	56	36	43

Source Marina Borboën, Etude des livres opératoires de l'Hôpital Cantonal de Lausanne de 1891 à 1930. Contexte et évolution de l'anesthésiologie, University of Lausanne, doctoral thesis in medicine, 1996

Note Only the years presented here were available for the Roux period

present a multitude of cases to his students and to undertake a large number of operations. According to the operating books that have been preserved, Roux occupied a dominant position in the operating room and only gradually gave way to his chiefs of clinic (see Table 4). He thus reproduced the organisation of work as he had known it in Kocher's department.[107]

The Creation of a New Surgical Clinic

The surgical clinic opened in 1883 was not satisfactory to Roux, because of its insufficient space and obsolete equipment. He demanded its transformation, at least after the 1900s. In a report sent to the hospital's management in 1906, he asked for the creation of new rooms to carry out specific tasks (preparation of patients, dressings, sterilisation, etc.). In 1910, he even obtained permission to use part of the administrative premises for the management of his overloaded department. In 1912, the political authorities agreed to Roux's request. The state architect, Eugène Bron, visited then German hospitals (Bonn, Cologne, Düsseldorf, Frankfurt, Mulhouse, Strasbourg, Wiesbaden), after which he and Roux drew up the plans for the new clinic together, the main part of which Roux financed with funds from his department.[108] The new surgical clinic was opened in 1914. It was equipped with the latest medical innovations (infrastructure of the Schaerer company), including an X-ray system for his department and a laboratory for analysis. It reflects the German organisational model in which the diagnostic infrastructure is located within the clinics and not autonomously and centrally within the hospital.

[107] In 1882, Benjamin Baudraz counted 299 operations in Kocher's department. Kocher himself performed 212 (71%), Roux 70 (23%) and the other assistants 17 (6%). Allier and Baudraz, op. cit., p. 216.

[108] ACV, S 73, Files 1315–1316, New Surgical Clinic.

This new surgical clinic corresponds to a rationalised and centralised conception of surgical practice. Until then, the spatial organisation of the Surgical Department was very simple. The operating room was housed in the central rotunda, which formed an extension of the hospital building. The diagnostic infrastructure, which appeared after the construction of the Cantonal Hospital in 1883, was housed in various rooms of the Surgical Department (the whole of the ground floor), without any overall reflection on the spatial organisation of the department.

The same cannot be said of the new clinic built in 1913–1914 (see Fig. 2). The space was organised around the operating room—auditorium (A), the area in which Roux practised. In order to guarantee aseptic conditions and to avoid disrupting the work areas, students and visitors accessed the auditorium by the stairs provided for this purpose. The patient, arriving through a side corridor (F), followed a continuous progression towards the operating room, passing first through a waiting room (H, G), then an examination room (K) and finally an anaesthetic room (P). After the operation, the patient was evacuated to the dressing room (N), probably to the recovery room (J, H), and then to his room through the side corridor (F). This real "healing machine" had two more wings which included diagnostic and ancillary services, such as the laboratory (L), the teacher's and assistants' workrooms (M, Q, R), sterilisation (B), etc.

The organisation of work in this surgical clinic conceived by Roux thus responded to a need for rationalisation of production (care of patients) which was an essential technical element in the modernisation of hospital medicine. The division of labour was essentially vertical and corresponded to a hierarchical definition of tasks: at the top—in the operating room—was Roux, assisted by his chief of clinic, then the interns and the specialised nurses, who were in charge of anaesthesia and dressings, and finally the junior staff who transported the patients from their rooms to the surgical clinic.

The Importance of War Surgery in the Training of Surgeons

In a context of highly practice-oriented professional training and a hierarchical organisational structure, war surgery had a special place. As Roger Cooter and Steve Sturdy stated, the Great War provided "a crucial site for the development of new kinds of medical organisation and division of labour".[109] Because it offered the surgeon a considerable number of wounded, the war gave irreplaceable practical experience.[110] It allowed the doctor to get his hands on many cases and test certain surgical techniques, but also learn how to manage large work units. In 1929, César Roux spoke of "the civil ransom of the Great

[109] Roger Cooter and Steve Sturdy, "Introduction", in Roger Cooter, Mark Harrison, Steve Sturdy (eds), *War, Medicine and Modernity*, Thrup, Sutton Publishing, 1998, p. 12.

[110] Othmar Keel and Philippe Hudon, "L'essor de la pratique clinique dans les armées européennes (1750–1800)", *Gesnerus*, 1997, pp. 37–58.

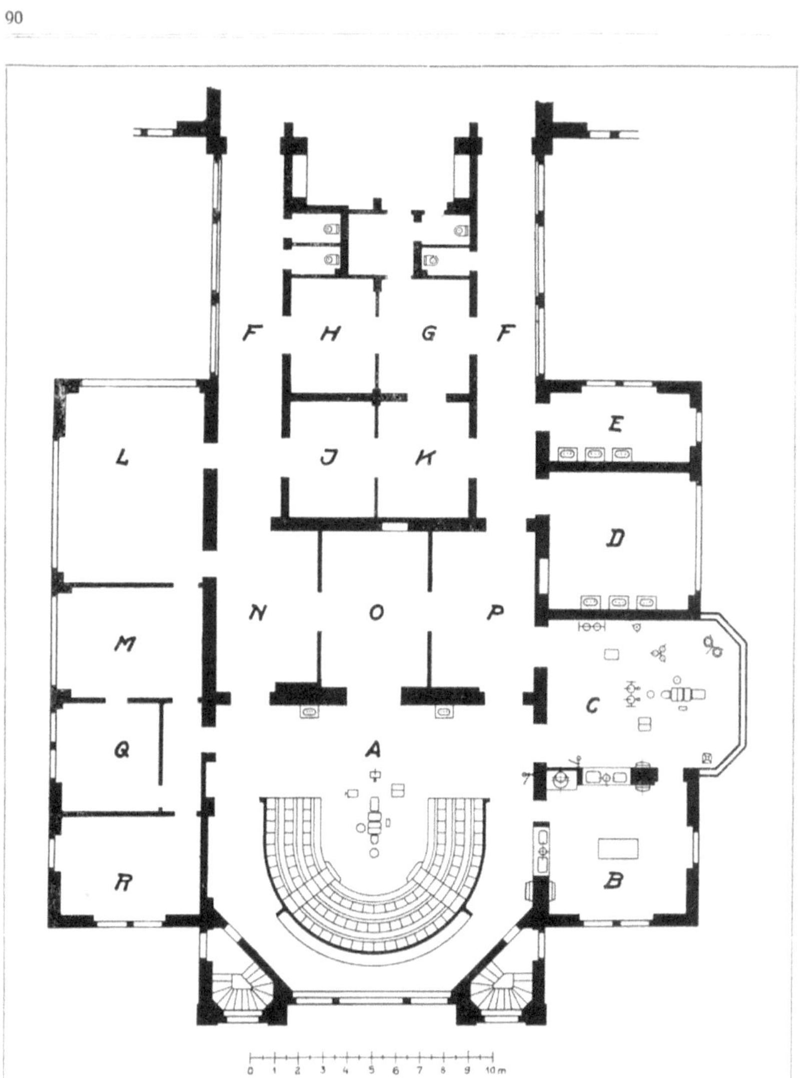

Fig. 85. Service d'opérations de la Clinique chirurgicale universitaire de l'Hôpital Cantonal de Lausanne, installé par la Maison M. Schaerer S. A. Berne.

A auditoire; *B* salle de stérilisation; *C* salle d'opérations; *D* salle d'examen et de pansement; *E* lavabos pour les opérateurs; *F* corridors; *G* et *H* salles d'attente; *I* salle des appareils plâtrés; *K* salle d'examen; *L* laboratoire; *M* appartement des assistants; *N* salle de pansement; *O* salle de cystoscopie; *P* salle d'anesthésie; *Q* bibliothèque; *R* cabinet réservé au professeur.

Fig. 2 Plan of the surgical clinic of the Cantonal Hospital, 1914 (*Source La construction* ..., op. cit., p. 90)

War"[111] and underlined the contributions of this conflict in terms of surgical knowledge: "The war put military surgeons in a position to recognise, with the help of the laboratory at hand, that the infection of wounds was not fatal afterwards and as soon as the so-called pathogenic germs penetrated. Delivering the most frightful and dreaded wounds a few minutes after the accident and in a proportion that forced the conclusions by the number, the war of position has shown that most accidental wounds can heal on occasion like that of an operation decided and practiced in our hospitals, provided that the toilet was made in time. This is a revolution in favour of civilian surgery".[112]

During the Great War, Swiss professors of surgery visited the hospitals of the belligerents on several occasions and exchanged their impressions. Kocher wrote to Roux in October 1914: "I have just returned from a tour myself to see the wounded and study war wounds. [...] I believe that pure asepsis is fine and good for small openings, as it is used a little too exclusively at the moment, but for large wounds some antisepsis is needed. Tell me your opinion".[113] In October 1914, Roux himself wrote to his wife from the military hospital in which he found himself that he "saw very interesting things".[114] This is why he wanted to bring his daughter Suzanne, who was then an intern in his Surgical Department, and wrote to his wife: "Even though it is terribly sad to see, I would be very happy if Suzanne could take a look: in 48 hours she would have seen more than in two years of books".[115] The various experiences of surgery and preventive medicine acquired during the war were shared in symposiums and specialised journals. Similarly, the Great War was an opportunity to test certain radiological innovations. The American historian Joel Howell stated that this conflict was the opportunity to use X-rays on a very large scale for the first time, to train doctors in this technology and to rationalise the costs (development of X-rays on film instead of on glass plates), which would benefit hospitals during the inter-war period.[116] This assertion is corroborated by two French doctors who published a brochure in 1921 in which they wrote, "the war enabled surgeons to become familiar with practices that were not only radiographic, but also and above all radioscopic. From this was born the idea - a natural one at that - of operations under the control of the fluorescent screen".[117] They cite Dr. Wullyamoz of Lausanne as one of

[111] Allier and Baudraz, op. cit., p. 394.

[112] Quoted by Allier and Baudraz, op. cit., p. 394.

[113] Cantonal and University Library (CUL), César Roux Papers, letter from Kocher to Roux, 30 October 1914.

[114] Letter from Roux to his wife Anna, 6 October 1914, quoted by Allier and Baudraz, op. cit., p. 310.

[115] Allier and Baudraz, op. cit., p. 106.

[116] Howell, *Technology* ..., op. cit., p. 7.

[117] ACV, César Roux Papers, Mauclaire et Bouchacourt, *Radioscopie chirurgicale*, Paris, Baillière et Fils, 1921, p. 7.

the forerunners of this practice. A copy of his radioscopic operating table was supplied by César Roux to the St-Jacques Hospital in Besançon in 1914.

It was not only scientific and technical considerations that prompted Swiss doctors to join French or German field hospitals. This pedagogical objective was in line with a humanitarian ideal that was widespread in the medical profession, in the wake of their involvement in military ambulances during the Franco-Prussian War of 1870. During the Balkan wars of 1912–1913, several of Roux's disciples, both Swiss and foreign, joined the various field hospitals; for example, Albert Reverdin was head of the Vaud-Geneva ambulance service. More than 80 Swiss doctors and nurses are said to have been involved with the various belligerents.[118] In Constantinople, two Turkish doctors who had graduated from the Faculty of Lausanne took over the medical management of the Swiss Hospital in Constantinople (150 beds) set up by the Swiss colony in that city.[119]

The extent of the Great War, and in particular the war of position in the trenches, made it possible to envisage the mass recruitment of young surgeons in the hospitals of the belligerents. The professors of surgery did not want to let such an opportunity arise and Kocher wrote to Roux in 1914: "I will not fail to make a request to the Federal Council as you wish to do, to get it to let our young surgeons take advantage of the opportunity that is too good only to learn war surgery instead of being bored at the frontier".[120] This was followed very quickly by the departure in numbers of surgeons to neighbouring countries—France for the French-speaking, Germany for the German-speaking. In October 1914, César Roux himself went to the St-Jacques Hospital in Besançon with some assistants and former students.

During World War II, professors of surgery were not as keen to send their students to military hospitals, partly because of the country's strategic situation—Switzerland was surrounded by the Axis powers—and partly because surgical training took a different turn. The four medical missions to the Eastern Front (1941–1943), led by Eugen Bircher and financed by Swiss companies working for Germany, were thus explained as much by ideological as by purely medical considerations.[121] Among the sixty or so doctors and nurses who took part in these missions alongside the Wehrmacht, there were a few surgeons active in Vaud hospitals, such as Frédéric Rodel, a graduate of the Faculty of Geneva and head of the surgery department of the Vevey-Samaritain Hospital (1943), and Hubert de Reynier, a former Decker intern

[118] According to Pierre Jeanneret, *Un itinéraire à travers le socialisme en Suisse romande: le Dr Maurice Jeanneret-Minkine (1886–1953)*, Lausanne Ed. de l'Aire, 1991, p. 65.

[119] ACV, César Roux Papers, *Rapport du Comité suisse de secours aux blessés ottomans sur son Action pendant la Guerre Balcanique 1912–1913*, Constantinople, 1914, 19 pp.

[120] CUL, César Roux Papers, letter from Kocher to Roux, 30 October 1914.

[121] Daniel Bourgeois, *Business helvétique et Troisième Reich. Milieux d'affaires, politique étrangère, antisémitisme*, Lausanne, Ed. Page Deux, 1998, pp. 109–131 and Daniel Heller, *Eugen Bircher. Artz, Militär, Politiker*, Zurich, NZZ Verlag, 1990.

and surgeon at the Rolle Hospital (1951). Similarly, some nurses from the Cantonal Hospital of Lausanne went to the Russian front in 1942 for reasons presented as professional by the director of the hospital: "The experience they would gain from the war could be useful".[122]

Training of Healthcare Personnel

The surgeon and his assistants were not the only ones in charge of the department. They were the senior staff and had a large number of nurses, assistants and servants under their command. In the hierarchical organisation of the hospital, these subordinate staff depended on their own management (senior deaconess, head nurse, etc.). In the Canton of Vaud, there were two professional training courses that could provide staff to fill these intermediate positions: the Saint-Loup deaconess house and the La Source nursing school. In each, the doctors were very present. They had direct control over the type of training given so it best met their work requirements.

The Deaconesses of Saint-Loup: Obedient Supervisors

Although they belonged to two apparently irreconcilable ideological families, the Institution of the Deaconesses of Saint-Loup, founded by conservative philanthropists involved in the Protestant Revival, and the Cantonal Hospital of Lausanne, the product of the radical-democratic state, have always had important medical relations. The chief physicians of Saint-Loup, generally surgeons, very often came from the Cantonal Hospital, or returned there after a few years of practice at Saint-Loup. Wishing to maintain their reputation for professional excellence, enabling them to occupy the nursing services of practically all the hospitals in the Canton of Vaud, the administrators of Saint-Loup poached young qualified doctors, both for the service of their hospital and for the training of deaconesses. Thus, two of Roux's disciples held the position of chief physician and professor at Saint-Loup Hospital after 1907: Henri Curchod (1907–1931) and Eugène Urech (1931–1962). Both were appointed to the Cantonal Hospital when they left Saint-Loup.[123]

The willingness to employ doctors from the most recognised fields does not imply that the deaconess house was subservient to the person of the doctor; quite the contrary. In his farewell speech in 1931, Curchod recalled the difficulties encountered at the beginning of his service: "I remind you that we have lived through difficult days. This young doctor [i.e., himself] had revolutionary ideas, and defended them with a fierceness that often forced you to resist him vigorously. I apologize for having been a bit violent at times: the years passed, I calmed down, and you gradually granted me what I asked

[122] ACV, K VIII D 32, letter from the Director of the Hospital to the State Council, 24 August 1942.

[123] Emile Bonard, *Histoire de l'Hôpital de Saint-Loup, 1852–1984*, Saint-Loup, Association des Amis de l'Hôpital de zone de Saint-Loup-Orbe, undated, pp. 36–40.

for: the telephone, electricity, assistants, and a magnificent enlargement of the hospital. Our conflicts came largely from prejudices which are now dissipated: the former directors of Saint-Loup looked down on the doctor; unfortunately, at that time, many doctors thought it was fashionable to profess atheism, and one understands the prudence which guided the directors of the establishment in their relations with them. The doctor was considered a necessary evil... This situation lasted for many years. The doctor, at Saint-Loup, was a character who was kept in the shadows. After a few years of mistrust, the director Béguin understood the role that the doctor should play. He placed his trust in me, and for several years I have had the pleasure of seeing him collaborate in the medical work of Saint-Loup. The fruit of this collaboration has been the magnificent development of our hospital".[124]

Since the middle of the nineteenth century, and even more so from the 1900s, doctors and surgeons working in hospitals have had direct control over the professional training of deaconesses. As Joëlle Droux has shown, an essential part of the training of deaconesses laid in the internalisation of the values of obedience, self-sacrifice, submission, etc.[125] Coupled with technical excellence, this behavioural characteristic suited perfectly to medical work in a hierarchical environment such as was found in the Roux Surgical Department or in the regional hospitals of Vaud after the arrival of the surgeon-modernisers. They accompanied the surgeons in the implementation of their new medicine. The administrators of the Nyon Hospital wrote in 1897 that "the presence of the deaconesses of Saint-Loup in the Infirmary, who were used to the requirements of antisepsis, made it possible to carry out even the most serious operations without fear".[126] As for Jean Morax, head of the Health Service, he explained the same year that "thanks to a solid scientific education, the deaconesses of Saint-Loup can serve as assistants to the most demanding surgeons and are often as skilled in this job as medical students".[127] In the regional hospitals, deaconesses thus occupied an important place alongside the medical profession during the years 1880–1930. In fact, before the arrival of interns in these establishments, it was the deaconesses who accompanied the surgeons in their daily work; they were in charge of the radiology and sterilisation facilities.

The place and role of deaconesses in hospitals changed over time. With the strong growth of the hospitals between the two World Wars, they could no longer take on all the tasks of the nursing staff (cooking, caring for the

[124] J. de Mestral Combremont, *Vies données... vies retrouvées. Les diaconesses de Saint-Loup*, Lausanne, Payot, 1932, pp. 141–142.

[125] Joëlle Droux, *L'attraction céleste. La construction de la profession d'infirmière en Suisse romande (19–20 ^ee^ siècles)*, University of Geneva, unpublished PhD thesis, 2000, 910 pp.

[126] Quoted by Gustave Piotet, *La médecine au service du malade*, Neuchâtel, La Baconnière, 1979, p. 30.

[127] Saint Loup Deaconess Institution, Annual Report 1896–1897, pp. 35–36.

sick, assisting the doctors, etc.). A conscious choice was made by the Saint-Loup authorities to reposition themselves in the internal management of the hospitals. This new strategy implied a redistribution of tasks within the hospitals and that priority be given to positions of responsibility. For example, the new agreement signed in 1921 between Saint-Loup and the Cantonal Hospital stipulated that the deaconesses were no longer responsible for major cleaning work. Between the wars, the deaconesses became hospital managers who held leading positions within the hospital, reporting to the administrative (bursar's office, kitchen, laundry, etc.) and medical (operating theatres, radiology, sterilisation, etc.) departments.

The Surgeons of Vaud and the La Source Nursing School

When the La Source Nursing School was reformed in 1890, several doctors were called to sit on its board of directors, including Victor Mercanton, former surgeon at the Cantonal Hospital and head doctor of the Children's Hospice, and Prof. César Roux.[128] Among the 69 people appointed as administrators between 1890 and 1930, there were a total of 14 doctors (20.3%).[129] They were generally men involved in the Swiss Red Cross and therefore directly involved in the training of nurses. There were also renowned surgeons—Kummer, head of the Surgical Clinic of the Cantonal Hospital of Geneva—and former students of Roux. The commitment of these doctors to La Source clearly illustrates the desire to control the training of nurses and to make it compatible with their expectations, even though the original aim of the school was not to train hospital nurses. On the contrary, the founder, Valérie de Gasparin, sought to promote the care of the sick in the family and not in a hospital environment.[130] Most of the girls trained in the 1860s and 1870s worked independently or for organisations supporting home care. Moreover, when there was a question of opening an infirmary within the school in 1903, William Barbey, nephew of the founder, recalled as guardian of the family traditions, "this institution was founded to develop the care of the sick 'in the family', the basis of the Christian Society, in opposition to infirmaries of all kinds and names".[131]

This position soon came up against the new hospital medicine which tended to concentrate on the care of patients. La Source had to reorient its offering towards the training of hospital nurses, which explains the 1890 reform and the arrival of doctors on the board of directors. Shortly after his appointment,

[128] Droux, op. cit.

[129] Archives of La Source Nursing School (ALS), D3-100.38, list of board members, 1890–1945.

[130] Denise Francillon, "L'œuvre sociale: la réalisation d'un idéal. De la charité pratique à la profession d'infirmière", in Denise Francillon (ed.), *Valérie de Gasparin, une conservatrice révolutionnaire*, Lausanne/Le Mont-sur-Lausanne, Ecole de La Source/Ed. Ouverture, 1994, pp. 100–136.

[131] ALS, F1-200.6, letter from William Barbey, 1er October 1903.

Roux wrote to the countess de Gasparin to demand practical training (1891): "When I accepted to be a member of the committee of the School of Nursing, I promised myself to make you aware of the impossibility that your director will always have – in my opinion – to train good nurses if he does not have a few beds at his disposal or a few patients to look after as in a hospital. The few moments that your students spend in the Cantonal Hospital can in no way represent the contact with the sick that is absolutely necessary for their education. And I am convinced that as long as you have not added a few sick rooms to the school or concluded an equivalent contract with a hospital, your pupils will infallibly remain in a state of obvious inferiority with regard to the deaconesses".[132]

These wishes were fulfilled the same year, with the appointment of a disciple of Roux as director of the school: Charles Krafft. In 1891, he opened the Beaulieu Clinic, as well as a free policlinic for the poor, which he used for the practical training of nurses. During the thirty years he spent at the head of the school (1891–1921), Krafft trained nurses with technical skills that met the expectations of the medical profession. To better affirm the necessity of training, he desacralised the surgical gesture and made it a collective act: "The best surgeon necessarily puts part of his power and a lot of his responsibility in the hands - more or less expert - of his operating guard, of the nurse who prepares the instruments, who controls them, who sterilizes them or who develops and draws his X-ray plates. The result of an operation depends on the asepsis of the silk, on the disinfection of the catgut; during the operation, success often depends on the composure of the aides [...]".[133] Here, as in Roux's surgical clinic, the division of labour remained vertical. The technical formation of La Source nurses did not in any way question the hierarchy of tasks and the predominance of the surgeon over the entire staff. Krafft explained his desire to train "interchangeable surgical assistants".[134]

Despite the attachment of the La Source School to traditional values that were ultimately very similar to those transmitted at Saint-Loup (the femininity of nursing, self-sacrifice, obedience, etc.), the nurses acquired practical training that opened the door to several private clinics with the most prominent doctors. All the renowned surgeons in French-speaking Switzerland (Krafft and Roux in Lausanne; de Quervain in La Chaux-de-Fonds; and Julliard and Kummer in Geneva) employed them, with the prize going to Roux, who engaged eight in his private clinic. However, many preferred to use deaconesses for the hospital services they managed. Thus, using the hospital archives alone can lead to confusion and give the impression that men like Roux were opposed to the La Source School because they did nothing to

[132] ALS, B1-1J, letter from Roux to Mrs. de Gasparin, 15 January 1891. Roux's emphasis.

[133] ACV, Charles Krafft Papers, PP 359/14, "Infirmière et chirurgie", *Extrait du Congrès français de chirurgie*, Paris, 1919, p. 6.

[134] Ibid., p. 7.

employ its nurses in their hospital departments. This apparent contradiction can be explained by a difference in organisation between private clinics and hospitals. The former were generally small and doctors needed nurses whose main quality was technical know-how. The direction and management of private clinics was usually entrusted to professional managers. Hospitals, on the other hand, were much larger in size, both in terms of number of beds and patients and in terms of junior staff (servants, nurses and various assistants). Doctors obviously needed trained and conscientious nursing staff but also, above all, staff who knew how to manage a work team and impose themselves with authority. Several testimonies show a significant difference between deaconesses and La Source nurses in this respect and that the quality of the professional training was not a determining factor.

4 The American Model: Decker and Saegesser (1930–1960)

When Roux retired in 1926, one of his disciples, a former chief of clinic almost sixty years old, was appointed head of the Surgical Department: Henri Vulliet (1926). He did not have time to train his own surgical school and numerous students; his professorship was, therefore, a moment of transition. Roux, retired, did not disappear from the Faculty; when it came to replacing his successor Vulliet, who died in 1932, his former colleagues asked him to assess the list of candidates proposed to the State Council. Their choices agreed and another of his disciples had to be appointed: Pierre Decker.[135]

The Decker period (1932–1957) was a transitional phase between the German generalist model brought in by César Roux and the American model of teamwork, which really took hold with the arrival of Frédéric Saegesser at the head of the Surgical Department (1957). Decker inherited from Roux a generalist and dominant conception of surgery which left little room for the full affirmation of emerging specialties (neurosurgery, cardiac surgery, anaesthesia, etc.). His farewell lecture was also an opportunity for Decker to return to "this new form of collaboration [that] would be magical teamwork"[136] and to express his scepticism about its application in medicine. He stated, "medicine must be based on specialisation. But this specialisation can only take place on a technical level. Above the technician must reign the man who has experience, the man who knows the things that technique cannot yet teach us, the man who is trained to judge beyond the numbers".[137] In his conception of surgery, Decker was not very favourable to the autonomy of some of the surgical specialities developed within his department by his chiefs of clinic

[135] AUNIL, minutes of the meetings of the Council of the Faculty of Medicine, 19 September and 10 October 1932.

[136] *Dernière leçon de M. le Dr. Pierre Decker, Professeur ordinaire de clinique chirurgicale à la Faculté de médecine*, Lausanne, University, 1957, p. 26.

[137] Ibid., p. 27.

and assistants. If he accepted and encouraged research, it was only under his authority and within the framework of his department. This desire to control emerging specialties led several of his students to leave the hospital and pursue their work in a private setting. Perpetuating the model of his master Roux at the time of specialisation, Decker acquired an image as a conservative surgeon, conveyed by many of his students.

Decker was not only the surgeon "who did a well-built work, more concerned with prudence than with innovation"[138] of which his successor Saegesser spoke. He also encouraged the research of his students and their stays in the United States, where he himself went on several occasions. Above all, Decker's greatest work was the new surgical clinic, opened in 1947 and inaugurated in 1949, which consecrated the division of surgical work, whatever Decker himself said, and contributed to the affirmation of specialities within surgery, all the more so as the saturation of the medical market encouraged the new generation of surgeons to envisage specialisation within their branch from the 1930s onwards.

Medical Plethora and the Birth of Specialist Titles

Although the position of the medical profession in the healthcare market was significantly strengthened at the end of the nineteenth century, doctors were very concerned about the deterioration of their material conditions during the inter-war period.[139] The feeling of a medical plethora was widespread, even if the phenomenon was never explicitly defined.

It is true that the number of physicians with the right to practice increased sharply since 1890–1900. This rise in the number of practitioners was much stronger than the constant demographic growth during the period 1920–1950 and it had a negative effect on the number of patients. The number of inhabitants per doctor fell from 2263 in 1880 to 989 in 1910 and 747 in 1920; i.e., an average annual decrease of 2.7% for the period 1880–1920. In the space of 40 years, the medical market in Vaud had become very dense. In this context, it is easy to understand the desire to fight against medical plethora during the inter-war period.

The challenge was considerable. The issue was to develop the healthcare market so that every doctor could find something to his or her liking, but also to protect this market against outside competition. The expansion of the market was achieved through the development of hospital infrastructure, the creation of private clinics and the emergence of specialties within medicine.

[138] Frédéric Saegesser, *César Roux. Son époque et la nôtre*, Lausanne, Ed. de l'Aire, 1999, p. 44.

[139] De Riedmatten Soun, Rosetti Daniel and Fussinger Catherine, "La création de l'assurance maladie, un danger pour le corps médical? (1893–1911)", *Revue historique* vaudoise, 1995, pp. 247–292.

The training of specialists was also strictly regulated and the number of designations was limited, so that within the healthcare market, specific healthcare niches were created and dominated by a group of doctors who were recognised by their peers. In 1929, the Swiss Medical Association (*Foederatio Medicorum Helveticorum*, FMH) set up a working group to consider the issue of regulating specialisations, in collaboration with the Cantonal medical societies and the existing specialist societies, such as the surgical society. In 1932, the title of FMH specialist was introduced for some fifteen branches, including surgery. It enabled doctors to control the fragmentation of the healthcare market and to reduce the accessibility of certain types of treatment.

The protection of the healthcare market from the outside world took place in three main directions. First of all, doctors fought against the development of a state-subsidised hospitalisation policy. During the inter-war period, the Vaud Medical Society (*Société Vaudoise de Médecine*, SVM) repeatedly accused the state of undercutting the market price with the low cost of hospitalisation at the Cantonal Hospital—or of other services such as laboratory fees, etc.—and thus exercising unfair competition with other hospitals, competing unfairly with doctors in the city. They did not hesitate to call into question the construction of the new surgical clinic at the Cantonal Hospital in 1942.[140] Secondly, doctors sought to restrict the number of practising doctors by limiting access to medical schools. During the revision of the health law in 1928, the commission in charge of the project, led by four doctors, expressed its desire "to limit the number of practitioners, given the plethora that reigns in certain professions, such as that of doctor and pharmacist; the plethora is a danger, the lack of a sufficient clientele being able to incite the creation of artificial work opportunities".[141] This position ultimately proved to be contrary to constitutional law guaranteeing the free exercise of a profession and the numerus clausus was not adopted at the Faculty of Lausanne. Finally, the medical profession tried to protect its market from foreign competition. The 1928 sanitary law introduced the only official recognition—with exceptions discussed on a case-by-case basis—granted to the federal diploma of medical doctor. During the Second World War, the doctors of the Health and Hospices Council and the SVM adopted a strict position of refusing to grant the right to practice to Jewish doctors who had taken refuge in the Canton.[142]

It is obviously difficult to measure the impact of all these measures. If we look at the density of the medical market, i.e., the number of inhabitants per doctor, we can see that the decline has slowed considerably. Whereas there were 747 inhabitants per doctor in 1920, there were 641 in 1930, 561 in 1940

[140] ACV, S 54, 1942, 42/24, letter from the Vaud Medical Society to the State Council, 4 May 1942.

[141] Bulletin of the Grand Council meetings (BGC), Explanatory Memorandum to the Bill to Replace the Sanitary Organisation Act of 14 September 1897, Spring 1928, pp. 12–13.

[142] ACV, S 73, minutes of the Health and Hospices Council.

and 559 in 1950; i.e., an average annual decline of 0.9% for the years 1920–1950. Despite this slowdown, the market was much more competitive for Decker's students than for Roux's, especially as the number of surgical positions in the Canton's regional hospitals was difficult to expand. This economic context explains to a large extent why young doctors began to show an interest in specialist training, which had been regulated by the Swiss Medical Association since the mid-1930s. In addition, in the early 1940s, new research incentives were introduced, encouraging young doctors to specialise in new areas.

The Beginnings of Research Support

In the 1940s and 1950s, scientific research in the medical field received new support through the foundation of new funding bodies, such as the Swiss Academy of Medical Sciences (SAMS, 1943) and the Swiss National Science Foundation (SNSF, 1952). Launched in the early 1940s by Alfred Gigon, from the Basel Faculty of Medicine, the idea of the SAMS was to bring together biologists and physicians active in the field of research in Switzerland in order to coordinate the various projects and benefit from broader support from private companies. In 1941, the Basel chemical industry and Nestlé agreed to create a donation fund and commit 400,000 francs to it during the first three years.[143] The promoters of the SAMS came from all the Swiss universities. The representatives of the Faculty of Medicine in Lausanne were professors from the Medical Clinic, the Radiology Department and the Orthopaedics Department. The absence of Decker, who was the head of the largest university clinic in Lausanne, should be noted but can probably be explained by his lack of interest in experimental research in the early 1940s. Following in the footsteps of his master César Roux, Decker was still essentially a practitioner. It was during the 1940s that research developed in his department, under the impetus of young assistants wishing to specialise.

In particular, the SAMS promoted educational trips abroad, mainly to the USA. In 1945 it founded a *Swiss American Center of medical exchange and information* in New York.[144] The aim was clearly to acquire new know-how developed in the United States and to transfer it to Swiss hospitals, as in the case of new anaesthesia techniques, for which the SAMS awarded a grant in 1946: "At present, it is necessary for many young Swiss surgeons to improve their skills in the United States. [...] Thanks to the awarding of scholarships of various amounts, ten Swiss doctors, among them five privatdozents, have been able to benefit from a more or less long study stay. In addition, the American

[143] ACV, S 54, 1943, 42/30, Swiss Academy of Medical Sciences, *Rapport sur les travaux préparatoires en vue de sa création*, 1949. On the beginnings of the federal research policy and the role of the SAMS in this process, see Antoine Fleury and Frédéric Joye, *Les débuts de la politique de la recherche en Suisse. Histoire de la création du Fonds national de la recherche scientifique*, Geneva: Droz, 2002.

[144] ACV, S 54, 1946, 42/20.

Swiss Foundation granted a sum of 2000 dollars for the training of a specialist in anaesthesia. As is well known, the technique of anaesthesia has reached a very high level in the United States, and the opportunity is now offered to a young Swiss doctor to become familiar with these methods".[145] In addition to the scholarships offered by the SAMS, there was at the same time support from private foundations, such as the Rockefeller Foundation or the American Swiss Foundation for scientific exchange, based in Boston and supported by Swiss industrialists.[146]

Several of Decker's students went across the Atlantic to train in a particular field, such as Buffat in neurosurgery, Naef and Francioli in thoracic surgery or Hahn in cardiac surgery, some thanks to a grant from the SAMS. Beyond the scientific training, the American model fascinated Swiss doctors by what it brought in terms of new working methods (high technical quality of the equipment, large financial investments, teamwork, etc.). In 1952, the Faculty of Medicine in Geneva declared that René Mach "had spent three months in the United States of America, not so much to complete his knowledge as to learn about the successful working methods of the scientific institutes in the New World".[147] Decker himself made a month-long study trip to the United States in 1948: despite his initial scepticism, he wanted to see with his own eyes this new medicine that his students were so enthusiastic about.

The Surgical Department Under Decker: The Emergence of Teamwork and Surgical Specialties (1936–1957)

Decker's entry into office took place in a socio-economic context of greater competitiveness in the healthcare market and easier access to specialised courses of study. The Cantonal Hospital itself reflects the "medical plethora" and the need to reposition itself in the market. The number of medical staff grew rapidly. While the number of senior doctors remained broadly the same from 1900 to the 1950s—that is, about ten senior professors—there was a real explosion in the number of assistants (interns, chiefs of clinic and assistant doctors). Unfortunately, the sources do not allow us to isolate the figures for the Department of Surgery, which is fully in line with the general trend of the hospital (see Table 5). Under Decker's leadership, the Surgical Department moved from a hierarchical organisation (vertical division of labour) to teamwork and diversification of individual skills (horizontal division of labour).

Decker did not want to be an omnipotent generalist. He quickly sought to subcontract certain courses to other doctors, such as children's surgery

[145] ACV, S 54, 1947, 42/7.

[146] Mireille Lador, "Institution et sciences: modèles et réformes à la Faculté de médecine de Genève (1930–1973)", in *La formation des médecins (19-20ᵉᵉ siècles)*, Bulletin du Centre Pierre Léon d'histoire économique et sociale, 1998, pp. 88–89.

[147] Ibid., quoted on p. 88.

Table 5 Doctors working at the Cantonal Hospital, 1900–1960

	1900	*1910*	*1920*	*1930*	*1940*	*1950*	*1960*
Heads of department	7	7	9	10	10	10	11
Assistants	10	11	11	11	36	66	82
Average number of assistants per department	1.4	1.6	1.2	1.1	3.6	6.6	7.5

Source Official yearbook of the Canton of Vaud, 1900–1960

Table 6 Careers of Decker's main chiefs of clinic, 1937–1958

Date	*Name*	*Specialties*	*Career*
1937–1942	Jean Rossier	Neurosurgery	Privatdozent (1941), premature death at 36 (1942)
1942–1947	Jean-David Buffat	Neurosurgery	Privatdozent (1942), assistant surgeon (1947), private practice (1947)
1947–1953	Pierre Francioli	Cardiovascular surgery, urology	Privatdozent (1952), lecturer (1957), professor (1979)
1953–1956	Frédéric Saegesser	General surgery	Privatdozent (1956), professor (1957)
1956–1958	Roger Mosimann	Vascular surgery	Privatdozent (1961), professor (1966)

Source ACV, Dossiers ATS, Rossier Jean; Olivier Robert and Franceso Panese, *Dictionnaire...*, op. cit.

(1935) and operating medicine (1936). The surgical team grew and diversified during the 1940s and 1950s, with the appointment of Jean Rossier as a privatdozent (1941), Théodore Ott as a special assistant in neurosurgery (1943), Jean-David Buffat as an assistant surgeon (1947), Eugène Urech as an extraordinary professor (1951), Pierre Francioli as a privatdozent (1952), Christian Reymond as chief anaesthetist (1954) and, finally, Frédéric Saegesser as a privatdozent (1956).[148]

Decker's training policy was fundamentally different from that of Roux. His main chiefs of clinic made their careers in the university environment rather than at the head of a regional hospital department (see Table 6). With the exception of Rossier, who died prematurely, and Buffat, who continued his career in the private sector, Decker's chiefs of clinic ended their careers as professors.

[148] RSC, Department of the Interior, various years.

The same applies to the assistant doctors who appeared in the Surgical Department during the Decker period. As State Councillor Despland recalled in 1956, "assistant doctors are doctors who have their own clientele in the city but are specialists in certain branches of medicine, whom the professor of certain departments - surgery, paediatrics, medicine, for example - calls upon because of their special knowledge. The assistant surgeon is a doctor in practice who comes to the Cantonal Hospital as needed to deal with cases from a specific specialty. He replaces the professor in certain particular cases which fall within his specialty".[149] These practitioners play an important role in the specialisation and diversification of skills within the department. They appear as central actors in the horizontal division of labour. Very often from the Surgical Department, sometimes former chiefs of clinic, they all had a career in medical research or university teaching.

Maurice Vulliet, assistant surgeon in 1943–1947, was head physician of the Children's Hospice (1949–1966) and professor of occupational health (1945–1966). As for Jean-David Buffat, assistant in 1947–1951, he became a private doctor of surgical therapeutics, distinguished himself in neurological research and spent most of his career developing the La Source Clinic, of which he has been chairman of the board of directors since 1955. Finally, Pierre Francioli, assistant in 1953–1959, moved away from pure research towards the teaching of general branches; a privatdozent of surgical semiology (1952–1957), in 1957 he became a lecturer of propaedeutic surgical clinic and of surgical anatomy from 1966, then professor (1979).[150]

There were also former students of Decker who distinguished themselves outside the Surgical Department and made a career in another medical specialty. However, the influence of their surgical training is obvious as they imported surgical methods into their preferred branches (ENT, paediatrics, urology, etc.). In these cases, the fusion of know-how allowed new specialties to emerge. The development of ENT surgery owes much to Jean-Pierre Taillens, a former Decker intern, who succeeded Prof. Barraud as head of the ENT Department in 1943. When Decker retired, he showed his gratitude by writing to him: "As a young surgeon, decided, according to the evolution of ENT, to launch my clinic on the surgical level and not only on the medical level which was the rule before, I applied at all times the teaching that you had given me".[151] It is also necessary to mention the case of paediatric surgery in which several doctors became interested in the post-war period. Contrary to what one might imagine, the Children's Hospice was not the main setting for the affirmation of paediatric surgery. Neither Henri Vulliet, surgeon of this establishment in 1910–1926, nor his son Maurice Vulliet, assistant surgeon and then head surgeon in 1926–1966, tried to establish themselves as specialists in paediatric surgery. Although they both held professorial positions, Henri

[149] BGC, 22 May 1956.

[150] Robert and Panese, op. cit.

[151] CUL, Pierre Decker Papers, letter from Taillens to Decker, 3 July 1956.

Vulliet as head of the chair of surgery and Maurice Vulliet as professor of occupational health, neither tried to make paediatric surgery a speciality attached to a university clinic, even though the latter gave courses in paediatric surgery as a private doctor from 1935.

It was a student of Decker's, Noël Genton, who made paediatric surgery independent. After internships at the Nyon Hospital and then in the Surgical Department of the Cantonal Hospital, he went to Zurich in 1956, where there was a children's surgery clinic, and trained for five years in this branch. On his return to Lausanne in 1961, he joined the Saegesser Surgical Service, where he founded a Department of Paediatric Surgery.[152] In the post-war period, doctors with basic training in general surgery were employed in departments dealing with other branches of medicine. This import of surgical methods was greatly encouraged by the regulation of the various FMH titles since 1932 which obliged candidates for a specialist title to spend one or two years in another branch of medicine after obtaining their medical diploma, generally without specifying the branch, in addition to the time necessary for their own speciality.[153] This measure strongly encouraged technological transfers between the various branches.

Finally, several of Decker's disciples made a career as heads of Surgical Departments in hospitals in French-speaking Switzerland. Following in the footsteps of their predecessors trained by Roux, they participated in the development of hospitals during the 1950s and 1960s. In the Canton of Vaud, for example, we find Paul-Henri Thélin at Sainte-Croix Hospital (1944) and then at Montreux Hospital (1948), Marcel Croisier at Sainte-Croix Hospital (1948), Hubert de Reynier at Rolle Hospital (1951) or Albert Dentan at Lavaux Hospital. Outside the Canton of Vaud, we should mention the case of Marcel Quéloz, who trained with Decker in the 1930s and then in the Netherlands and who was head of the Surgical Department of the Fribourg Cantonal Hospital for twenty-five years (1951–1975). Several other Decker students set up private practices in the Lausanne or Geneva region and operated on their patients in private clinics, sometimes with partial access to the Cantonal Hospital as consultants.

Let us return to the new generation of surgeons who, under Decker's authority, began to specialise in a particular organ or part of the body, at a time when the medical market in Vaud was becoming saturated with general surgeons during the 1930s. The regional hospitals had almost all been modernised and were headed by surgeons in their prime, notably those trained by Roux. Similarly, the large general clinics open to the medical profession, such as the Cecil Clinic or La Source, already had many licensed physicians. The opportunities for Decker's students to work and pursue a career in a hospital environment were thus greatly reduced. It is understandable that

[152] Robert and Panese, op. cit.

[153] *Bulletin professionnel des médecins suisses*, 1935, pp. 654–655.

these young surgeons were attracted by medical research and did not hesitate to undertake study and training trips to surgical clinics active in specialties, mainly in the United States and the Netherlands. By empowering certain fields of research, Decker's students created niches of activity in which their dominant position as specialists was recognised. This empowerment came up against Decker's ambiguous position. He was fully aware of the need to diversify surgical activities in Lausanne in the direction of new specialities, in particular for the reputation of his department and its position on the healthcare market. On the other hand, Decker had a hard time seeing his students escape his control when they returned to Lausanne. His students did not hold this against him: they left the Cantonal Hospital and moved to private clinics, or even to the Cantonal Hospital in Geneva, and continued their work as specialist surgeons in complete independence. This happened in particular in the cases of neurosurgery, cardiovascular surgery and hand surgery.

Neurosurgery

At the end of the 1930s, a talented young doctor spotted by Decker, Jean Rossier, travelled twice to the United States to attend the classes of a famous student of Kocher, Prof. Harvey Cushing, considered one of the founders of neurosurgery. Cushing gave Rossier his moral support, authorising him to translate into French one of his major works entitled *Intracranial Tumors*. He then found an attractive surgical niche, but his premature death at the age of 36 put an end to a promising career (1942).[154]

The Surgical Department did not give up its desire to break into this new discipline. Decker hired an intern, Theodore Ott, whom he had appointed as a special assistant in neurology (1942). Ott became a privatdozent in 1951 and then head of the Centre for Electroencephalography in the Internal Medicine Department in 1954. He made neurology a world-renowned specialty in Lausanne.[155] At the same time, Decker sent Jean-David Buffat, who had just returned from a three-month internship with one of the first Swiss surgeons to engage in neurosurgery, Prof. Krayenbuhl of Zurich, in the United States (1947). The stay on the other side of the Atlantic gradually became an obligatory step in the building of a surgical career and Decker had to explain to a rather sceptical Health and Hospices Council that "Dr. Buffat's study trip to the USA is not a personal matter, but a necessity for the Surgical Department".[156] On his return to Lausanne, Buffat participated in research in neurosurgery until his departure for the private sector in the early 1950s.[157] He was then replaced by Roger Campiche, assistant of neurosurgery (1955), then chief of clinic in this branch (1961), professor (1975) and head of the autonomous neurosurgery service (1983). However, the real promoter of

[154] ACV, ATS Files, Rossier Jean.

[155] Robert and Panese, op. cit.

[156] ACV, S 73, minutes of the Health and Hospices Council, 29 October 1946.

[157] Information kindly provided by Denise Francillon, archivist of La Source.

neurosurgery at the Cantonal Hospital was Eric Zander, former assistant and chief of clinic to Krayenbuhl in the neurosurgery department of the Cantonal Hospital in Zurich. He was hired by Saegesser in 1958 as a neurosurgical assistant and became a professor in 1963. In the 1960s, he developed this branch into an independent department.[158]

The Beginnings of Cardiovascular Surgery

Heart diseases were usually the responsibility of internal medicine before young assistants from Lausanne made the heart a surgical object. Cardiology was first taught within the framework of the Internal Medicine Service by Ivan Mahaim, who was a privatdozent of heart diseases from 1931 and professor of cardiology at the beginning of the 1960s, and then by Pierre Desbaillet, chief of clinic (1952–1957) and privatdozent of cardiology from 1963.[159]

Some of the doctors on Decker's team also considered the possibilities of heart surgery. The first assistant to be trained in this specialty was Andreas Naef, who had graduated from the Faculty of Zurich and joined Decker's department in 1943. His interest initially led him to an emerging specialty not yet present in French-speaking Switzerland, thoracic surgery, which was then essentially lung surgery. In his memoirs, Naef highlights the difficulty of the professional opportunities available to young doctors at the end of the inter-war period.[160] The desire to specialise corresponded with a wish to establish a niche in the healthcare market and to make a career of it. Stating that he wanted to "secure [his] future in the Lausanne service",[161] Naef obtained permission from Decker in 1946 to travel to the United States "to learn this surgery".[162] During his hospital internships in Baltimore, Boston, Chicago and New York, he witnessed the beginnings of cardiac surgery and, on his return to Lausanne, undertook the first operations on cardiac malformations, with the collaboration of cardiologists such as Ivan Mahaim (1947–1948).[163] However, difficulties with Decker, who did not grant his assistant the requested autonomy, put an end to Naef's collaboration with the Cantonal Hospital (1949). On his return from a second trip to the United States, where he pursued his training in cardiac surgery, he moved to the private clinic La Source (1950) where, since 1951, he has been performing cardiac operations. During the 1950s, La Source became the centre of cardiac surgery in French-speaking Switzerland, to which cardiologists from Lausanne (Prof. Mahaim) and Geneva (Prof. Duchosal) sent

[158] Robert and Panese, op. cit.

[159] Ibid.

[160] Andreas Naef, *From tuberculosis to heart transplantation. 1940–1990. Parcours d'un chirurgien*, Geneva, Médecine & Hygiène, 1995.

[161] Ibid., pp. 19–20.

[162] Ibid., p. 19.

[163] Ibid., p. 44.

their patients who needed to be operated on. On the strength of this experience, Naef was appointed assistant surgeon at the Cantonal Hospital of Geneva (1956) where he continued his career before being hired in 1964 by Yverdon Hospital, whose administrators wished to acquire a leading surgeon.

In the meantime, other Decker students began specialising in cardiac surgery. Pierre Francioli gave his first lecture as a privatdozent on heart surgery (1953), a branch in which he had specialised during his years as a senior physician. In particular, he made several trips to the most renowned hospitals over the years 1951–1953 (France, the Netherlands, USA) for further training in heart and thoracic surgery. However, after Decker's departure, Francioli took over part of the teaching of general surgery and abandoned research into cardiovascular surgery.

It was then Charles Hahn developed this specialty, after numerous trips to the United States and the Netherlands.[164] He was commissioned by Decker, and later by his successor Saegesser, to develop this speciality at the Cantonal Hospital with a small team at his service and obtained a teaching position as a privatdozent. However, towards the end of the 1950s, Hahn fell out with the management of the hospital and the faculty, who were reluctant to provide him with all the equipment he required. He then turned to the private clinics in Lausanne and joined Naef in la Source. Until the early 1970s, private clinics in Lausanne invested massively in open-heart surgery.

Hand Surgery[165]

After graduating from the Faculty of Lausanne (1933), Claude Verdan began his surgical specialisation at the Surgical Department of the Faculty of Zurich. He was an assistant to Prof. Paul Clairmont (1937–1938) and then to Decker in Lausanne from 1944. He developed his knowledge of ambulatory surgery at the Surgical Polyclinic, which was under the control of Decker. Verdan was appointed privatdozent (1951) and professor (1961). In parallel to his university activity, he opened a private business, Longeraie Clinic (1946), to which the Surgical Polyclinic was transferred in 1964. This alliance between the private and public sectors was conducive to the development of surgical specialties, such as hand surgery, of which Verdan became one of the world's leading specialists, alongside plastic and reconstructive surgery, developed in collaboration with other surgeons after 1967. The specific knowledge developed in this field enabled Verdan to obtain a place in Decker's succession (1957). The case of hand surgery, and more broadly reconstructive surgery, shows it was not impossible to develop a surgical specialty in Decker's department. The agreement of the "boss", as well as the autonomy resulting from the juxtaposition of several workplaces (private clinic + public policlinic), explain

[164] Charles Hahn, *Chirurgien du cœur. L'une des conquêtes médicales du siècle par un grand patron de Suisse romande*, Lausanne, 24 Heures, 1987.

[165] Claude Verdan, *Mémoires d'un chirugien*, Lausanne: Fondation Claude Verdan, 5 volumes, 1999–2001.

the success of the subtle path taken by Verdan in his specialisation. It was no coincidence that he became the head of a chair at the Lausanne Faculty of Medicine—something that neither Buffat, Hahn nor Naef had achieved.

The New Surgical Clinic of the Cantonal Hospital: "Science in the Service of Humanity"[166]

The strong increase in the number of doctors making up the surgical team and the diversification of specialisations did not find the material conditions conducive to their realisation in the university surgical clinic which dated from 1916. Moreover, this hospital service could not compete with the new operating theatres of the regional hospitals and private clinics in Lausanne. Decker's impatience to see the hospital acquire a new surgical clinic was due as much to a strategy of repositioning himself in the hospital care market as to a scientific and educational necessity.

In 1936, he made a first report to the Health and Hospices Council in which he exposed the shortcomings of his department in terms of equipment (radiology, operating room furniture), organisation of space and flows (narcosis room separated from the rest, access corridor between the various rooms, enlargement of the assistants' offices), nursing staff (increase in their number) and the well-being of the patients (increase in the number of wards, creation of a recovery room, etc.).[167] However, the years of crisis were not very conducive to fulfilling such demands, although the public authorities recognised the validity of the request. It was not until 1942 that the Grand Council unanimously accepted a credit of 1.2 million francs for the construction of a new surgical clinic. The Vaud authorities wanted to provide themselves with the best possible infrastructure and called on the services of renowned hospital architects, William Vetter and Jean-Pierre Vouga (see Chapter 5).

Conceived by its designers as "the heart of the hospital",[168] the clinic has four operating theatres, each with a series of adjoining rooms (waiting, preparation and narcosis, dressing, and recovery). This new infrastructure allowed the implementation of a surgery which was split up with the appearance of numerous specialities, as well as the passage to longer interventions thanks to the control of shock and narcosis. The new surgical clinic was the product of a collaboration between Decker and the architects; it reflects the will of the chief physician to move to a new type of organisation, based on teamwork and continuous work.

The organisation of work took a further step forward. Whereas the division of labour was previously mainly vertical, in the new Decker Clinic it was

[166] ACV, S 73, *L'Illustré*, 1949, no. 48, p. 13.

[167] ACV, K VIII B 213/15, Decker's report on the Surgical Service, 26 February 1936.

[168] William Vetter and Jean-Pierre Vouga, "Hôpitaux et cliniques du Canton de Vaud. Bases d'un plan de santé", *Bulletin technique de la Suisse romande*, 1948, p. 177.

also horizontal. The head surgeon can no longer directly control everything that happens in his clinic and its four independent operating rooms. He has become an organiser and distributor of tasks among his ever-growing team. Of course, the hierarchy remains and Decker is still the boss in his surgical clinic. But he was assisted by a host of assistant doctors and deputies who were involved in the care of patients at a specific stage, according to their speciality. Moreover, aseptic standards were reinforced in the inter-war period (masks and gloves became widespread) and asepsis was made a ritual, in the ethnological sense of the term, allowing for a strict separation between the surgeons who intervened directly on the sterile operating field and the other people present in the operating room who did not have access to it (assistants, nursing staff, visitors, students, etc.), which reinforced and clarified the division of labour[169] (Fig. 3).

The spatial organisation of the new surgical clinic had itself undergone a profound modification that reflects these new ways of working. Everything was designed to allow for the simultaneous care of several patients, without these different flows interfering with each other. One of the aims was to "avoid any external influence on the working conditions in the operating rooms".[170] Apart from the operating room for policlinic procedures in the old part of the building (21), this clinic has three operating rooms (28 I, II and III) which are independent but combined in one operating group. Patients arrive on their beds in the hall (43), coming from the hospital ward (right) or from the emergency room (main entrance, left). They are taken to the waiting room (37 I, II and III) and then to the anaesthesia room (34 I, II and III) where they are transferred to a mobile operating table which is brought into the operating room (28 I, II and III). During this first phase, the surgeon and his assistants are in the preparatory room (36) where they "put on their boots, aprons and masks and wash". In this room, observation windows allow them to "monitor [...] the preparation of the patient and the operating room, as well as the work in the sterilisation room. Once their preparation is complete, the surgeons access the operating rooms through a passageway that connects the two rooms and also serves as access to bring sterilized instruments from the sterilisation room [33] to the operating rooms".[171] After the operation, the patients are transferred to the dressing room (35 I, II and III), where they find their bed, and then back to the hospital ward.[172]

The operating group was thus designed to allow the simultaneous and continuous management of several operations. The hierarchical organisation

[169] Pearl Katz, "Ritual in Operating Room", *Ethnology*, 1981, pp. 335–350 and Stefan Hirschauer, "The Manufacture of Bodies in Surgery", *Social Studies of Science*, 1991, pp. 279–319.

[170] Vetter and Vouga, op. cit.

[171] Ibid.

[172] Ibid.

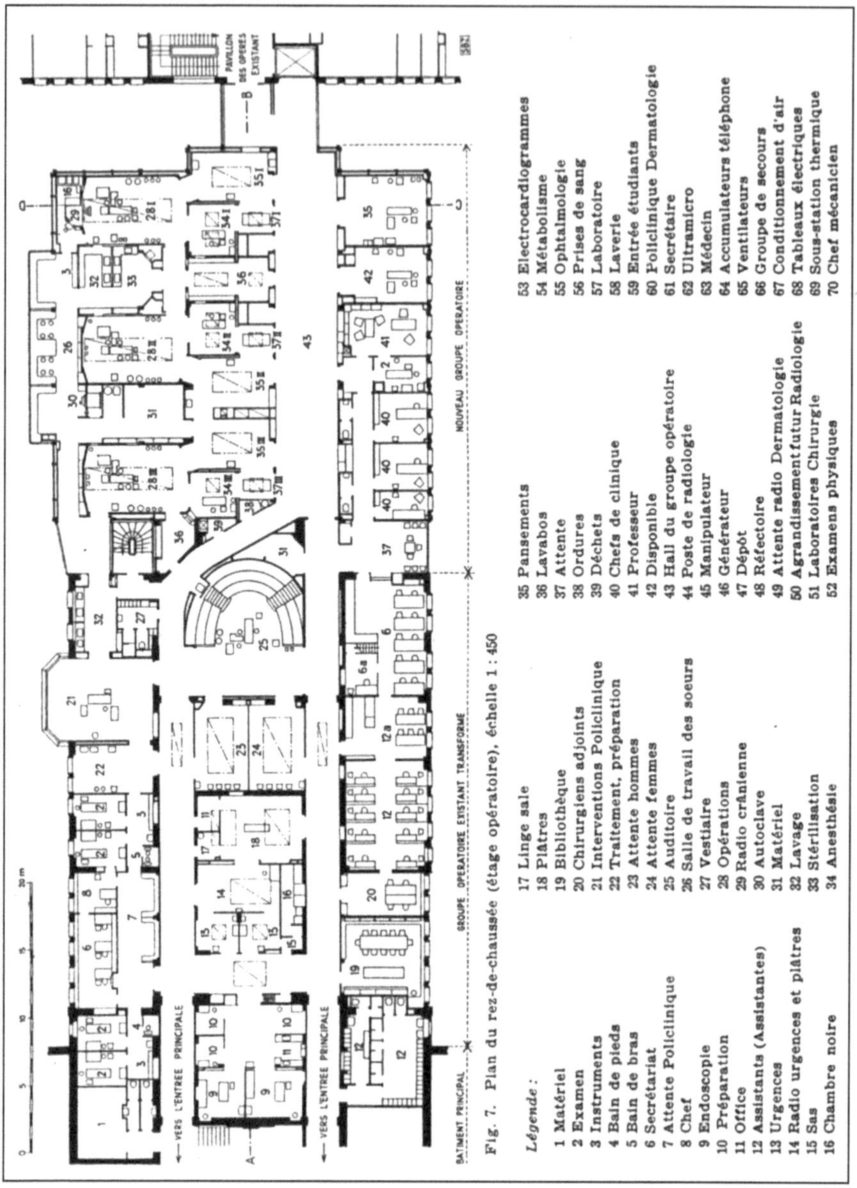

Fig. 3 Plan of the surgical clinic of the Cantonal Hospital of Lausanne, 1947 (*Source* William Vetter and Jean-Pierre Vouga, "Le nouveau groupe opératoire de l'hôpital Cantonal de Lausanne [Clinique de Chirurgie]", *Schweizerische Bauzeitung*, 8 May 1948, p. 263)

of the surgical clinic as it existed at Roux disappeared in favour of an organisational model based on the desire to ensure maximum fluidity in the care of patients by a team of surgeons. In Decker's conception, "concentration allows for more efficient care at an extremely low cost. You only have to compare it to what is happening in the car industry to be convinced of the validity of these arguments".[173] By the time Decker retired in 1957, the Surgical Department had grown from 2100 to 2200 patients in 1900 to almost 4000 annually. Although this new establishment had a very high cost—the overall cost estimated at 4.2 million francs in 1949, compared to 1.2 million in 1942—it did not raise any controversy in the Grand Council, mainly because the State did not do it to the detriment of regional hospitals.

After Decker, the Consecration of Team Surgery

The question of Decker's succession is a delicate one. There was no medical personality who had the necessary knowledge in all the fields that had been explored since the 1940s. The Faculty Council decided to replace Decker with three surgeons: a general practitioner, Saegesser, who was appointed professor and head of the Surgical Department, as well as two specialists as lecturers, Verdan, in hand surgery, and Francioli, in urology. Finally, the new team was completed with Auguste Jost as assistant surgeon and an intern, Pierre Desbaillet, as assistant cardiologist.[174]

Saegesser's appointment broke with a certain surgical tradition which, with the Kocher-Roux-Decker lineage, had made the German model the reference for the practice of surgery in Lausanne. Frédéric Saegesser was highly representative of the new generation of surgeons who emerged around Decker from the end of the 1930s onwards, launching themselves into various surgical specialities and acquiring their knowledge in the United States. Although he remained a general surgeon, despite a marked interest in thoracic surgery, Saegesser built his training on a truly international scale. After obtaining his medical degree at the Faculty of Geneva (1942), he undertook further training in Leyden (Prof. Bromm), London (Prof. Brock) and Denver (Prof. Swann), before being hired by Decker as assistant head of clinic in 1947.[175]

From the outset, Saegesser called for the continuation and extension of teamwork, as well as the development of scientific research. In his installation speech (1959), he insisted on "the complexity of the problems to be solved [which] makes the assistance of numerous collaborators indispensable",[176] among whom were anaesthetists, physiologists, specialised nurses and various

[173] Archives of the Federation of Hospitals in Canton Vaud, Letter from Charles Rochat to François Cuénoud, November 6, 1957.

[174] AUNIL, minutes of the meetings of the Council of the Faculty of Medicine, 1957.

[175] Robert and Panese, op. cit., pp. 1127–1128.

[176] *Installation des professeurs ordinaires H. Badoux, Ch. Jéquier, P. Collart, D. Bonnard, G. Vincent, F. Saegesser*, Lausanne: Payot, 1960, p. 54.

technicians. This public discourse was a way of demanding and justifying the granting of financial means and a policy of strong growth of the Surgical Department. Very quickly, Saegesser completed his team and sought to add young doctors in the various emerging specialities, such as neurosurgery (Eric Zander, 1957), vascular surgery (Roger Mosimann, 1959) or musculoskeletal surgery (Bernard de Montmollin, 1962). Very often, they acquired international experience in the most renowned clinics in the world (Great Britain, The Netherlands, France and The United States) and created autonomous chairs within the Surgical Department. Zander was appointed professor in 1964 and Mosimann in 1966.

Saegesser was supported in his endeavours by the SNSF, which granted him a sum of 70,000 francs in 1958 to found a centre for experimental surgery. An active international collaboration was set up, among others with prof. Bromm of the University of Leyden (1959) with whom Saegesser had stayed in the mid-1940s, for "experimental surgery and in particular for the preparation of a whole series of open-heart operations".[177] On the other hand, relations were more difficult with his colleagues in the Faculty, who feared that the strong growth of the Surgical Department would be to their detriment. In 1959, when the Faculty Council refused to grant the title of assistant physician to one of his disciples, Francioli, Saegesser explained that he "would like to choose his collaborators himself. He considered it abnormal for the Faculty to interfere in the affairs of a department head".[178]

Teamwork and the empowerment of parts of the surgery were not only the result of the organisational will of the department head and his followers. They were also made possible by the strong growth in hospitalisations for surgery. Between 1957 and 1960, there were nearly 4000 hospitalisations per year in this department alone, which was more than 28% of all the patients of the Cantonal Hospital.[179] The Surgical Department was thoroughly restructured in the years 1969–1974 in order to give larger autonomy to the various specialties which were now recognised. As a young retiree, Saegesser declared that "in a free, efficient and developing surgery, no hierarchy [...] is possible. We need to create a spirit of understanding".[180]

5 Conclusion

The development of the technical medical system, characterised by new working methods, developed by César Roux (German model) and then by

[177] RSC, Department of the Interior, 1959, p. 51.

[178] AUNIL, minutes of the meetings of the Council of the Faculty of Medicine, 6 June 1959.

[179] RSC, Department of the Interior. The total number of patients hospitalised at the Cantonal Hospital was 11,716 in 1940 and 14,389 in 1960.

[180] Frédéric Saegesser, "The future of surgery as I see it", in *Swiss Society of Surgery, 1963–1988*, Basel, Schwabe & Co, 1990, p. 81.

Pierre Decker and Frédéric Saegesser (American model), resembled a real industrialisation of hospital medicine (double movement of mechanisation and concentration) followed by a division of labour. This transformation had a decisive impact on the growth, organisation and management of hospitals. The new surgery, which was not confined to the surgical clinic of the Cantonal Hospital, implies a profound change of the means of production that are hospitals. The mutation of the medical-technical system implies that of the hospital system.

Indeed, surgical innovations were not adopted automatically in the various institutions of the Canton. Their implementation implied a profound restructuring of management methods, the aim of which was to control expenses, increase resources and adopt a rationalised organisation. As in the industrial sector, the surgeon-modernisers worked in close collaboration with the administrative management of the hospital, which also tended to become more professional in the inter-war period. The transformation of the hospital system was thus not a natural phenomenon resulting from the discoveries of medical science. Their large-scale application required a profound structural and managerial reorganisation that took a particular form depending on the type of institution. The next two chapters of this work attempt to show how the various reorganisations made possible and accompanied the development of hospital medicine, firstly in the case of the Cantonal Hospital of Lausanne and then in private philanthropic hospitals.

CHAPTER 3

Management and Organisation at the Cantonal Hospital of Lausanne

1 Introduction

The Cantonal Hospital of Lausanne is at the heart of the Vaud hospital system. The special position it occupies in relation to other healthcare institutions (regional hospitals, specialized hospitals and private clinics) is explained by three factors, its function, size and legal status. First of all, the Cantonal Hospital's sole purpose is not to care for and treat patients, as in most other hospitals in the canton; the Cantonal Hospital is also, and above all, a university centre attached to a Faculty of Medicine where teaching and research activities are carried out. The example of surgery discussed in the previous chapter is highly revealing in respect of the training role of the Hospital. As the main place of study for the canton's doctors, it is where they build their medical knowledge. The Cantonal Hospital maintains special relations with other establishments in the hospital system and there is a clear link of dependence between the latter and the former with regard to medical know-how.

Secondly, the Cantonal Hospital occupies a dominant position due to its size. Since the end of the nineteenth century, it has accounted for about half of the hospital system's capacity, a proportion that has remained roughly the same throughout the twentieth century. Although the legal need for a medical facility for the entire indigent population in the Canton is a factor in explaining this size, it seems that the academic nature of the institution is the main cause. As the Hospital hosted the clinics of the Faculty of Medicine, it had to offer a minimum range of hospital services and have a critical mass of patients. In addition, the various professors in charge of each clinical service used it as a personal work tool, both for hospitalising their private clientele and for their research activities, two factors that strongly accentuated the growth trend of the establishment. It is also necessary to take into account the demographic

P.-Y. Donzé, *The Formation of the Swiss Hospital System (1840–1960)*,
https://doi.org/10.1007/978-981-19-3911-2_3

growth and urbanisation of the canton, which saw an increase in the population of the city of Lausanne from 29,356 inhabitants in 1880 to 126,328 in 1960.[1] The cantonal authorities faced constant demographic pressure and were required to provide the population with a constantly developing hospital infrastructure.

Finally, the Cantonal Hospital is the only public institution in the Vaud hospital system. It belongs to the State of Vaud and is attached to the cantonal administration, whereas all other hospitals in the system are private institutions. This does not mean the hospital's financial resources are unlimited. On the contrary, periods of relative affluence (1870–1914 and 1945–1960) and periods of crisis (1914–1945) followed one another and influenced the development of the hospital. However, the question of hospital revenues was not solely dependent on the state of public finances. In order to better control the development of the institution, the management of the Hospital constantly sought to make its sources of income independent.

2 The Cantonal Hospital Before the New Buildings of 1883

Despite a change of ownership, there was no abrupt break of service between the Lausanne City Hospital and the Cantonal Hospital which took its place in 1806. The transformation of this establishment took place in stages, with increasing intervention by the cantonal administration which led to the construction of new buildings in the early 1880s.

A Hospital that Focuses on the Sick (1806–1870)

In the first part of the nineteenth century, the Cantonal Hospital refocused on the curable sick. When the State bought the establishment from the city of Lausanne (in 1806), it took in a very disparate indigent population made up of the sick, the elderly, the insane, prisoners, abandoned children, prostitutes, etc.[2] It was a multifunctional social institution like those found elsewhere under the Ancien Régime. The insane were the first to leave the hospital, entering instead a separate establishment dedicated to them (in 1811). They were followed by prisoners (in 1826), boys' discipline (in 1846) and girls' discipline (in 1869).[3]

[1] *Annuaire statistique du canton de Vaud—1985*, Lausanne, Service cantonal de recherche et d'information statistiques, 1985.

[2] Vincent Barras and Cécile Lacharme, "L'Hospice cantonal", in *Vaud sous l'Acte de Médiation, 1803–1813: la naissance d'un canton confédéré*, Lausanne: Bibliothèque historique vaudoise, 2002, pp. 176–181.

[3] Geneviève Heller, "Les lieux de la maladie: quelques repères historiques", in Hermann-Michel Hagmann and Jean-Pierre Fragnière (eds), *Maintien à domicile. Le temps de l'affirmation*, Lausanne: Réalités sociales, 1997, pp. 15–25.

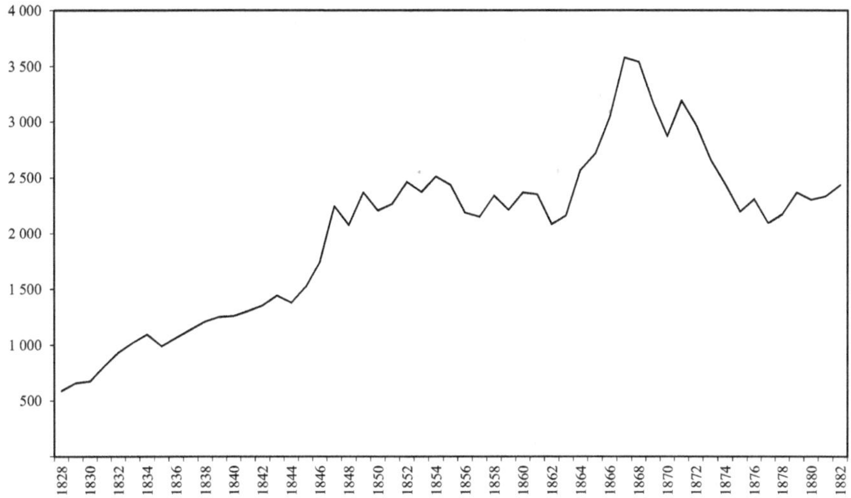

Fig. 1 Number of patients hospitalised at the Cantonal Hospital of Lausanne, 1828–1882 (*Source* RSC, Department of the Interior, 1828–1882)

These successive departures made it possible to broaden the types of care offered, "to give more room to the patients and to create separate wards for certain disgusting or dangerous diseases, because of their contagious nature",[4] as with syphilis, where prostitutes were confined to the Hospital, at least from the end of the 1840s. In addition, the Hospital opened up to the free hospitalisation of non-Vaudois with the signing in 1849 of an agreement with the canton of Berne, whose subjects were numerous in the canton of Vaud. In fact, they represented nearly 7% of the patients hospitalised in 1847–1848.[5] Similar arrangements were signed with several foreign states from the mid-1850s (Belgium in 1855, Italy in 1856, Austria in 1859, Prussia in 1862, Bavaria in 1862, etc.), in order to guarantee reciprocal free hospitalisation for their various nationals. The first part of the nineteenth century was, therefore, a period of refocusing and opening up; the Hospital became an establishment for curable somatic patients, whatever their origin, and thus began a dynamic growth in hospitalisations that statistical analysis confirms (Fig. 1).

The Hospital reached its maximum inpatient capacity at the end of the 1840s. While the average annual growth in admissions was 6.9% for the period 1828–1847, it entered a phase of stagnation for the period 1848–1882, providing we do not take include the exceptional years from 1865 to 1873, when many patients with scabies were admitted for short periods of treatment. The average length of stay was similar, falling sharply between 1836

[4] RSC, Department of the Interior, 1845.

[5] ACV, K VIII A 42/1, Hospice protocol, 1849.

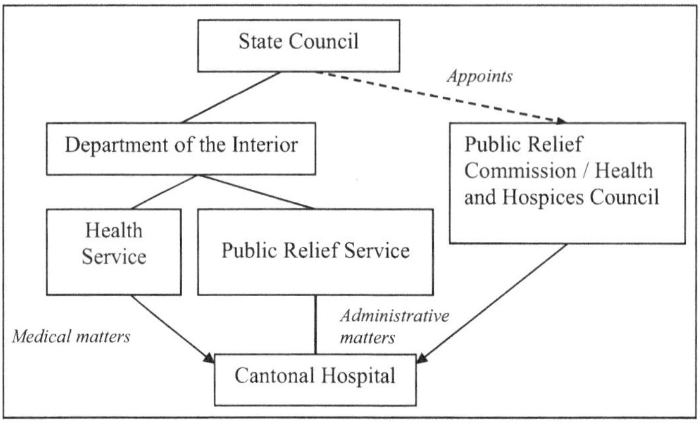

Fig. 2 Administrative bodies governing the Cantonal Hospital of Lausanne

and 1849, from 36.9 to 24.9 days (a decrease of 32.5%).[6] For the period 1849–1882, the length of stay fluctuated between 20 and 25 days (annual average of 22.4 days), if we do not take into account the years 1865–1873.

The Hospital as a Service of the Cantonal Administration

The Cantonal Hospital was not organised like similar establishments elsewhere in Switzerland or abroad where public hospitals were generally administered by ad hoc administrative commissions. It was not managed autonomously but was integrated, since being bought from the city in 1806, into a public administration department with other institutions (Public Relief Service). Many actors were directly involved in the administration of the institution from this time (see Fig. 2).

First of all, the State Council was involved at the top of the hierarchy. The head of the Department of the Interior intervened personally on many occasions, among other things in matters of employee appointments or the extension of certain services. Since 1845, the Cantonal Hospital has been a hotbed of clientelism by the Radical-Democratic Party. In 1873, for example, Dr. Rouge recalled, "the State Council made all the appointments, right down to the kitchen girls".[7] In the 1890s and 1900s, the hospital became an important channel for careers in the cantonal administration. In the day-to-day management of the hospital, the State was present through several other administrative actors.

First of all, there were two services of the Department of the Interior which operated at different levels: The Health Service and the Public Relief Service.

[6] Figures unknown before 1836.

[7] Louis Rouge, "Etude sur l'assistance des malades et sur les hôpitaux", *RMSR*, 1873, p. 213.

The Health Service dealt with questions of public health and the practice of medicine; therefore, it was the main point of contact for questions concerning the organisation of the medical service within the hospital. As for the Public Relief Service, this was responsible for financial and organisational matters relating to the Hospital which was officially attached to it. Finally, the Public Relief Commission—renamed the Health and Hospices Council (HHC) in 1885—performed, among many other functions, the role of the administrative commission of the Cantonal Hospital, although it never sat as such. At each meeting, matters concerning the Cantonal Hospital were discussed along with other issues (care of the insane, the elderly, tuberculosis patients, etc.), in a context that remained very general. This commission essentially played a supervisory role and intervened very little when there were no problems to be solved. It was even suspended in the years 1862–1875 and temporarily replaced by civil servants from the Public Relief Service. From 1885 onwards, the Health and Hospices Council played the role of the Hospital's administrative commission, in addition to its traditional role of supervising the practice of medicine. Finally, other official actors intervened more sporadically in the management of the establishment, such as the Department of Public Instruction for questions of university education or the Grand Council for various points of detail addressed in interpellations or motions.

The fragmentation of the management and control authority of the Cantonal Hospital favoured a broad autonomy of the institution and gave real decision-making power to its management; however, this organisational structure was not conducive to financial independence. The Hospital's assets, as well as most of the donations it received, were held in a Hospice fund which allowed part financing of the institutions grouped in this service (placement of the insane and the elderly, thermal baths, etc.), the balance being paid from the State budget. The Cantonal Hospital, therefore, had no control over a large part of its income. While this shortcoming was not felt to be particularly burdensome in the first half of the nineteenth century, this changed when it came to financing the medical innovations at the end of the century. At this point, the management of the Cantonal Hospital sought to diversify its income.

The Public Relief Service and Commission were already present in the 1850s and 1860s; however, their interventions were limited to the acceptance of women in childbirth and non-Vaudois, the control of the length of stay and questions relating to the management of personnel (discipline, dismissals, holidays, appointments, etc.). With the introduction of a Public Relief Commission with a wider remit, there remained only a bursar with little power at the head of the hospital's administrative service. The bursar was mainly concerned with keeping the books and maintaining order in the establishment; he had no power over the staff of the institution and was under the orders of the council.

The Crisis of the 1870s and the Construction of the New Hospital in 1883

In the 1870s, the Cantonal Hospital experienced a growth crisis. It was an establishment that had refocused its concern on the sick but it did not have the means to respond to this new function: how could it hospitalise and cure the sick of a canton with a growing population in an establishment dating from the 1760s and originally intended to take in the canton's floating poor population (old and sick people without families, prisoners, abandoned children, etc.)? In the end, it was the government's proactive intervention in the early 1870s that made the change possible. The decision to build a new hospital in 1874 and the appointment of Samuel Cuénoud as director in 1876 are indicative of the importance the Cantonal Hospital had acquired in the eyes of the radical-democratic modernising elites.

The Old Hospital Is Encumbered

Statistics showing the number of patients admitted to the hospital indicate its maximum capacity was reached at the end of the 1840s; however, it was not until about fifteen years later that the political authorities became aware of the need for a larger hospital. In 1866, the Grand Council appointed a commission to consider the need for a new hospital. Initially, the commission recommended various changes to improve the technical environment (e.g., kitchens, staircases, latrines, etc.),[8] although this policy was not sufficient to meet the growing demand for hospitalisation.

The construction of a new institution for the insane raised the question of the use of the old buildings, the State Council preferring to use these as a dependency of the Cantonal Hospital (1872).[9] Despite the opposition of several deputies who demanded the construction of a new hospital, this solution received the support of several doctors directly involved in hospital medicine who saw it as an opportunity to test the pavilion model. The Grand Council agreed and decreed the relocation of part of the surgical department to these old buildings, pending the opening of a new hospital the State Council requested to be built in 1874.[10] Before this new establishment was available, other annexed installations were set up such as a lazaretto for children with ringworm and women in childbirth (1872–1884), isolation pavilions (1875) and a small infirmary for convalescents (1876–1881). Finally, the State decided, for similar reasons, to financially support the patients admitted to the local infirmaries from 1875 on (see Chapter 5).

[8] RSC, Department of the Interior, 1866.

[9] Catherine Fussinger and Deodaat Tevaearai, *Lieux de folie, monuments de raison. Architecture et psychiatrie en Suisse romande, 1830–1930*, Lausanne: Presses polytechniques et universitaires romandes, 1998, pp. 59–67.

[10] BGC, 10 February 1872.

The Introduction of the German Model (1883)

The new hospital buildings were constructed by the state architect Henri Assinare in 1882–1883. First of all, this prestigious establishment was built according to a hotel concept in which climatic concerns (sunshine, pure air, etc.), medical concerns and the beauty of the site were combined. The new hospital was also a source of pride for Lausanne's councillors, as Marc Dufour stated in 1882, "it is always with a certain pride that I pass by the building that is now completed. […] When the new hospital is occupied, we shall have a building which, from the point of view of location, will be one of the best placed and most favourably situated hospitals in Europe at the present time".[11] Referring to the location of the future hospital, Dupont had already written in 1876 that it was "in a situation which, from the hygienic point of view, could not be surpassed. The air circulates there without encountering any obstacle, not a single ray of sunlight is lost, and one enjoys a splendid view".[12] This quest for clean air and sunlight also played a role in the adoption of certain principles of the suburban model, more conducive to the circulation of air between buildings isolated from each other. The monumental hospital model was increasingly rejected because it favoured the presence of large areas of shade and humidity and prevented optimal air circulation in the hospital space, all of which the hygienists of the mid-nineteenth century sought to avoid.[13] In 1873, Louis Rouge published a long article in which he condemned monumental hospitals and pleaded in favour of the pavilion model for health reasons.[14] The same year, the Health Council mandated Recordon, a medical doctor and the architect Assinare for a study trip to Germany. In particular, they were asked to visit the city of Leipzig, where one of the first German hospitals designed according to the pavilion model had been opened in 1871.[15] The Leipziger Krankenhaus St. Jakob, which benefited from the expertise of Rudolf Virchow, became an important model for the reconstruction of many hospitals in Germany.[16] The German experts Recordon and Assinare met during their trip recommended the adoption of a model halfway between the block hospital and the pavilion hospital, that is, the construction of a central building flanked by several pavilions.[17] The committee of the Grand Council in charge of this project wrote in 1875, "the assistance of Messrs. the experts was very valuable, because in addition to several detailed

[11] BGC, 20 January 1882.

[12] Dupont, "Le service de chirurgie…", op. cit., p. 254.

[13] Alain Corbin, *Le miasme et la jonquille. L'odorat et l'imaginaire social, XVIIIe–XIXe siècles*, Paris: Flammarion, 1986.

[14] Louis Rouge, op. cit.

[15] ACV, K VIII B 18.

[16] Axel Hinrich Murken, "Das deutsche Baracken- und Pavillon-Krankenhaus von 1866 bis 1906", in *Studien zur Krankenhausgeschichte im 19. Jahrhundert im Hinblick auf die Entwicklung in Deutschland*, Göttingen: Vandenhoeck & Ruprecht, 1976, pp. 72–104.

[17] BGC, 1875.

advices which were taken into account, these eminent men, by approving the system which served as a basis for the project of our committee, confirmed the State Council in the idea that the plan which we have the honour of submitting to the Grand Council, meets all the modern requirements of hospitals".[18] The Cantonal Hospital of Lausanne was thus built on the model of the Leipziger Krankenhaus St. Jakob.

As for the organisation of the medical infrastructure, this corresponded with the affirmation of a new hospital medicine focused on surgery. Here too, the German influence is obvious. The central building had an apse with a glass rotunda housing the operating theatre. This south-facing extension of the main building provided optimal light conditions for surgical work. These rotundas, present in many hospitals of the Belle Epoque, disappeared during the inter-war period, with the arrival of artificial lighting. By giving the operating room the central place traditionally given to the chapel, the designers of the Hospital made it the temple of a new triumphalist medicine.[19]

Financing the Cantonal Hospital (1850–1883)

The crisis of the 1870s involved not only real estate but also finances. Until the beginning of the decade, the financial needs of the hospital were extremely stable: about 100,000 francs were enough to keep the establishment running. At around 1872, expenses began to rise sharply; they exceeded 150,000 francs in 1876 and 200,000 francs in 1882. This upsurge reflects more than the quantitative development of the establishment.

The increase in the cost of caring for patients, whose numbers are relatively stable, largely explains this growth in operating expenses (see Fig. 3). The average cost of a day of hospitalisation shows a very similar trend to that of operating expenses, both being characterised by an accelerated rise during the 1870s. The cost per day rose from less than 0.88 francs in 1850 to 1.88 francs in 1860, 2.18 francs in 1870 and 3.11 francs in 1880. This increase reflects the changes in the hospital environment as revealed by the evolution of the structure of expenditure.

The structure of expenditure varied considerably over time (see Table 1). As is generally the case in mid-nineteenth-century hospitals, food expenses predominated, accounting for more than a third of hospital expenses (37.3% on average) and the wage bill was relatively low (14.2%). The most notable development in the case of Lausanne is the sharp rise in expenditure on drugs in the second half of the 1870s. While its value fluctuated around 15% until 1875, its share increased to almost a quarter of the expenditures in 1880. The declared cause of this sharp growth was the adoption of the antiseptic method around 1875–1876 by the head of the surgical department, Emile Dupont,

[18] ACV, K XIII 35, draft decree concerning the construction of the new hospital, 21 January 1875.

[19] Jean Imbert, "L'évolution de l'architecture hospitalière: piété, salubrité, bien-être", *Bulletin de la Société française d'histoire des hôpitaux*, 1984, n°49, pp. 25–38.

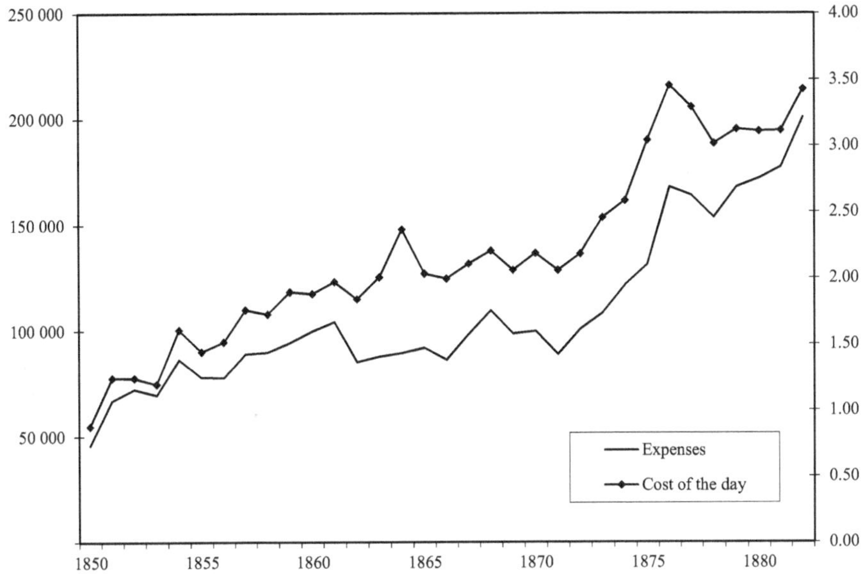

Fig. 3 Operating expenses of the Cantonal Hospital and average cost per day of hospitalisation, in current francs, 1850–1882 (*Source* RSC, Department of the Interior, 1850–1882)

Table 1 Main expenditures of the Hospital, in %, 1855–1880

	1855	*1860*	*1865*	*1870*	*1875*	*1880*	*Average (1855–1880)*
Salaries	15.0	12.0	15.5	14.7	13.9	15.0	14.2
Food	48.8	36.1	34.6	34.0	29.9	37.7	37.3
Drugs	12.8	14.5	15.5	15.2	16.6	24.8	16.7
Various	23.4	27.4	34.4	36.1	39.6	22.5	31.8
Total	100.0	100.0	100.0	100.0	100.0	100.0	100.0

Source RSC, Department of the Interior, 1855–1880
Note "Miscellaneous" includes mainly building maintenance

which involved abandoning reusable cloths in favour of single-use flannel. This was the first medical innovation in the nineteenth century to have an impact on finances.

The Hospital's own income (from patients' pensions, income from assets, etc.) remained extremely stable, amounting to an average of 10,690 francs per year. This covered 5–13% of expenditure depending on the period. Such a low proportion can be explained by two factors. Firstly, in a phenomenon not specific to Lausanne, the hospitalised population was largely indigent

Table 2 Deficit compared to operating expenses, in %, 1856–1882

Period	*1856–1860*	*1861–1865*	*1866–1870*	*1871–1875*	*1876–1880*	*1881–1882*
Deficit	87.7	88.0	87.4	90.8	94.1	94.3

Source RSC, Department of the Interior, 1856–1882

and could not bear an increase in the cost of hospitalisation. The profitable patients—the middle and upper classes—were still largely treated at home. During the period 1850–1880, the proportion of free stays amounted to 90.1% of the total number of hospital days, with no significant change over time.[20] Secondly, specific to Lausanne, the integration of the Cantonal Hospital into the Public Relief Service played a negative role in the financial independence of the establishment. Most of its assets—essentially the assets of the former Villeneuve Hospital, nationalised in the 1800s[21] and donations—were capitalised in the Public Relief Service fund and used for the development of the entire service, not just the Hospital. Organisations similar to the Cantonal Hospital of Lausanne in other cantons were essentially self-financing at that time. The Bourgeois Hospital in Fribourg had a self-financing rate of 88.4% in its 1887 budget, while the Bourgeois Hospital in Porrentruy was 83.0% dependent on income from its assets for the years 1815–1870.[22] Therefore, the particular structure of the Public Relief Service meant the Cantonal Hospital was not financially autonomous at a time when self-financing was the rule elsewhere. Moreover, the increasing dependency on the Public Relief Service rose over time, as shown by the evolution of its deficit in relation to its operating expenses (Table 2).

The Cantonal Hospital was consequently in a situation of extreme financial dependence on the State when the first surgeon-modernisers appeared. Such a mode of financing was undoubtedly appropriate for multifunctional hospitals with a minimalist and non-progressive infrastructure. On the other hand, the modernisation of the medical-technical equipment and the growth of the institution required new types of resources that were put in place in the 1890s–1900s.

Strengthening Administrative Authority

Finally, the mid-1870s were characterised by the intervention of the political-administrative power and the strengthening of the management. Whereas until then the director of the hospital depended on the commission or the Public Relief Service, this position took on new importance with the appointment

[20] RSC, Department of the Interior, 1850–1880.

[21] Eugène Olivier, *Médecine et santé dans le Pays de Vaud. 2nd part: Au XVIIIe siècle: 1675–1798*, Lausanne: Payot, 1962, p. 793.

[22] Pierre-Yves Donzé, *Bâtir*..., op. cit., p. 47.

in 1876 of a close friend of Louis Ruchonnet as head of the establishment: Samuel Cuénoud.[23] The former director, Georges Neyret, became the bursar under his successor.[24] Cuénoud came from the world of engineers, bringing with him their modernist and rationalising ideology. A graduate of the Special School of Lausanne—the future Swiss Federal Institute of Technology—he taught mathematics at Lausanne College (1857–1869) before becoming director of the Lausanne Cantonal Industrial School (1870–1874). This establishment, which was the result of Ruchonnet's public education policy, was a pure product of radical-democratic positivism that aimed to facilitate the training of engineers.[25] Inaugurated in 1869, this school was placed under the direction of Cuénoud, followed by the successive direction of two brothers of César Roux, Louis (1874–1882) and Félix (1882–1898). In addition, at the time of his appointment as head of the hospital, Samuel Cuénoud was a member of the General Board of the Banque Cantonale Vaudoise and of the committee of the Industrial and Commercial Society of Vaud. Finally, he was closely involved in the Vaud Society of Mutual Aid, of which he was president from 1870. Overall, he was a man who combined scientific rationalism with the management of public goods when he took over the Cantonal Hospital in 1876. Although his stay at the head of this establishment was short (1876–1882), it was nevertheless decisive because it was at a turning point in the modernisation of the hospital. It was during these few years that the organisation of the new Cantonal Hospital, which opened in 1883, was set up and decided upon. After his departure for the post of mayor of Lausanne (1882) where he was noticed for his talents in reorganising the municipal administration, Cuénoud did not abandon hospital affairs. As a deputy in the Grand Council (1882–1905), he was an important political intermediary and was appointed, at the age of more than seventy, a member of the Health and Hospices Council, where he succeeded his friend Louis Roux (1909).

3 The Integration of the Cantonal Hospital into the Faculty of Medicine (1883–1914)

The new hospital was a decisive step in the process leading to the opening of the University in 1890. The Academy lacked a medical faculty to transform itself into a university and the Cantonal Hospital provided the basic infrastructure for the organisation of university clinics from 1883 onwards. It is difficult to imagine that the cantonal authorities—who were already thinking about a university in the 1870s—did not have the university objective in mind when they intervened in hospital affairs in the mid-1870s. In 1872, Louis Ruchonnet himself proposed to the State Council that a two-year preparatory

[23] Erich Gruner (ed.), *L'Assemblée fédérale suisse, 1848–1920. Biographies*, Berne: Francke, 1966, pp. 795–796.

[24] ODCV, 1876.

[25] *L'Ecole industrielle de Lausanne. Notice historique*, Lausanne: Payot, 1902, 234 p.

Table 3 Directors of the Cantonal Hospital, 1883–1929

Name	*Period of office*
Charles Delorme (1826–1894)	1883–1894
Louis Borgeaud (1849–1910)	1895–1909
Louis Mermoud (1861–1945)	1909–1929

Source Official Directory of the Canton of Vaud, 1883–1929 and AVC, ATS files

medical school be set up within the framework of the Academy to make it easier for young people to become interested in the medical professions and prepare for the transition to university. Eager to make his idea a reality, he contacted professors in Strasbourg who would accept a chair in Lausanne.[26] In 1873, the project was submitted to the Health Council, but it did not survive the departure of Ruchonnet from the State Council (1874). When the Faculty of Medicine was created (1890), the Cantonal Hospital was entrusted with the practical training of medical students. By hosting the various university clinics, it saw the arrival or assertion of new branches of medicine (dermatology, paediatrics, laryngology, etc.) for which the chief physicians requested the development of the hospital infrastructure. The Faculty appears to have been a decisive growth factor.

Empowerment of Hospital Management

The management of the Hospital and the administrative authority continued to be strengthened. This was both a question of financial necessity and the organisation of an institution whose structure became more complex with the creation of new medical services. The state alone could not afford the high capital costs and the increasing operating deficits that would follow. The task of the hospital administration was therefore to release the new resources necessary for the transformation of the hospital.

At the Head of the Hospital: Directors from the Public Administration

Three men succeeded each other at the head of the establishment between 1883 and 1914. Although all of them were Radical-Democratic Party members experienced in the management of public administration, there was a significant change in the recruitment process (Table 3).

Charles Delorme was a pastor of the National Church close to the State. He was a deputy in the Constituent Assembly of 1861 who campaigned for the maintenance of the links between the Church and the State, with the result that the National Church could influence public education.[27] He himself was

[26] ACV, K XIII 38, letter from Louis Ruchonnet to the State Council, 17 January 1872.

[27] Robert Centlivres and Jean-Jacques Fleury, *De l'Eglise d'Etat à l'Eglise nationale (1839–1863)*, Lausanne: Eglise nationale vaudoise, 1963, pp. 87–107.

the director of the teacher training college between 1876 and 1882. He distinguished himself by the development of practical teaching, in particular thanks to the addition of an application school to perfect the theoretical training of future regents.[28] After Delorme's death, the State Council appointed Louis Borgeaud, director of the Morges Arsenal since 1878. He also served on the municipal councils of Morges and Lausanne. His career culminated in 1909 with his appointment to the Lausanne prefecture. Finally, the third director of the Hospital during this period was a civil servant from the Department of the Interior, Louis Mermoud.[29] He joined the Hospital at the age of 17 years as an accountant (1878) and was appointed head of the Public Relief Service in 1907, thus becoming Director Borgeaud's right-hand man in the Department, whom he succeeded in 1909. Throughout his career, Mermoud enjoyed the support of the Radical-Democratic Party, being the brother of National Councillor John Mermoud. His appointment opened up a new channel for the recruitment of hospital directors which dominated until the mid-1950s. It was no longer enough to be a member of the Radical-Democratic Party and to have proven oneself at the head of a public administration. The State Council favoured men from the Department of the Interior and, more specifically, from the Health Service or the Public Relief Service; that is, managers who were already familiar with the administrative functioning of the Cantonal Hospital and who ensured a certain continuity between the various hierarchical levels of the health administration (Cantonal Hospital, Health and Public Relief Services, Department of the Interior). This mode of operation attenuated the possible negative effects for the cantonal administration and the State Council of the increasing autonomy of the Hospital's management.

The administrative team working alongside the director grew quickly.[30] In the 1880s, there was only a secretary-accountant to assist the director. Later, a second secretary was appointed (1891), an assistant accountant (1896), a third secretary (1903), an office assistant (1914), a secretary for the maternity ward/infant clinic (1916) and a telephone operator (1917) so, by 1918, there were eight administrative officers at the head of the Hospital. The hospital bureaucracy still appeared limited; however, by 1914 the Hospital had more administrative staff than the Public Relief Service responsible for overseeing its management, which had only five officials in total. This trend continued and became more pronounced in the following decades. This does not mean the Department of the Interior became less involved in hospital affairs. The Health Service and the Health and Hospice Council supported generally the Hospital's management—in fact, individuals moving from one administration to the other, at all levels of the hierarchy, were frequent in the course of a

[28] *Une école pour l'école. 150 ans d'Ecole normale dans le Canton de Vaud*, Lausanne: Ecoles normales du canton de Vaud, 1983, pp. 99–102.

[29] ACV, ATS files, Mermoud Louis.

[30] ODCV, 1880–1920.

career. The career of Director Mermoud reveals this trend, assisting in establishing administrative control over the establishment, particularly in the face of the rapidly growing medical profession.

A New Financial System: The Hospital Creates Its Own Resources

The main management innovation adopted in the early 1880s consisted of the search for the Hospital's own resources in order to ensure the financial development of the establishment. Indeed, the Public Relief Service was increasingly busy following the opening of the Cery Psychiatric Asylum in 1873, among other developments. The annual deficit of the Hospices reached an average of 288,107 francs for the years 1883–1900 and then increased to 468,337 francs in 1905, 751,598 francs in 1910 and more than one million francs in 1914. On average, this represented 4.7% of the State's expenditure for the whole period.

In the 1870s, the Hospital was more than 90% dependent on public aid to cover its expenses. It was not possible to modernise the hospital with such little control over resources. The new revenues generated by the hospital administration allowed for a sharp increase in expenses—from nearly 275,000 francs in 1883 to about 600,000 francs in 1914—with a relatively constant deficit of about 300,000 francs per year. The coverage of the expenses by the Hospital's own revenues increased strongly from 7.2% in 1883 to 27.4% in 1900 and 34.9% in 1914, which limited its dependence on the State.

The new revenues were of several types. Most came from the pensions paid by patients. The hospital authorities decided to make the patients who were not indigent pay for themselves. The new establishment opened in 1883 attracted more and more members of the middle classes who had previously been reluctant to be hospitalised, a phenomenon the State Council had foreseen in 1881: "The population of the Hospital tends constantly to increase, in spite of the numerous refusals of admission caused by periods of overcrowding and the sending of patients to the local infirmaries. It is a fact now well noted that the treatment of diseases in hospitals meets with less and less repugnance, even among persons who, by their social position, would seem to have to resort to hospital care only as a last resource".[31] The proportion of free days for the indigent thus fell from 86.8% of total days in 1883 to 50.6% in 1914. The total pensions paid by the patients amounted to 88.9% of the receipts for the years 1886–1914.[32]

A special category of patients also appeared; that of the private clientele of the chief physicians. Dr. Dupont was the first to ask the HHS in 1883 "for authorisation to have a resident's room at his disposal to perform an operation on a patient [...]".[33] The request was granted but on an exceptional

[31] RSC, Department of the Interior, 1881, p. 76.

[32] RSC, Department of the Interior, 1886–1914. Figures unavailable prior to 1886. This figure includes pensions paid by the indigent as well as those paid by private patients.

[33] ACV, K VIII B 61, protocol of the Hospice Commission, 5 May 1883.

basis. This type of practice evolved very quickly, under pressure from doctors who wanted to use the hospital infrastructure for their private practice, so that by 1892 there were nine private boarding rooms, comprising a total of 16 beds.[34] This practice developed, in particular after the creation of the Faculty of Medicine, contributing to the reputation of the Hospital in the context of strong development of medical tourism in Lausanne. The private clientele of the medical professors had a particularly beneficial effect on the operation of the establishment. The amount of these private pensions is known from 1895. Until 1914, their participation brought in nearly 37,800 francs each year; i.e., 27.1% of the revenue—a proportion which was far from being reached in the inter-war period. In addition, from 1910 onwards, the private clientele often made donations to the medical professors when satisfied with the treatment they received. These donations were capitalised in special funds intended for the development of the infrastructure of the university clinics.

In addition, the private clientele that came to the Cantonal Hospital for hospitalisation made use of the high-end medical and technical equipment installed in the establishment (X-rays, operating room, etc.). The use of this infrastructure thus generated financial resources for the hospital. X-rays were taxed from 1904 onwards and very quickly became a profitable investment, bringing in 2875 francs in the first year, up to 19,567 francs in 1910. During the years 1910–1913, this service provided nearly 10% of the Hospital's income. The second area of substantial profit was surgery, for which the Hospital collected operating fees from 1898 onwards. These amounts were modest and relatively stable, averaging 4242 francs per year for the period 1898–1914; however, they played an important role in the development of the Hospital. They were not included in the operating revenues but were kept in a Cantonal Hospital Fund which allowed for certain investments outside the budget of the Public Relief Service—another sign of the desire for autonomy on the part of the Hospital's managers.

Organisation of the Various Hospital Services

Despite the diversification of hospital revenues, the new resources generated by the opening of the establishment to non-indigent patients were not sufficient to finance the development of the University Hospital. Moreover, as the State did not want to go into debt, original solutions had to be found such as subcontracting certain clinical courses to pre-existing private institutions and attempting centralisation in the 1910s.

The Impact of the Faculty of Medicine

The new hospital was a decisive step towards the creation of a Faculty of Medicine in 1890, for which it provided clinical teaching. When it opened in 1883, the Cantonal Hospital had two separate departments—surgery

[34] RSC, Department of the Interior, 1892.

and internal medicine—that were each divided into two divisions—men and women—employing four doctors and four assistants. The nursing service was provided by the deaconesses of Saint-Loup, who used the hospital as their main training ground. From 1883 onwards, the hospital's management sought to control the development of the establishment and to limit its financial impact. Shortly after the inauguration of the buildings, the HHS asked the chief physicians to think about the economical use of antiseptic bands and heating in the wards, as well as a rational hospitalisation policy, focusing in particular on the discharge of convalescents and incurables.[35] In 1890, an admission commission was set up by the Department of the Interior. It was made up of the hospital director, the head of the Health Service and the chief doctors of the surgical and medical departments. Its aim was to direct patients to the various departments. The growth in the number of hospitalisations was remarkable from the opening of the new Hospital. The arrival of the university clinics in 1890 only reinforced the upward trend that had been apparent since 1883. The number of patients rose from 2723 in 1883 to 6634 in 1914—an increase of almost 143%.[36] This growth was not a result of certain medical and technical innovations that would allow patients to be treated more quickly as their average length of stay remained stable at around 25–30 days; it was simply a consequence of the development of its capacity. The number of hospital days thus increased from 71,398 in 1883 to 195,541 in 1914.

Apart from these statistical data on the evolution of the number of patients, it is difficult to establish exactly what influence the new Faculty of Medicine had on the development of the Cantonal Hospital. The recruitment of professors shows a certain bipolarisation between clinical and non-clinical (laboratory) professorships. The former were local practitioners from Lausanne or the canton of Vaud, close to the ruling elite. They were in charge of the hospital department corresponding to their chair and had private clinics or practices in addition to their university hospital work.[37] As for the non-clinical chairs (physiology, histology and pathology), the Vaud cantonal authorities appointed scientists of foreign origin to head them.[38] Physiology was awarded to Alexandre Herzen, a Russian by birth and a graduate of the University of Geneva where he had been an assistant to Prof. Schiff. Histology went to Nathan Loewenthal, a graduate of the University of Berne, also Russian and a pupil of Schiff who had been his assistant and successor at the Institute of Advanced Studies in Florence; finally, pathology went to Henri Stilling, a German and former private doctor at the Faculty of Strasbourg. All three were

[35] ACV, K VIII B 61, protocol of the Hospice Commission, 1883.

[36] RSC, Department of the Interior, 1883–1914.

[37] According to the *Annuaire lausannois* or the *Indicateur vaudois* of the 1890s, eight of the twelve professors appointed in 1890 had a clinic or a private practice.

[38] The biographical information quoted below is taken from Olivier Robert and Franceso Panese, op. cit.

essential for the research activities at the Faculty of Medicine, of which they were the scientific showcase. They had neither a practice nor a clinic in the city so they were not in competition with their Vaud colleagues who headed the clinical chairs.

As soon as the Faculty opened in 1890, the Hospital was reorganised to accommodate the new clinics required for university teaching. In order to have more space, the surgery and internal medicine departments, which had been split since 1883, were placed under the sole authority of professors César Roux and Edouard de Cérenville. The space thus freed up allowed for the addition of dermato-venereology services in 1890 (Prof. Emile Dind), laryngology in 1894 (Prof. Louis Secrétan) and paediatrics in 1898 (Prof. Adolphe Combe). Despite the arrival of the Faculty of Medicine, certain hospital services largely dominated the Cantonal Hospital. Predominance was given to surgery, while internal medicine and dermato-venereology can be explained both by the very general character of these branches and the proximity of their chief physicians to political authorities. When it came to the question of fitting out the Cantonal Hospital to accommodate university clinics, it was indeed Roux and de Cérenville who discussed the reorganisation of the establishment with the State Councillor Eugène Ruffy.[39] As for Dind, he had long-standing relationships within the Radical-Democratic Party. As head of the Health Service (1885) and professor of forensic medicine at the Academy following the departure of César Roux (1888), he took the opportunity of the creation of a Faculty of Medicine to take up the chair of dermato-venereology, a field in which he did not possess any specific knowledge or technique but where his experience as a public health practitioner enabled him to impose himself. These three departments alone accounted for almost 80% of the hospital's beds.

The years 1904–1916 saw the construction of three new buildings, one of which—the expansion of the surgical department from 1913 to 1914—only accentuated the imbalance between the various hospital services. The first of these was the new university policlinic, built in 1904. The policlinic was traditionally of considerable importance in the university hospital facilities inspired by the German model, based on the alliance of a medium-sized hospital, laboratories and a policlinic which played a social role (treating the poor) as well as an educational one (training doctors). This double function explains the importance the authorities gave to the development of this establishment. Moreover, the Central Dispensary of the city of Lausanne, directed since 1892 by Paul Demiéville, a former assistant of Theodor Kocher and friend of César Roux, was a dazzling success.[40] In 1898, the Grand Council, at the request of the liberal deputy Adrien Demiéville, Paul's brother, granted a credit of 490,000 francs, increased by a contribution of 200,000 francs from the municipality of Lausanne, for a new building. The latter was inaugurated in 1904

[39] ACV, K VIII B 6, HHS protocol, 4 October 1888.

[40] Guy Saudan, "Dispensary and policlinic in Lausanne: 100 years of medicine and society", *RMSR*, 1989, pp. 267–277.

and included, in addition to the policlinic services, various laboratories of the Department of the Interior and the University (control of foodstuffs in beverages, dairy station, zoology, comparative anatomy, mineralogy).[41] The second important hospital construction was the enlargement of the surgical clinic of César Roux from 1913 to 1914 which confirmed the overwhelming domination of surgery in the establishment (see Chapter 2). The maternity ward, opened in 1883 in one of the four pavilions built behind the hospital, experienced strong development (81 women in childbirth in 1885; 136 in 1890; 290 in 1900)[42] under the direction of Oscar Rapin but only succeeded with difficulty to impose itself in front of the surgical department which kept the upper hand on gynaecological cases. The infrastructure of the maternity ward no longer corresponded to the medical criteria of the 1890s. It did not have an isolation room and it was difficult to perform deliveries under satisfactory aseptic conditions; however, financial difficulties delayed the construction of a new building. Equipped with 140 beds and medical-technical equipment from the Schaerer company, the new maternity ward was inaugurated in 1916.

The new maternity hospital truly launched the expansion of Lausanne's hospital complex which took place during the 1920s and 1930s. Because of its financing, it belongs to the first generation of public hospital buildings (1883–1916). In fact, during the inter-war period, most new hospital construction was based on a system of mixed financing between the state and the private sector. This policy was not completely new. It was the continuation of a policy of subcontracting certain hospital activities to the private sector that had been put in place with the creation of the Faculty of Medicine.

Subcontracting of Some Clinics to Private Philanthropic Institutions

During the transformation of the Academy of Lausanne into a University, the State Council came up against the hostility of certain deputies and notables, generally liberals, who were opposed to this project they considered too costly, as well as from country doctors who feared that a Faculty of Medicine would lead to a medical plethora (see Chapter 2).[43] The financial question was of primary importance and had a strong influence on the structure of the Cantonal University Hospital. State Councillor Ruffy, the main political promoter of the University, declared in 1890 that, "in order to spare the peasant deputation and taking into account the financial capacities of the canton, the creation of the University should not appear as a costly undertaking nor as a prestige operation [...]".[44] The cantonal authorities then considered using existing private institutions to subcontract certain clinical courses.

[41] Ibidem.

[42] RSC, Department of the Interior, various years.

[43] Laurent Tissot, *Politique...*, op. cit., p. 62.

[44] Quoted in Laurent Tissot, *Politique...*, op. cit., p. 90.

Rather than fighting a particularly dense network of philanthropic institutions, the State Council proposed the networking of public and private medical establishments in Lausanne. This rapprochement was greatly facilitated by the reconciliation movement between liberals and radicals, against the background of the rise of socialism. The personal relationships between the doctors working in these various establishments undoubtedly played an essential role in bringing them together. The consultative commission for the creation of a Faculty of Medicine, set up by Ruffy in 1887, brought together six doctors involved in various establishments and all in favour of the University. Three of them were liberals: Edouard Bugnion, Edouard de Cérenville and Marc Dufour; and the other three were radicals: Emile Dind, Frédéric Paschoud and César Roux.[45] Their divergent political commitments were not synonymous with distinct professional paths—quite the contrary. The commission included representatives of the Cantonal Hospital (Roux and de Cérenville) but also of the private sector, such as the Blind People's Asylum (Dufour) or the Central Dispensary (de Cérenville and Dind). Edouard de Cérenville was a key figure in this network[46]: head of the medical department of the Cantonal Hospital on two occasions (1870–1883 and 1888–1898), he was one of the founders of the Central Dispensary of Lausanne (1887) and sat on the board of directors of the Blind People's Asylum (1884–1900). He was also one of the founders of the Leysin Climate Society and the Vaud League against Tuberculosis. Finally, several members of his family (his brother Henri and his nephew Roger) sat on the committee of the Institution of Deaconesses of Saint-Loup which took over the nursing service of the Cantonal Hospital in 1883.

The first institution in which university teaching was decentralised was the Blind People's Asylum which had been home to the ophthalmology clinic since 1890. This represented the continuation of a long tradition of collaboration between the Department of the Interior and Frédéric Recordon, the first specialist in ophthalmology in the canton of Vaud. The latter became interested in this branch of medicine as soon as he completed his internship at the Cantonal Hospital in 1837 and became the first head doctor of the Asylum (1843–1880).[47] At the same time, he made a career in the cantonal administration as a member of the Health Council (1863–1882) and the Public Relief Commission which managed the Cantonal Hospital (1858–1861). He was also head of the Health Service (1857–1885) and professor of forensic medicine (1862–1869) and hygiene (1869–1874) at the Academy. The links between the private and public sectors were maintained and developed by his successor, Marc Dufour, assistant physician (1869) and then chief physician (1880) of the Asylum. As a promoter of the Faculty of Medicine, he made his

[45] Laurent Tissot, *Politique...*, op. cit., p. 62.

[46] ACV, ATS files; Olivier Robert and Franceso Panese, *Dictionnaire...*, op. cit.

[47] ACV, K VIII B 18, letter from the Hospice Commission to the Health Council, 12 September 1837.

Asylum the ophthalmic clinic of the Faculty, with the support of the administrative commission of this establishment which stated in 1888, "the creation in Lausanne of a University comprising the complete cycle of medical studies imposed on us a duty, that of offering the State the possibility of having in our hospital an ophthalmic clinic".[48] In addition to the gains in terms of prestige and university recognition, the State made a financial contribution.

A second agreement was signed in 1892 with the Central Dispensary for the teaching of the policlinic but there was no plan to organise home visits for the students "in order not to encroach on the private clientele of the doctors".[49] This institution became the University Policlinic and was entrusted to a friend of César Roux, Paul Demiéville. It was both an important place for social and preventive medicine in Lausanne—with the arrival of Charlotte Olivier at the head of the Anti-Tuberculosis Dispensary (1911)[50]—and a place for teaching ambulatory medicine to students.

Finally, the question of the Orthopaedic Hospice as a place of university education has already been widely discussed (cf. Chapter 2). It should be remembered that it was under the medical direction of Placide Nicod that a real collaboration between this establishment and the State was established and this was strengthened at the end of the 1920s with the construction of a new building near the Cantonal Hospital.

Attempted Centralisation (1910–1920)

The subcontracting of certain courses and the desire for the growth of the new medical services created with the Faculty of Medicine made the hospital authorities fear a certain dispersion of the establishment or even its break-up. After twenty years of strong growth, the political and university authorities tried to control this centripetal trend. The 1910s saw an effort to centralise the hospital within the Cantonal Hospital.

In 1913, the hospital authorities introduced the post of an assistant physician for the Internal Medicine Department.[51] This was a qualified doctor, more experienced than an intern, who assisted and relieved the head doctor. This function made it possible to maintain the unity of the department, which is not the case with the creation of second departments of medicine and surgery, these leading to the appointment of several senior doctors in the same branch with the relational and organisational problems this can entail. Despite some voices in favour of setting up second departments in Lausanne, essentially to reinforce the freedom of teaching, the Grand Council chose the solution of assistant doctors in order to avoid the multiplication of

[48] Foundation of the Asylum for the Blind, annual report, 1888, p. 15.

[49] Archives of the University of Lausanne, minutes of the meetings of the Council of the Faculty of Medicine, 2 February 1892.

[50] Geneviève Heller, *Charlotte Olivier*..., op. cit.

[51] BGC, 12 November 1913.

departments. In this way, "administrative centralisation and unity of scientific doctrine [...] ensured order and stability".[52]

The various hospital laboratories were centralised at the end of the 1910s.[53] When Louis Michaud was appointed as professor of the medical clinic to replace Bourget (1913), the situation of the analysis laboratories was disorganised. Each hospital department had a minimal facility and collaboration between them was non-existent. Michaud had been trained in the German school and was a fervent supporter of bacteriology.[54] He studied at the Faculty of Berne and did his thesis in medicine and biology with Prof. Sahli and Prof. Langhans as their assistant (1902–1906). He then continued his studies with Prof. Lüthje in Frankfurt and Prof. Krehl in Heidelberg (1906–1910). When he was appointed to Lausanne, the HHS promised him the direction of a central laboratory for his medical research but things were slow to materialise, especially since the laboratory assistants of the medical clinic had left for the Faculty of Sciences after Bourget's death.[55] While waiting for a solution, the analyses were carried out within the framework of the Food Control Service, under the authority of the Department of the Interior and this occasionally led to conflicts with the Confederation which subsidised the laboratory.

Finally, in 1916, the State Council decided to create a joint chemistry laboratory for the Faculties of Science and Medicine, headed by a chemist directly under the authority of a professor of chemistry. In compensation, the various departments of the hospital were allowed to keep their facilities for routine analyses. This laboratory was partly financed by the Department of Public Education but soon found most of its funding from private clients: Lausanne doctors used it for their private analyses. Michaud himself also used this laboratory for the medical clinic's analyses, which quickly led to unforeseen additional costs. Despite several attempts to reorganise the laboratories in the 1920s and 1930s, the chemical institute continued to carry out analyses for the Cantonal Hospital until 1942 when the bacteriology laboratory of the Faculty of Medicine took over.

These various centralising attempts were aimed at controlling the development of hospital medicine. In the inter-war period, this desire came up against material difficulties that prevented the State from taking sole charge of the growth of the hospital infrastructure. It was the contribution of the private sector that proved decisive in the redeployment of the Cantonal Hospital.

[52] Laurent Tissot, *Politique...*, op. cit., p. 173.

[53] ACV, K VIII B 113 and S 73.

[54] Olivier Robert and Franceso Panese, *Dictionnaire...*, op. cit., pp. 860–861 and the booklet *Louis Michaud, 1880–1956*, Basel: Benno Schwab & Cie, 1957.

[55] ACV, K VIII B 6, HHS protocol, 1916.

4 Privatisation and Rationalisation (1920–1950)

The period between the two world wars was a period of fragmentation of the Cantonal Hospital into multiple specialised medical establishments. The diversification of hospital medicine took place in the direction of a horizontal division of work, materialised by the construction of new buildings. Although each of these units underwent a strong rationalisation of work, they all belonged to a common institutional unit: the Cantonal Hospital. The administrative management and the Department of the Interior worked to rationalise this polymorphous organisation, with the aim of ensuring its functioning and releasing the necessary financial resources.

Strengthening the Administrative Control

During the inter-war period, the Cantonal Hospital underwent a change in scale that can be described as a real explosion. The capacity of the hospital is a good indicator of its general development: between 1910 and 1950, the number of beds rose from 525 to 1158—an increase of 120%. Growth is also measured in terms of autonomous care units. The various hospital services moved out of the hospital walls and were organised within their own buildings. A veritable "hospital city" was created in the heights of Lausanne, in the immediate vicinity of the Cantonal Hospital. While there were only three main buildings in 1916 (the Hospital, Polyclinic and Maternity Ward), by 1950 there were ten (the Hospital, Polyclinic, Maternity Ward, Bourget Pavilion, Institute of Physiology, Orthopaedic Hospice, Sandoz Hospice, Isolation Pavilions, Nestlé Hospital and Institute of Pathology), to which must be added a few consequential extensions (the Surgical Clinic and Rossier Hospital).

Looking in detail at hospitalisations, its growth was no longer as dynamic as it had been during the period 1883–1914. The number of patients stagnated at around 8000 per year until around 1935, then increased sharply at the end of the 1930s, reaching almost 14,000 hospitalisations per year after 1945.[56] The difficult years between 1920 and 1935 can be explained as much by the socio-economic context as by data specific to the hospital system. On the one hand, the Cantonal Hospital was overcrowded and could only increase its capacity by constructing new buildings, which mainly took place in the 1930s. On the other hand, the regional hospitals and private clinics in Lausanne, which experienced major modernisation of their infrastructure during the inter-war period, were increasingly competing with each other.

The management of the Cantonal Hospital became more complex as it grew. The administration of a constantly growing and, above all, increasingly heterogeneous establishment in a highly competitive environment had to be ensured. As a consequence of this evolution, the administrative team working alongside the director grew. Remaining relatively stable until the end of the

[56] RSC, Department of the Interior, 1920–1950.

Table 4 Directors of the Cantonal Hospital, 1909–1953

Name	*Period of office*
Louis Mermoud (1861–1945)	1909–1929
Jules Nicoud	1930–1938
Rodolphe Rubattel (1896–1961)	1939–1945
Emile Cottier (1890–1981)	1946–1953

Source Official Directory of the Canton of Vaud, 1909–1953

1930s (between six and 10 people), the administrative department developed considerably thereafter. There were 33 officials working alongside the director in 1950 and 50 in 1960. The administrative management was itself rationalised at the end of the 1940s, with the empowerment of the bursar's office, the accounts department, the personnel department and the legal department. The development of the hospital bureaucracy thus responded as much to an increased need for personnel to cope with the increase in hospitalisations, particularly in the 1940s, as to the need to ensure the functioning of an institution whose administrative tasks were becoming increasingly complex.

This growth allowed the Hospital to become much more independent of the Department of the Interior. Indeed, the Public Relief Service—called the Hospices Service from 1938 onwards—remained small in size.[57] Until 1945, it consisted of only five civil servants, a number that had not changed since the 1860s. Their number increased somewhat during the period 1945–1960, with eight officials in 1950 and 11 in 1960. However, their primary task was to organise a new hospitalisation policy (see Chapter 5); they had very little involvement in the internal affairs of the Cantonal Hospital.

Relations between the Department of the Interior and the Hospital were excellent and were maintained by the choice of directors, all of whom came from a service or commission of the Department of the Interior.[58] Apart from the case of Louis Mermoud mentioned above, it should be noted that Jules Nicoud began his career as a secretary in the Department of the Interior, before becoming head of office in the Health Service (1919) and deputy director of the Hospital (1928). Additionally, Rodolphe Rubattel, a law graduate and director of the newspaper companies *Feuille d'avis de Lausanne* (1925) and then *La Revue* (1932), had been a member of the HHS since 1932, being chosen seven years later to manage the Hospital. Finally, Emile Cottier began his administrative career at the age of 18 as an employee at the Orbe Land Registry (1908), then as a secretary in the Federal Military Department (1909), before joining the Vaud cantonal administration in the Commercial Police Office (1919). He became secretary (1933) and later head (1937) of the Public Relief Service (Table 4).

57 ODCV, 1860–1960.

58 ACV, ATS files.

New Competition from Private Clinics

In the 1880s–1920s, private clinics were mainly owned by professors of medicine. In the city of Lausanne, this was notably the case for Bourget, Dufour, Roux and Nicod who all owned at least one clinic in which they admitted their private clientele and from which they derived most of their income.[59] Hospitals were still poorly organised for receiving the private clientele of the professors—the Cantonal Hospital had only 15 beds for them in 1901—and the private clinic was complementary to the Cantonal public establishment.

During the inter-war period, the Cantonal Hospital opened up to private clients and the private clinics were redeployed, putting an end to their complementarity. The private clinics changed their nature during the 1920s and 1930s: they became the place of work for doctors who did not have access to the modernised hospitals and needed the new medical-technical infrastructure. In Lausanne, there was no emergence of large collective private clinics set up by the medical profession as a whole; however, several clinics were modernised or created during this period, characterised by their openness to a large number of doctors. They became real competitors for the Cantonal Hospital in the race to hospitalize wealthy and therefore profitable patients. The examples of the clinics of La Source and Cecil illustrate this evolution perfectly.

Reorganisation of La Source

The Clinique Beaulieu is a private establishment that Charles Krafft, a disciple of Roux, founded when he became head of the nursing school at La Source in 1891. The purpose of this private clinic was to offer practical training to nursing students. However, the juxtaposition of these two establishments was not without confusion. In 1896, Krafft explained to the administrators of the school that this clinic was his and that the pensions paid by his patients should not be given to La Source, saying the clinic "is a private property, it is installed in a house for which I pay a rent, it was created at my expense, at my peril and risk, it is furnished and maintained completely at my expense, it is directed by a person who is in my pay, it is occupied by the patients of my particular clientele; there is therefore no reason whatsoever for La Source to take any benefit from the Clinique de Beaulieu".[60]

After the death of Krafft (1921), the La Source school was completely restructured. In 1922, it bought the Clinique Beaulieu from Krafft's heirs. On an organisational level, the functions of the administrative director and head doctor were separated. As for the medical service, it was divided between a person in charge of surgery and gynaecology, Henry-César Krafft, son of the

[59] Dominique Dirlewanger and Catherine Fussinger, "Les nécrologies des médecins romands: une autopsie du corps medical", *Revue historique vaudoise*, 1995, p. 229.

[60] ALS, D3-200 1/2, Delegation Minutes, 28 April 1896.

deceased, and another for internal medicine, Henri Tecoz. However, the real change in the clinic lies in its opening to the medical profession: 33 doctors treated their patients in 1923, 42 in 1925 and 57 in 1926. The number of hospital days started at 1390 in 1896, rose to 4551 in 1922 and 7965 in 1925. This opening of the clinic to the medical profession was intended to create new resources to finance the school. In 1924, the director already stated that it was the clinic that allowed the organisation to be financially balanced: "The clinic alone has protected us from large deficits".[61] In fact, the clinic's income represented 23.7% of total operating resources in 1930, 40.1% in 1940 and 77.6% in 1950.[62] The competition with the Cantonal Hospital became more intense in the 1940s and 1950s. Several former assistants of Prof. Decker developed surgical specialties—in particular open-heart surgery—for which they did not obtain the resources required at the hospital. One of them, Jean-David Buffat, even became chairman of the board of directors of La Source in 1955.

Opening of the Cecil Clinic

The Cecil Clinic is, without doubt, the private establishment that competed most with the Cantonal Hospital. It was opened in 1931 in the former Hotel Cecil, which had gone bankrupt two years earlier. The redevelopment of a former luxury hotel into a clinic illustrates the decisive importance of medical tourism in Lausanne. The administrative director of the establishment between 1935 and 1968, H. Platel, was also the former director of the Leysin Grand Hôtel and in 1938 he was also president of the Society of Hoteliers of Lausanne-Ouchy.[63]

The interest and originality of the Cecil Clinic lie in its openness to the medical profession. It allowed many doctors who did not have access to the medical and technical infrastructure of the Cantonal Hospital to hospitalize their private clientele in a modern setting, first and foremost the owner of the clinic, Charles Thélin. After his medical studies in Lausanne, Thélin specialised in gynaecology during his internships and gave courses in this field as a privatdozent but he did not have access to the Cantonal Hospital for the hospitalisation of his patients. Thélin was very involved in the defence of the professional interests of the medical profession and was president of the Lausanne Doctors' Association. After having practised during the 1920s in the small Mont-Riant Clinic, he wished to modernise his working environment and, in 1930, bought the Hotel Cecil which he transformed into a clinic by a specialist in hospital matters, the Lausanne architect Georges Epitaux (see Chapter 4).[64] Shortly after the opening of the establishment, he sent a circular to his fellow doctors in which he specified:

[61] ALS, Report of the Director for the year 1924, *The Source*, 1925/4.

[62] ALS, *The Source* newspaper, 1930, p. 23; 1940, p. 18; 1950, p. 17.

[63] ALS, E1-7, letter from Director Vuilleumier to Platel, Director of Cecil, 31 August 1938.

[64] *FOSC*, 1930.

> Our X-ray room is always at your disposal for all bone, lung and gastrointestinal radiology. We are also conveniently located for various investigations introduced in recent years: pyelographies, hystero-salpingographies, gall bladder investigations, demonstration of cerebral ventricles, determination of the permeability of the spinal canal. The Clinic has the necessary instrumentation for these examinations. [...] We would also like to remind you of our physiotherapy facilities: radiotherapy, diathermy, quartz lamp, galvanisation and faradisation. Our equipment is of good quality and safe to use. [...] Finally, it may be useful for you to know that we have a cystoscope and a rectoscope of very good brands. These instruments, of relatively rare use in private practice, seemed to us to have a natural place in the instrumentation of a general clinic.[65]

The modernity of the Cecil Clinic and its openness to the medical profession quickly made it an establishment that was in direct competition with the Cantonal Hospital. The latter had to adapt its tariffs for private patients and renovate its radiological installation in order to remain competitive in the private care market. However, as paradoxical as it may seem, the head doctors of the Cantonal Hospital also occasionally practised at Cecil, like Prof. Rosselet, head of the radiology department of the Cantonal Hospital, who also looked after Cecil's X-ray installation in the 1930s and 1940s.[66]

Hospital Financing: The Affirmation of a New Management System

The Cantonal Hospital was in a highly competitive market during the inter-war period. The strategy pursued by its management since the 1880s, namely the financial autonomy of the hospital, was fully in line with this perspective. The Hospital could amortise its investments and release new operating resources by engaging in the care of profitable patients.

The development of expenditure is similar to that of hospital admissions and remained relatively stable until the end of the 1930s. The operation of the hospital required almost two million francs per year. The sharp rise in expenditure from the 1940s onwards reflects both high inflation and the extensive development of the establishment, until an annual expenditure of around 3.9 million francs was reached in 1945 and 8.9 million francs in 1950. This growth was not to the detriment of the Hospital's autonomy, since the coverage of expenses by its own resources increased from 30.4% in 1920 to 49.8% in 1930. For the period 1930–1945, the average proportion of self-financing was 50.2%.

This management success was the direct result of the transformation of the hospital care market, whose clientele became solvent. Indeed, among the main new resources created during the inter-war period were pensions paid by patients, as well as revenues from the radiology department.

[65] Cecil Clinic Archives, undated circular [1931–1935].

[66] ACV, K VIII D 84, letter to Rosselet, 5 August 1948.

Boarders in Common Rooms Replace Wealthy Clientele

Until the 1914–1918 war, the Cantonal Hospital benefited from the international reputation of Lausanne's medicine. A large number of private patients sought treatment from professors such as Roux and Bourget, not only in their private clinics but also in the private departments of the Cantonal Hospital. The pensions they paid to the hospital increased steadily from nearly 20,000 francs per year in the mid-1890s to 57,980 francs in 1913. This resource represented an average of 27.1% of the total operating income for the years 1895–1914[67]; the private borders were, therefore, essential to the running of the establishment.

The situation was different in the inter-war period. On the one hand, the international clientele became more discreet, "largely because certain doctors and surgeons wanted to surf the prices, on a par with those of the great practitioners of Paris or elsewhere",[68] according to the health authorities, but also because the Swiss tourist industry was less dynamic during the inter-war period than before 1914. On the other hand, the Cantonal Hospital saw itself competing more and more seriously with the regional hospitals and private clinics of Lausanne. As a result of this competition, income from private clients fell sharply from 26.3% of total operating income in 1910 to 14.6% in 1930 and 8.1% in 1950.

The situation of the Cantonal Hospital in the face of competition from private clinics was ambiguous. First of all, there was a need to invest permanently in medical and technical equipment in order to remain a modern establishment in the eyes of the public. For example, considerations of this type explain, to a large extent, the modernisation of the radiology laboratory. However, these investments had a cost and the Hospital, which could not constantly increase its pension prices at the risk of seeing its private clientele flee, had to increase its capacity to receive this clientele. However, in the 1940s, the Hospital's management came up against the powerful medical lobby which also demanded an end to free consultations in the policlinic. In a 1943 letter addressed to the Department of Finance which proposed an increase in the number of rooms for private residents, the director of the Hospital expressed his scepticism, as "the doctors of Lausanne are strongly opposed to any increase in the volume of the Hospital's private services; they believe that the State should not compete with private clinics [...]".[69]

Under these conditions, the hospital management decided to put more pressure on the patients hospitalised in common rooms (middle and working classes). The number of free days for indigent patients fell from 50.6% of total days in 1914 to 34.6% in 1922; this trend would probably have been confirmed thereafter, but the data were no longer published after that date. In fact, the pensions paid by these patients show a strong upward trend, rising

[67] RSC, Department of the Interior, 1895–1914.

[68] ACV, S 73, HHS minutes, 3 December 1930.

[69] ACV, K VIII D 37, letter from Rubattel to the Department of Finance, 9 April 1943.

from 400,512 francs in 1920 to 684,270 francs in 1935 and 1.9 million francs in 1950. These pensions represent an extremely stable share of hospital resources: 71.9% on average for the period 1920–1947. In conclusion, it was the pensions of the so-called "ordinary" patients that allowed the rate of self-financing to increase, not the wealthy clientele. On the other hand, it was not only the patients themselves who paid the cost of the pension; in the 1920s and 1930s, health insurance was introduced.

The lack of general statistical data on health insurance companies makes it impossible to obtain an overall view of the phenomenon; however, the Vaud Society for Mutual Assistance (*Société vaudoise des secours mutuels*, SVSM), which had a large number of branches throughout the canton and many members, is a good example of the interaction between insurance companies and hospitals. Originally, the purpose of the mutual aid societies was not to cover the costs of hospitalisation—which were not charged in the event of indigence—but to make up for the loss of earnings resulting from an employee's inability to work (illness or accident). However, during the inter-war period, several insurance companies and mutual benefit funds signed agreements with hospitals to guarantee agreed rates for their members. The SVSM signed such an agreement with the Cantonal Hospital in 1930.[70]

By facilitating access to the hospital in the event of illness, the SVSM attracted a very large number of new members, from 5223 in 1916 to 9562 in 1935 and 25,697 in 1950.[71] This increase was necessary to replenish the society's funds which were being undermined by rapidly rising expenses. Medical and pharmaceutical expenses amounted to less than 10,000 francs per year until 1924, then rose to 212,301 francs in 1935 and 1.3 million francs in 1950.[72]

The leaders of the SVSM foresaw the financial impact of the 1930 convention. They wrote in their 1931 report, "there is no doubt that medicine has made and is still making real progress, but this progress is being made only at the cost of great sacrifices which are reflected in our ever-increasing expenses. X-rays, fluoroscopy, radiation, diathermy, complicated analyses, all these factors unknown 25 years ago are bleeding our funds [...]".[73] SVSM's reserve funds thus decreased by more than half between 1930 and 1943. The financial salvation of the society was found in the increase in the volume of membership fees (299,674 francs in 1930; 492,783 francs in 1940; and 1.9 million francs in 1950), due both to the increase in the number of members and to the increase in the average fee (32.8 francs per person in 1930–1944; 41.6 francs in 1945; and 55.4 francs in 1950).

[70] *Bulletin de la Société vaudoise des secours mutuels*, n°15, May 1931, p. 11.

[71] *Bulletin de la Société vaudoise des secours mutuels*, n°38, May 1954, p. 19.

[72] Ibid.

[73] *Bulletin de la Société vaudoise des secours mutuels*, n°16, December 1932, p. 6.

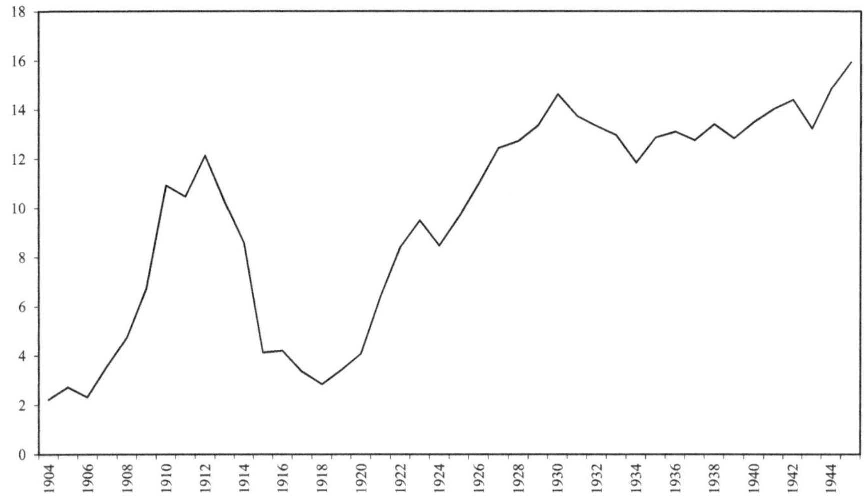

Fig. 4 Radiological service revenue as a percentage of operating revenue, 1904–1945 (*Source* RSC, Department of the Interior, 1904–1945)

Insurance companies thus became essential financial partners in the development of hospitals. Their privileged position made them key players in cantonal hospital policy after 1945 (see Chapter 5).

Radiology: A Profitable Innovation

The X-ray facility is a diagnostic and therapeutic tool that symbolises the modernity of medicine. As Howell has shown for the United States, the possession of a high-tech radiological infrastructure enables hospitals to occupy a dominant position in the healthcare market: radiology is not only used to see inside bodies in order to treat them better, but also to attract private clients seduced by the scientific aspects of this new medicine.[74] The debates on the modernisation of this service at the Cantonal Hospital in Lausanne show that the situation there was similar.

Before the 1920s, there was hardly any serious competitor to the Radiology Laboratory of the Cantonal Hospital and it quickly benefited from the international clientele hospitalised in Lausanne's clinics and palaces who came to take X-ray photographs. The hospital's management quickly realised the financial implications of this new technology, which already represented 10% of operating revenue in 1910 (see Fig. 4). The 1914–1918 war and the absence of international clients was a hard blow. In 1917, the Health Service explained the drop in radiological revenue by the fact that "since the war, the number of foreign patients coming to be examined with X-rays has greatly diminished".[75]

[74] Joel Howell, *Technology in the Hospital...*, op. cit.

[75] RSC, Department of the Interior, 1917, p. 102.

The creation of the Central Radiological Laboratory in 1916, which centralised the Hospital's various radiological facilities under a single management, was a response to both practical and financial considerations. The hospital authorities stated, "there is no doubt that by organising the service in a rational manner, we will be able to contribute a certain amount each year to the administration of the Hospital".[76] These are the same considerations that led the HHS to accept in 1920 the modernisation proposed by Isenegger, head of the Laboratory. The HHS explained, "it was important that the service be profitable, despite the ever-increasing number of private laboratories in the city".[77] The aim was to capture the private client market of the city's doctors. The appointment of a widely recognised medical specialist to head the radiology department was as much a scientific as a marketing decision. In 1922, the HHS hired Alfred Rosselet, assistant to Rollier in the tuberculosis clinics of Leysin and a privatdozent at the University of Geneva, who was offered an annual salary of 10,000 francs as well as a share in the profits of the Radiology Department.[78] Rosselet's arrival at the Cantonal Hospital enabled the latter to adopt a dominant position in the field of hospital radiology. He was indeed part of the new generation of radiologists who took over the radiology laboratories of the major Swiss hospitals during the inter-war period and established themselves as the undisputed specialists in the field.[79]

In the 1930s, competition in the Lausanne market became more intense, especially with the Cecil Clinic, which inaugurated a new X-ray installation in 1931. The HHS decided to purchase two new X-ray machines, although they were expensive, stating, "the X-ray installation of the Cantonal Hospital must be the first in the canton"[80] so the private doctors in Lausanne and its region would continue to send their patients there. As for the radio-diagnostic division of the Cantonal Hospital, it was completely modernised and reorganised in 1934 and again in 1938 when the development of anti-cancer treatments required more powerful and precise equipment.

The Radiology Department became profitable in the 1920s. The profits from this service were partly used to finance special funds. In addition to a contribution of 6–8000 francs, depending on the year, granted to Rosselet, part of the income from radiology was paid into a "special risk fund" from 1924 onwards which enabled compensation to potential accident victims (e.g., burns, hair loss, etc.); however, most of this money was used to keep the hospital running. The constant technical modernisation was a real commercial success. In the mid-1920s, the peak of the 1910–1913 period was reached again. In the 1930s, the share of income from radiology stabilised at an average

[76] ACV, K VIII B 113, Organisation of a radiological and radiotherapy service at the Cantonal Hospital, undated [1916].

[77] ACV, S 73, HHS minutes, 20 October 1920.

[78] ACV, S 73, minutes of the HHS, 1921.

[79] Monika Dommann, op. cit.

[80] ACV, S 73, HHS minutes, 16 July 1931.

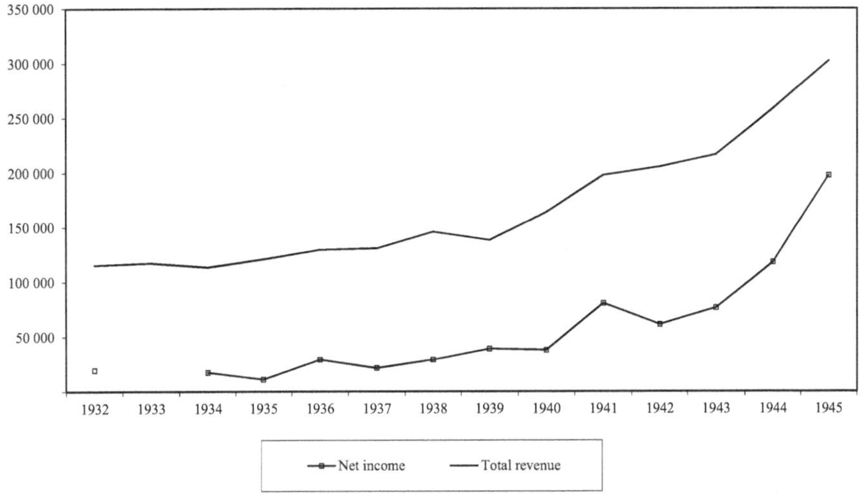

Fig. 5 Total income and net profits of the radiological service, in current francs, 1932–1945 (*Source* RSC, Department of the Interior, 1932–1945 and ACV, K VIII D, various years)

of 13.1% of the hospital's income. The net profit of the department also increased sharply, amounting to 16.8% of the revenues in 1932, 23.2% in 1940 and 65.4% in 1945 (see Figs. 4 and 5). This trend was confirmed in the immediate post-war period with a sharp increase in the number of X-rays: 18,895 in 1945 and 30,399 in 1950. In 1951, the Grand Council granted a credit of 1.2 million francs without opposition for the expansion and transformation of the Radiology Department, with the aim of maintaining an attractive offer and responding to a growing demand. The parliamentary committee in charge of this investment stated, "this is a hospital service which, far from costing the state money, is in fact an interesting source of income".[81] The gross income of this service passed the 400,000 francs mark in 1948 and the 600,000 francs mark in 1953.[82]

Private Sector Intervention in Hospital Infrastructure Development

Private resources not only played a role in financing the operation of the hospital, through patient pensions and radiology fees but also intervened directly in the development of the hospital infrastructure. From 1918 to 1949, all the important buildings put into service within the Lausanne hospital complex were the result of a partnership between the private and public sectors. This collaboration was the result of the strengthening, in the 1920s,

[81] BGC, 21 May 1951.

[82] Ibidem.

of the alliance between liberals—urban elites defending economic liberalism and private interests—and radicals—a pragmatic statist right-wing—which led to a turn in government policy illustrated by a fight against the development of the social state and public spending. In the 1930s, the climate of corporatism only increased the tendency to bring the public and private sectors closer together.[83]

Development of Hospital Services

During the 1930s, several hospital wards saw the creation of new buildings following the intervention of private funds. During the decade 1932–1942, no less than four departments inaugurated new edifices as a result of such interventions. The first of these was a bequest of 500,000 francs from the industrialist Edouard Sandoz-David, founder of the chemical company Sandoz SA (merged into Novartis in 1996), to the State of Vaud for the creation of a hospice for the chronically ill. This establishment was opened in 1932. The opening of this building enabled the Cantonal Hospital to be relieved of some of the chronically ill patients who were crowding it but did not in itself solve the problem of hospitalisation for this type of patient. For Sandoz SA, this participation strengthened the links with the Cantonal Hospital and the Faculty of Medicine. It also helped to secure the loyalty of an important pharmaceutical customer and facilitated the entry of private research into the university clinics.

The second service opened in this context was also the result of industrial support. The new medical clinic was opened in 1935 thanks to a donation of one million francs from the Nestlé and Anglo-Swiss Holding Company, on the occasion of the merger with the chocolate manufacturer Peter, Cailler and Kohler (1929). The new building, designed by the architect Georges Epitaux, reflects the presence of a doctor trained in the German school at the head of the clinic, Prof. Louis Michaud. The Nestlé Hospital, built in an L shape, was organised in two distinct and complementary wings: to the south, a hospital unit, including the patients' rooms, and to the north-west, a scientific unit, grouping the laboratories and the teaching rooms. Michaud also had a medical clinic with laboratories which became a centre of medical research, thanks in particular to its links with the Swiss Academy of Medical Sciences of which he was the main promoter at the University of Lausanne. The Nestlé company, beyond the highly symbolic benefit of such a donation, derived an obvious economic profit. The inter-war period appeared to be a phase of diversification of its production towards vitamin and dietary products developed in its own laboratories in collaboration with outside doctors.[84] Similarly, some Nestlé directors benefited symbolically from this collaboration.

[83] Olivier Meuwly, *La politique vaudoise au 20e siècle*, Lausanne: PPUR, 2003, pp. 23–59.

[84] Jean Heer, *Nestlé, Cent vingt-cinq ans de 1866 à 1991*, Vevey: Nestlé SA, 1991, pp. 171–172.

In 1933, the Chairman of the Board of Directors, Louis Dapples, was awarded an honorary doctorate by the Faculty of Medicine in Lausanne. Together with two other Nestlé directors, Jean-Constant Corthésy and Enrico Bignami, who were awarded the same title in 1960, he was the only non-scientist to receive such a distinction until 1975.[85]

Finally, two buildings owe their existence to donations from medical professors. The Rossier Hospital, an annex of the maternity ward including the gynaecological clinic which opened in 1937, owed its origin to a bequest of 30,000 francs from Prof. Guillaume Rossier.[86] Head doctor of the maternity ward and professor of obstetrics (1903–1928), he could not develop his establishment by taking in gynaecological cases, which were the prerogative of César Roux's surgery department. His donation increased in the years 1930–1934 by a sum of 250,000 paid by his brother Alfred Rossier. Similarly, the new Institute of Pathological Anatomy, opened in 1942, owed its creation to a legacy of 900,000 francs from a former professor of forensic medicine, Georges Spengler.[87] Until then, the institute had been housed in a small pavilion behind the Cantonal Hospital, opened in 1890. This building soon proved to be too small to handle the various demands of the Cantonal Hospital, especially since it was already home to private cancer research in the early 1920s. Prof. Jean de Meyenburg (1919–1925), followed by his successor Jean-Louis Nicod (1925–1965), made several requests to the HHS for the modernisation of their institute. Spengler, who was a member of the HHS was sensitive to this request and bequeathed his fortune to the State in order to build a new Institute of Pathology.

Strengthening Links with Private Specialist Hospitals

The political context of public–private partnership was also very favourable to the development of links between the Cantonal Hospital and the Faculty of Medicine on the one hand and the private specialist hospitals on the other. First of all, the repatriation of the ophthalmology clinic to the Cantonal Hospital did not survive Prof. Eperon. Following his death (in 1920), the president of the Blind People's Asylum, Gaston Boiceau, approached the State Councillor Thélin to consider resuming relations. The government, preferring to play the card of complementarity between Lausanne hospitals rather than that of competition, accepted this offer. In the same year, the State and the Blind People's Asylum signed an agreement whereby the Asylum undertook to make an ophthalmological clinic available to the Faculty for an annual sum of 8000 francs.[88] The professor and head of the department were appointed by mutual agreement between the two partners. Jules Gonin, former head of Marc Dufour's clinic, assistant physician (1901–1918) and head physician

[85] Guy Saudan, *La médecine à Lausanne...*, op. cit., p. 256.

[86] ACV, K VIII D 62 and S 73.

[87] ACV, K VIII D 64 and S 73.

[88] ACV, S 73, HHS minutes, 1920.

at the Asylum from 1918, was appointed to the chair of ophthalmology in 1920.[89]

Similarly, the Orthopaedic Hospice became closer to the Cantonal Hospital in the 1920s as it reoriented itself towards surgical activity. The State gave its financial support to this institution by making available a plot of land near the maternity hospital, in order to build a new building, which was opened in 1927. In exchange for this support, the state was given the right to appoint the head doctor of the institution, who was also in charge of the chair of orthopaedics.

Special Funds for Clinics: A Step Towards the Privatisation of Hospital Services?

The organisation of the Cantonal Hospital as it was conceived in 1883 did not provide an independent budget for each medical service. Depending on their needs, the chief physicians had to turn to the hospital management or to the Department of Public Education (university teaching) and the Interior (hospital service) to acquire the necessary equipment. Such a system was administratively complicated and, in the 1900s, special funds were set up. They were dependent only on the heads of the department. These funds were donated by private individuals—companies, patrons or professors' clients—to maintain the infrastructure of the university clinics.

The special funds of the Cantonal Hospital experienced a strong development in the inter-war period. The hospital authorities, who at that time largely favoured the intervention of the private sector in the development of the hospital, could not but be pleased with this. The first special funds attached to clinics were those of the paediatric professor Adolphe Combe (1907) and the surgical professor César Roux (1910). From 1910 onwards, each department head had his own fund and used it for various investments outside the budget. The total value of these funds increased from 183,591 francs in 1920 to 362,484 francs in 1940.[90]

The chief physicians were entirely responsible for these funds, the management of which they were not accountable for. The HHS thus learnt in 1921 that Prof. Dind had developed a blood analysis service and subcontracted it to private doctors, with the profit from this operation being used to develop the laboratory. An assistant managed this fund without reporting to anyone. In fact, the Reports of the Council of State often only present an annual balance sheet of these various funds; therefore, we know their value on 31 December of each year but very little about how they were used. The hospital authorities themselves were in the dark. The director of the Hospital wrote in 1937 about gifts received from the pharmaceutical industry: "the donations referred to, and made in favour of our hospital services, reach a significant

[89] Olivier Robert and Franceso Panese, *Dictionary...*, op. cit., pp. 528–529.

[90] RSC, 1920–1940.

figure, and we do not know all of them".[91] This ignorance could sometimes be dangerous because it allowed the development of practices that bordered on legality. Thus, in the years 1923–1924, the HHS suspected certain pharmaceutical companies of providing special funds in exchange for drug tests carried out by favoured chief physicians.[92] While there was no question of abandoning the clinical testing of drugs carried out within a specific scientific framework, i.e., under the responsibility of the chief physician, the HHS refused to accept any donation from the pharmaceutical industry in compensation.[93]

Cancer Research: A Private Initiative

The Institute of Pathology took a further step in its relationship with the private sector. In the 1920s, it saw the development of research financed by an industrial company. In 1920, Marcel Aubert, a friend and business associate of Prof. Dind, director of the Cossonay cable factory, proposed to pay the Cantonal Hospital a sum of 120,000 francs over ten years to finance cancer research. Despite the reluctance of some members of the HHS, such as Alfred Carrard who "saw this as a gesture by a private individual who provides the necessary money, but at the same time intends to designate the doctor for the work; this would be a precedent which other people could also use in the future to request a laboratory",[94] an agreement was signed. Indeed, a protégé of Aubert and a former intern of César Roux, Alfred Renaud, was hired as a special assistant.

Cancer research was institutionalised in 1924 with the creation of a research centre (*Centre anti-cancéreux romand*, CACR), all the French-speaking cantons participating except Geneva which founded its own organisation the same year. The difficulties encountered by Renaud at the Pathological Institute largely explain the creation of a private institution recognized as being of public utility and therefore subsidised. When it was founded, the CACR received private donations amounting to more than 112,000 francs from both industrial companies and medical circles.[95] Thereafter, the CACR could count on the constant financial support of the Cossonay cable factory, whose directors Rodolphe Stadler and Jean-Louis de Coulon held the positions of president and vice-president of the foundation board from 1951 onwards.

The CACR combined experimental research and clinical application. Located in the pavilion that housed the maternity ward until 1916, the research laboratories were placed under the scientific direction of André de Coulon in 1924. Holding a Ph.D. in science from the University of Geneva, he worked previously as a bacteriologist in prestigious institutions such as

[91] ACV, K VIII B 63/2, letter from Nicoud to the Health Service, 19 June 1937.

[92] RSC, Department of the Interior, 1920.

[93] ACV, S 73, minutes of the HHS, 1924.

[94] ACV, S 73, HHS minutes, 7 September 1920.

[95] *Centre anti-cancéreux romand des cantons de Fribourg, Neuchâtel, Valais et Vaud*, Lausanne: Imprimeries réunies SA, 1929, p. 14.

the Panthéon Hospital in Paris and Pasteur Institutes in Paris and Strasbourg (1917–1924). He was head of the experimental research department of the CACR for more than 10 years (1924–1935). With his appointment, the anchoring of medical research in experimental science was confirmed. When he died in 1935, he was replaced by a physicist, Pierre Mercier, who had worked at the Marie Curie laboratory in Paris. In addition to these experimental research activities, the CACR developed clinical applications in the various departments of the Cantonal Hospital and also in certain regional hospitals in French-speaking Switzerland.[96]

Conclusion

The privatisation of many of the functions of the Cantonal Hospital (e.g., equipment, research, operating income, etc.) had a strongly positive impact on the canton's finances. The share of the hospital's deficit in the total expenditure of the Hospices Service fell sharply from 58.6% in 1920 to 54.0% in 1930 and 51.4% in 1940.[97] However, this privatisation had negative effects in terms of organisation. During the 1930s, the Cantonal Hospital became a veritable city whose development and growth were not thought through in their entirety. The lack of planning and coordination led to a policy of rationalisation of the hospital, which aimed at economies of scale as well as better organisation of the establishment.

Rationalisations

The rationalisation of large production units was a phenomenon that affected the entire economic world of the inter-war period (including industrial companies, banks, public administration, etc.) and hospitals were no exception. The first aim was to reorganise organisations that had become larger and more complex, often split into several divisions, in order to improve the fluidity of production. The second major goal of rationalisation was to achieve economies of scale through centralisation and standardisation. When applied to the hospital world, rationalisation simply reiterated the major principles of centralisation and hierarchisation, directly derived from the underlying ideology of corporatism and the cult of leadership.[98] An association was even set up in 1930 to ensure the dissemination of rationalisation among hospital managers: the Veska Association.

[96] *Cancer Centre*..., op. cit., p. 7.

[97] RSC, Department of the Interior, 1920–1940.

[98] Matthieu Leimgruber, *Taylorism*..., op. cit.

Veska: "Simplifying, Saving and Improving Everything That Can Be Done in the Operation of a Hospital"[99]

Founded in 1930, the Association of Swiss Hospitals (*Verbandes Schweizerische Krankenanstalten*, Veska) played a decisive role in the rationalisation of healthcare institutions. On the one hand, it proposed the standardisation of accounting and the way in which the price per day of hospitalisation could be calculated, as well as the rational reorganisation of hospitals. This association was a member of the International Management Institute in the early 1930s.[100] The engineer Alfred Carrard wrote in 1944 in the *Revue Veska* that "industry was the first to realise the advantages it could gain from a methodical application of the science of work. These same advantages could and should be used in state enterprises [i.e. cantonal hospitals]".[101] On the other hand, Veska acted as a hospital trade union and as a single point of contact in major hospital issues that affected all institutions in the country, in order to unify and negotiate collective agreements with various partners (negotiations with health insurance companies and doctors, training of nursing staff, etc.).

In particular, Veska sought to rationalise hospitals by standardising equipment (room furniture, linen, cotton wool, dressings, etc.). This rationalisation, coupled with a new organisation of hospital space, led to the creation of a model hospital which Veska presented to the public at the 1939 National Exhibition. It was organised around an operating room equipped with high-tech equipment.[102] The operating room was placed at the heart of the hospital organisation. Veska was a strong promoter of the transformation of hospital medicine through its intervention in favour of an organised and rationalised environment aimed at optimising flows.

Cost control was another important concern in the 1930s. As early as 1937, Veska organised the bulk purchase of supplies for its members in order to achieve economies of scale. In 1938, Hans Frei, a physician from Berne, wrote an article in the *Veska magazine* entitled, "How to increase income and reduce expenditure in the hospital without affecting its activities?"[103] He reviewed the various means used to increase resources (e.g., the creation of reserve funds, public aid, radiological services, etc.) and limit expenses (e.g., rationalisation of equipment, centralisation of technical services, single management, etc.), all of which have been implemented in the hospitals of Vaud.

Finally, this association was very active in the training of hospital administrative staff. It organised advanced courses or trips to international congresses and provided information in its magazine on the hospital systems of other countries. For example, in 1949, the assistant director of the Cantonal Hospital,

[99] *Veska magazine*, 1937, p. 1.

[100] Matthieu Leimgruber, op. cit., p. 154.

[101] *Veska magazine*, 1944, p. 253.

[102] Jules Wagner (ed.), *The Golden Book of the 1939 National Exhibition*, Zurich: Verkehrsverlag, 1940, pp. 231–233.

[103] *Veska magazine*, 1938, pp. 209–213.

Alfred Chevalier, took part in a week-long course that familiarised him with the problems of nutrition, personnel, hospital economics, law, etc.[104] Courses were intended for administrators as well as for junior employees, such as the laundresses for whom courses were set up in Lausanne in 1937 and 1938.

At the Cantonal Hospital in Lausanne, the rationalisation that took place at the end of the 1930s was fully in line with Veska's concerns. The aim was to make budgetary savings but also to coordinate the operation of the hospital, whose buildings had multiplied. When the Nestlé Hospital was designed in 1930, the HHS stated, for example, that this new construction would require "a second X-ray department, new kitchens, etc.",[105] which suggested that costs would increase and there would be organisational problems between the various hospital buildings. Indeed, managing the flow of food, linen, patients, etc. between the various components of the hospital complex was a major issue. In 1940, the hospital management set up a weekly meeting with the bursar, the sister director, the head of the Nestlé Hospital, the linen room manager, the heads of the workshops, the head of the kitchens and the head gardener with the declared aim of "intensifying collaboration between the various departments".[106] Similarly, in February 1940 a member of the management visited the Montreux-Palace, the Buffet de la Gare in Lausanne and the cantonal hospitals in Geneva and Basel, with a view to improving the operation of the bursar on the basis of what was being done elsewhere (centralisation of the control of deliveries and distribution in the departments). Similarly, the standardisation and development of the technical environment (unification of the three telephone lines in 1924, increase in the number of gas meters in 1937, etc.) were aimed at better cost control.

The rationalisation projects implemented by the hospital's management affected various departments within the establishment, whether medical, administrative or hotel. However, the success of these reforms varied greatly as they encountered difficulties that reveal the financial and power issues at stake within the hospital departments.

Rationalisation of the Pharmacy Service

The cost of drugs became a real problem in the 1920s, with the mass-market introduction of specialties; i.e., synthetic products manufactured by the pharmaceutical industry. During the years 1890–1914, the increase in the expenditure of the Pharmacy Service was limited, rising from 37,076 francs to 83,509 francs with an average annual growth of 3.3%; this largely reflects the general development of the establishment.[107] The increase in expenditure accelerated during the inter-war period, mainly during the years 1925–1940 which showed an average annual growth of 4.1%. In absolute figures, the

[104] ACV, K VIII D 89.

[105] ACV, S 73, HHS minutes, 28 May 1930.

[106] ACV, K VIII D 24, circular of 15 January 1940.

[107] RSC, Department of the Interior, 1890–1914.

expenditure of the Pharmacy Service amounted to 121,699 francs in 1925 and 231,989 francs in 1940.[108]

The profiles of the two pharmacists who headed the department in 1923–1935 were not, however, conducive to questioning the sales policy of the pharmaceutical industry, to which they were both close. Samuel Mercanton (1923–1925) had worked for fifteen years as a chemist-pharmacist in a chocolate factory before joining the pharmacy department of the Cantonal Hospital as an assistant (1917) and then head of the department (1923). Henri Golaz (1926–1935) came from a largely corporatist private pharmacist background. He practised independently for thirty years in Vevey (1896–1926) and was president of the Association of Vevey Pharmacists. In 1925, he was appointed lecturer in galenic pharmacy at the University and the following year he became professor and head of the hospital pharmacy. He was known in the scientific world for the development of a synthesis allowing the preservation of the active principles of plants. The Golaz dials were produced by the company Golaz & Cie, founded in 1896. In 1905, this company merged with Zyma SA to become the most important pharmaceutical company in the canton of Vaud (integrated into Ciba-Geigy in the early 1980s).[109]

Under these conditions, it is easy to understand the reluctance of the chief pharmacists to question the dependence of the Cantonal Hospital on the pharmaceutical industry, to which they were closely linked. The people who were blamed for the rising cost of drugs were first and foremost the doctors who prescribed them. Between 1929 and 1934, Golaz repeatedly accused doctors of prescribing too many expensive pharmaceutical specialities but did not intervene in favour of a reorganisation of his own department.

In the end, the arrival of Roger Freudweiler changed the situation (1935). He was the first pharmacist to obtain a doctorate in this field at the University of Lausanne (1932) and came from a research background with no direct personal links to industry. In collaboration with the hospital's management and the Health Service, in 1937 he embarked on the rationalisation of his department, including the desire to limit the number of specialities used and to produce certain medicines himself in order to reduce the increasing costs arising from their use. He explained in a report: "To illustrate, from a budgetary point of view, the necessity of using our 'loco' [i.e. homemade] products, we will give only one example, that of Algine suppositories in strong doses replacing Cibalgine suppositories in strong doses. Our monthly production is of 600 pieces on average, which we sell at Fr. 3.32 per cent, i.e. Fr. 19.92 per 600. The purchase price of the speciality is Fr. 22.40 per cent (wholesale price!). Our production thus enables us to make monthly savings

108 RSC, Department of the Interior, 1925–1940.

109 Pierre Germond, *Chronique des Pharmacies de la région veveysanne de 1326 à 1989*, Vevey: P. Germond, 1989, pp. 47–48.

of Fr. 114.50, i.e. Fr. 1,374 per year for this activity alone".[110] Rationalisation efforts also included cooperation with the medical profession. Freudweiler drew up a complete list of the products used in the whole of the Cantonal Hospital in 1937 and submitted this 27-page document containing more than 400 names of medicines to the various heads of department for examination, "asking you to kindly note the important specialities which are in common use in your department, and instead of which it would be advisable to create original magistral formulae which could replace the specialities in question, as well as all those with similar therapeutic indications. For the creation of these original formulas, we ask you to indicate the constituents that you wish to see included, possibly with their dosage, with a view to the development and presentation of these preparations in their most appropriate form. On the other hand, we are struck by the fact that certain products of the Pharmacopoeia are not used in the Hospital. This is the case, for example, for Bromisovalum (fancy name Bromuval) which could replace specialities such as Sedormid".[111]

These plans soon met with hostility from the pharmaceutical companies, in particular from the Basel-based companies in the Association of Swiss Pharmaceutical Chemical Manufacturers.[112] In a letter addressed to the chief physicians of the Cantonal Hospital, this association protested against the plans of the Pharmacy Department (1937). The Hoffmann-LaRoche company in particular was dissuasive: it threatened to abolish the special conditions granted to the Cantonal Hospital (discount on the wholesale price) in case Freudweiler continued the in-house production of competing Alyba tablets. It also threatened to break off all relations with the State of Vaud and pointed out that its donations had recently enabled the acquisition of a cardiograph. This was all it took for the hospital authorities to intervene with the pharmacist, who was aware that "the preparation of all these products in our laboratories is not to the liking of the large manufacturers, in particular Ciba and especially Hoffmann-LaRoche",[113] but who was determined to see his reform through. The director of the Hospital intervened energetically with the Health Service to whom he wrote: "As far as we are concerned, we will add that the donations to which it is alluded, and made in favour of our hospital services, reach a significant figure, and we do not know all of them. It would therefore seem advisable, in the interest of the State's finances, to renounce the above-mentioned substitution, and to stick to the original remedies, at least for those from Hoffmann-LaRoche".[114]

[110] ACV, K VIII B 63/2, report by Freudweiler to the HHS, 20 January 1938.

[111] ACV, K VIII B 63/2, letter from the Health Service to heads of department, 30 April 1938.

[112] Sandoz, Hoffmann-La Roche, Wander, Society for the Chemical Industry.

[113] ACV, K VIII B 63/2, report by Freudweiler to the HHS, 20 January 1938.

[114] ACV, K VIII B 63/2, letter from Nicoud to the Health Service, 19 June 1937.

Freudweiler was therefore unable to compete with the pharmaceutical industry in the production of medicines. He tried to intervene again in 1947 by denouncing the use of the first antibiotics, which he considered abusive. But penicillin reduced the length of hospitalisation from three weeks to 2–3 days; the medical effectiveness of this new product was coupled with a limitation in the care of patients that corresponded to the expectations of the hospital administration. Faced with the therapeutic revolution brought about by the adoption of antibiotics, Freudweiler's reforms seemed anachronistic.

When the Interests of the Hospital Meet Those of the Doctors: The End of Free Ambulatory Consultations (1944–1950)

The rationalisation of outpatient care was successful because it was not carried out against the lobbies affected by this measure—the insurance companies and private practitioners—but with them. With the development of health insurance in the 1930s, the University Polyclinic and the outpatient consultations at the Cantonal Hospital lost their charitable character and led to demands from the insurance companies and the medical profession, both of which, for their own reasons, wanted to put an end to the general free provision of outpatient care.

In 1944, the Vaud Society for Mutual Assistance (SVSM) complained that only its members were billed for outpatient care, which was subsequently reimbursed. Since outpatient care was free for uninsured patients, the SVSM considered this to be an inequality of treatment that was detrimental to the expansion of health insurance among the population. Doctors, for their part, complained about the loss of income resulting from free consultations. Prof. Maurice Jaccottet was their spokesman and declared that "reduced-price consultations seem to me to be unfair competition with independent doctors".[115] He was supported by several of his colleagues, such as Prof. Jaeger, head of the dermatology clinic, who wrote to the hospital management in 1948: "We have noticed that certain categories of patients who are not without financial means are increasingly coming to our free consultations and are thus exploiting the cantonal hospital to some extent".[116] Chief doctors complained about the preferential hospitalisation conditions for those insured by the National Insurance Fund (*Caisse nationale suisse d'assurance en cas d'accidents*, CNA). The agreement signed with this state organisation in 1918 provided for lower medical fees than those of the cantonal tariff. Denouncing unfair competition for the medical profession, they obtained its termination in 1947.

The political authorities took account of the doctors' demands in the case of the agreement with the CNA. As for the abandonment of free outpatient consultations, the Department of the Interior declared itself in favour of this

[115] ACV, K VIII B 213/15, letter from Jaccottet to HHS, 17 November 1946.

[116] ACV, K VIII D 68, 30 June 1948.

measure, essentially for reasons of financial profitability, but proposed consultations at reduced prices for social reasons.[117] The outpatient consultations of the ENT, surgery and dermatology departments were reformed, in this sense, in 1946. In that year they brought in a total of 15,862 francs which was still a derisory amount compared to the general budget of the Hospital (0.75% of the operating revenue in 1946). However, the income from the policlinic increased rapidly, amounting to 64,198 francs in 1950 (1.6% of operating income) and 126,739 francs in 1953 (2.6%).[118] It was mainly a question of responding to the demands of the doctors and denouncing abuses, as the HHS declared in 1947, "we have even seen ladies in fur coats going up to the Children's Clinic in taxis to present their children for free consultations".[119] However, this financial logic alone could not meet the expectations of the Health Service. Indeed, the abandonment of free outpatient care risked compromising social and preventive medicine, particularly with regard to the fight against venereal diseases. The HHS, in 1948, refused to abandon free care in dermatology policlinics, citing the principle that "priority should be given to the social cost of the problem".[120] Moreover, the policlinics had a function of regulating hospitalisations and limiting the congestion of the Cantonal Hospital. Vannotti explained, in 1949, that the aim of the medical policlinic was "to make precise diagnoses in order to avoid unnecessary hospitalisations. This way of proceeding [allows us] to make substantial savings".[121] It was during the Jequier-Doge period (1950–1977) that the Policlinic was truly modernised. In 1957, the Grand Council adopted a decree which gave the establishment a new legal status and opened it to solvent patients, in particular those sent for more in-depth analyses by doctors established in the city.[122] From then on, outpatient consultations were put on an equal footing with hospitalisations, since only the indigent were reimbursed for their expenses.

Reorganisation of the Accounting Department (1938–1941)

The first attempts to restructure the Hospital's accounting system were made at the beginning of the 1920s in a climate of crisis in public finances and reorganisation of the cantonal administration.[123] In 1921, the director Mermoud complained to the HHS about the chief doctors who placed orders for instruments without taking into account the hospital's budget. He wanted the management to have control over expenditure and obtained a statement from

[117] ACV, K VIII B 213/15, files of Me Henri Rapin, member of the HHS.

[118] RSC, Department of the Interior, 1946–1953. This figure is no longer mentioned in subsequent reports.

[119] ACV, S 73, HHS minutes, 22 January 1947.

[120] ACV, S 73, HHS minutes, 26 July 1948.

[121] ACV, S 73, HHS minutes, 8 December 1949.

[122] BGC, 6 May 1957.

[123] François Wisard, op. cit., pp. 249–266.

the HHS that the heads of departments should have an autonomous budget but must request authorisation above an amount fixed by the Department of the Interior. The chief doctors largely circumvented this measure through the private funds attached to their departments, over which they had complete control but which were not dependent on public finances and were accounted for outside the hospital's budget.

It was not until the end of the 1930s that the hospital's administration and accounting were truly reformed.[124] At this time, the HHS called on professional managers as experts for the restructuring. The reorganisation of the administrative services was entrusted to an accountant-controller from the Finance Department and to an independent chartered accountant from Lausanne. They introduced centralised control of the bursar's office and proposed the reorganisation of the legal department.

In fact, the Hospital's accounts only included, under the heading "patients' pensions", the sums actually collected and not those invoiced.[125] This method resulted in a larger than expected accounting deficit, as well as a significant loss of income; in 1938, the two experts spoke of approximately 2500 disputed claims per year. At the time, patients' pensions were an essential resource for the operation of the Hospital, representing 84.3% of the establishment's income in the 1930s. It is easy to understand the urgent need to remedy this dysfunction. The hospital's management was aware of this issue. As early as 1936, it appointed a new official in charge of legal affairs. When he arrived, the administrative documents relating to patients were neither classified, dated, numbered nor arranged in personalised files.[126] The systematic organisation of these patient files was not enough to bring in the unpaid bills. In 1943, the hospital administration put forward the figure of 6000 disputed claims per year; i.e., a sum of about 300,000 francs that corresponded to nearly 17% of invoiced pensions and 10% of operating expenses.[127]

The main problem was the inability of a large number of patients to pay for their hospitalisation. Director Rubattel wrote to the Department of Finance, which was studying the possibility of increasing pensions to solve the problem of litigation, that "the majority of the Hospital's patients (Vaudois, Confederates and foreigners) were from very modest backgrounds"[128] and that it was not possible to charge them more. In the long run, the development of health insurance would solve this problem (see Chapter 5).

[124] ACV, K VIII D 65.

[125] ACV, K VIII D 37.

[126] ACV, K VIII D 64.

[127] ACV, K VIII D 37.

[128] ACV, K VIII D 37, letter from Rubattel to the Department of Finance, 9 April 1943.

Conclusion

The various reorganisations of the Cantonal Hospital show they can only be carried out with the agreement of the lobbies affected by the reform projects (free outpatient care). In the absence of a structured lobby, the attempt to rationalise the pharmacy illustrates, on the contrary, the case of reform attempted against an overly powerful lobby. These considerations are not limited to the rationalisation that took place in the 1930s and 1940s. During this phase, the hospital authorities (management, Hospices Service, Health Service, and Department of the Interior) experienced the growing intervention of organised lobbies in the hospital system that had to be reckoned with in the construction of a new hospital policy after 1945.

The period 1920–1950 was also the first stage in the hospital authorities' awareness of the need to organise the hospital system, not only single organisations. At that time, these considerations were essentially limited to the Cantonal Hospital as a conglomerate of buildings and partners that was undergoing rapid expansion. The will to coordinate the various care units that make up the Cantonal Hospital, to evaluate future needs and to plan the territory became the main impetus of a hospital policy applied to the whole canton after 1945. Considering the Cantonal Hospital, it entered a new phase in the 1950s which saw the return of the State after three decades of partnership with the private sector. This phenomenon can be explained by the affirmation of a new cantonal hospital policy for which the State is the main guarantor and in which the Cantonal Hospital occupies a central place.

5 The Cantonal Hospital in the 1950s: The Return of the State

The 1950s were a transitional phase between a period of all-out development based on the intervention of the private sector and another of extraordinary growth which appeared in the 1960s. This phase of reorganisation of the hospital system was reflected in the affirmation of the State as a major player. The political authorities integrated the Cantonal Hospital into a much broader hospital policy that took into account all the hospitals in the canton. Under these conditions, the policy of rationalisation had to be carried out at the cantonal level and the changes made to the Cantonal Hospital can only be understood within this new political framework (see Chapter 5).

Measured in terms of capacity and number of hospitalisations, the Cantonal Hospital appears to be in a stagnation phase. The number of available beds remained stable (1158 in 1950 and 1133 in 1960) and the growth in the number of patients slowed down. The number of hospitalisations was 13,243 in 1950 and 14,389 in 1960, after it reached a peak of 16,953 patients in 1957.[129] The drop in the years 1958–1960 was only temporary, since the number of hospitalised patients exceeded 17,000 in 1963 and 20,000 in 1969.

[129] RSC, Department of the Interior, 1950–1960.

Moreover, this drop was seen as a positive effect of the agreement signed by the State in 1953 with = regional hospitals for the hospitalisation of indigent patients, whose real cost of care was paid by the State since 1955. Thus, indigent patients no longer had a material interest in coming to the Cantonal Hospital for treatment, which allowed a certain disengagement from the establishment.[130] The administrators of the hospital declared, in 1960, the decrease in the number of patients "corresponds perfectly to a more rational distribution of patients within the Vaud hospital system, which is one of the goals we are pursuing".[131]

It is rather at the level of equipment and the qualitative environment that we must look for the dynamism of the 1950s. As in the case of the surgical department (see Chapter 2), new medical specialities emerged for which facilities were needed. The development of the human environment is a good indicator of this transformation of medicine. The number of employees rose sharply from 805 in 1950 (including 66 assistant doctors and 10 senior doctors) to 1396 in 1960 (including 82 assistant doctors and 11 senior doctors). The staff also changed in nature, as the deaconess institution of Saint-Loup gradually withdrew its nuns in the years 1946–1958 in favour of lay and international staff. The human environment thus became denser during the 1950s. The number of employees per hundred patients is a good indicator of the human capital invested in the Hospital. It remained very stable during the first part of the twentieth century, with a slight upward trend from 2.4 employees per 100 patients in 1900 to 3.0 in 1920 and 3.6 in 1940. This index had already risen to 6.1 in 1950 and 9.7 in 1960, which meant that the density of personnel had practically tripled between 1940 and 1960.[132] As a consequence of this increase in density, salary costs accounted for a growing share of operating expenses. While they amounted to 28.9% of the total in 1930 and 32.2% in 1940, they reached 57.0% in 1950 and 60.7% in 1960.[133] The affirmation of human capital as the primary factor of production thus had a direct impact on hospital accounting.

The Resources of the Cantonal Hospital in the 1950s

Despite the general upward trend in expenditure, the Hospital managed to generate its own income, which meant that it was no longer dependent on the State for its development; the financial management of the Hospital was, therefore, in full continuity with the inter-war period. The coverage of expenditure by income even increased slightly (44.3% in 1950 and 48.4% in 1960). As for the structure of the establishment's income, this did not really change since the end of the 1930s, even though there was a decrease in patients'

[130] RSC, Department of the Interior, 1959.

[131] RSC, Department of the Interior, 1960, p. 57.

[132] RSC, Department of the Interior, 1900–1960.

[133] Louis-Samuel Prod'hom and others, op. cit., at 51.

pensions (75.5% of income in 1950 and 64.8% in 1958) to the benefit of income from technical services (radiology, laboratories, pharmacy), the share of which rose from 16.9% in 1950 to 29.0% in 1958.[134] The policy of making these services profitable by making them available to the medical profession outside the Hospital was bearing fruit.

Finally, the operating fees were still accounted for outside the operating budget and continued to be added to the Cantonal Hospital funds to finance capital expenditure. The evolution of this type of revenue perfectly illustrates the important break that took place in the Surgical Department with the opening of the new Decker Surgical Clinic in 1947. Before this date, the surgical fees collected were limited, which explains Prof. Decker's claims and protests about the obsolescence of his department in the years 1932–1945. The new surgical clinic enabled the clinic to enter a phase of strong growth. In 1948, the 40,000-franc mark in fees was passed for the first time, and the results from the 1950s confirmed this trend, with a peak of 181,385 francs in 1959. The division of labour in the Surgical Department and the multiplication of medical specialities had an eminently positive effect in terms of the development policy of the establishment. These taxes were of little importance to the operating budget—they represented an average of 0.7% of the expenses in the 1950s—but they contributed to a reserve for investment which allowed the Hospital's management to propose the provision of its own funds when investments were requested from the Grand Council.

Development of Hospital Equipment: The End of Partnerships with the Private Sector

The construction of the new surgical clinic was an opportunity for the State to return to financing the equipment of the Cantonal Hospital. It put an end to a policy of hospital development based on the private sector that had lasted for more than 25 years. The obsolescence of the surgical clinic in the early 1940s (it had not been renovated since 1914) highlighted the limits of this policy. Since he took up his post in 1932, Prof. Decker constantly called for improvements to his department for pedagogical (training of surgeons), scientific (development of surgical research) and financial reasons (competition with the surgical departments of private clinics and regional hospitals). The modernisation of this clinic was crucial for the Cantonal Hospital, but no philanthropist emerged to cover the cost. In the absence of private funding, the government decided to intervene in the early 1940s.

The various credits granted for the construction (1.35 million francs in 1942, 1.8 million francs in 1945, 934,500 francs in 1949) were an opportunity to point out the drawbacks of the hospital policy pursued between the wars. Maurice Jeanneret, a communist deputy, explained to the Grand Council

[134] RSC, Department of the Interior, 1950–1958. Detailed figures are not available after 1958.

in 1945, "what the State Council's technique was in recent years for improving our hospital buildings [...]. They were waiting for a millionaire, if possible a doctor and unmarried, to die bequeathing his fortune to the State".[135] The State Councillor responsible for health policy, Norbert Bosset, supported these statements by explaining, "these donations were themselves subject to certain conditions to which we had to submit. Thus, for example, when I had to discuss the question of the Rossier Hospice, that is to say the establishment annexed to the maternity hospital, Mr. Benjamin Rossier, who had come to see me in the name of the family, had set as a condition that the State should be able to provide the necessary sum and that the envisaged project should be immediately put into effect. It was the same during the talks with Mr. Dapples for the Nestlé donation. The condition imposed on us was to undertake this construction before any other".[136]

After 1945, the development of hospital facilities was conceived within a new political framework aiming to take into consideration the health needs of the whole canton. The State adopted a proactive, less passive position than before. If it wanted to make the Cantonal Hospital the hub of an organised and coordinated hospital system, it had to take charge of the development of its facilities itself.

The surgical clinic cost the State more than four million francs but it did not encounter any real opposition as the new hospital policy was based on a very broad political consensus. The same applies to all the credits granted by the Grand Council to the Cantonal Hospital until the end of the 1950s. In total, the State invested nearly 17 million in this establishment during the years 1942–1960.

During the period 1940–1960, the hospital system took on an increasingly important role within the cantonal administration. While the Hospices Service represented about 10% of the State budget in the inter-war period (10.7% in 1940), this share rose to 13.7% in 1950 and 15.0% in 1960. This growth was mainly due to the Cantonal Hospital which accounted for 40.1% of the expenditure of the Hospices Service in 1930, 54.5% in 1940, 59.1% in 1950 and 64.5% in 1960. The Cantonal Hospital alone accounted for 9.7% of the State's expenditure in 1960.[137]

6 Conclusion

The numerous reforms, adaptations and restructurings the Cantonal Hospital of Lausanne underwent were all aimed at improving its operation and providing it with sufficient financial resources. The strengthening of the administrative management in the 1870s, the diversification of resources during the years 1880–1914, the rapprochement with the private sector during

[135] BGC, 22 May 1945.

[136] Ibid.

[137] RSC, Department of the Interior, 1940–1960.

the inter-war period, the rationalisation during the period 1930–1950 and the return of the State after 1950 appear to be elements tending towards these goals, aimed at providing an adequate material framework for hospital growth.

The management of a larger, more complex and more expensive institution was only possible through a strengthening and empowering of the administrative structure. The role of this hospital management was not only to ensure order in the institution and its day-to-day operation but also to manage the hospital's growth and supply it with sufficient resources. The development of the hospital infrastructure required ever-increasing financial resources that the state alone could not provide. The hospital management was able to generate new income by opening up to profitable patient groups, mainly middle- and upper-class citizens and people with health insurance. Patients thus became the main source of funding in the last years of the nineteenth century which explains, to a large extent, the gradual affirmation of a true marketing-type logic in hospital management; it was a question of positioning the hospital in an increasingly competitive healthcare market. The example of the development of the Radiology Department is particularly telling in this respect. This is an extremely profitable service that tended to multiply within the hospital system and whose constant modernisation responded as much to the scientific needs of the head doctor as to the need to maintain a dominant position in the healthcare market. The Cantonal Hospital was not the only hospital in the canton. It was in direct competition with the regional hospitals, the specialised institutions in Lausanne and the private clinics which were themselves seeking to increase their market share in the hospitalisation of patients. The example of the regional hospitals, discussed in the next chapter, highlights the transformation of local institutions that complement the Cantonal Hospital into hospitals with a modernised and competitive medical-technical infrastructure.

CHAPTER 4

The Transformation of Regional Hospitals

1 Introduction

Hospitalisation in the Canton of Vaud was not the sole responsibility of the Cantonal Hospital of Lausanne. From the 1840s onwards, a large number of local infirmaries provided almost half of the hospital system's capacity in the Canton. At first, these small establishments, linked to philanthropic elites close to the Protestant Revival, depended largely on private generosity. They were not founded as the outcome of medical progress, but rather as a result of an awareness of social issues on the part of the traditional elites.[1]

In the last decades of the nineteenth century (1880–1900), philanthropic hospitals experienced a serious financial crisis stemming from a change in the scale of these establishments and their transformation into medico-technical platforms, intended both to care for the sick *en masse*, in order to respond to the increase in population, and to make them available to the medical profession as a working tool. Traditional charitable resources could no longer ensure the construction of new and better-equipped hospitals as well as the operation of organisations that had become larger and therefore more expensive. Additionally, this change of scale took place in a context of newly rationalised and standardised management methods that run counter to the personalised relationship between the philanthropist and "his" patients. Solutions and new financial resources had to be found to enable the operation of these private establishments—a phenomenon that has attracted much attention from historians abroad.

[1] This phenomenon is similar in the United States. Morris Vogel, "The transformation of American hospital, 1850–1920", in S. Reverby and D. Rosner (eds), *Health Care in America: Essays in Social History*, Philadelphia, 1979, p. 105.

P.-Y. Donzé, *The Formation of the Swiss Hospital System (1840–1960)*,
https://doi.org/10.1007/978-981-19-3911-2_4

Great Britain is an exemplary case of the limits of funding based on philanthropic resources. The British hospital system relied heavily on private institutions founded in the eighteenth and nineteenth centuries and supported by the aristocratic elite. In his study of London hospitals, Keir Waddington showed that the development and modernisation of this hospital system led to heavy deficits in the second half of the nineteenth century, along with a reduction in donations in hospital revenue (46% for all London hospitals in 1864 and 1.7% in 1910). The creation of the *Prince of Wales Hospital Fund* by aristocratic families in 1897 delayed the decline of the philanthropic model but did not prevent it.[2] The use of pensions for the sick became necessary after 1914, their share of total operating resources rising from 2% in 1900–1904 to 29% in 1920–1924 for London hospitals.[3] The transition from the private philanthropic model to a new model based on patients' pensions can be observed in most continental European countries. In some cases, such as Germany and several northern and eastern European states, the adoption of compulsory health insurance favoured this transfer of costs to the sick.[4]

Despite the adoption of different modalities in various countries, the transfer of the costs of hospital growth to inpatients seems to have taken place throughout the Western world. In the Canton of Vaud, the transformation of local charity infirmaries into modernised regional hospitals is an excellent illustration of this phenomenon.[5]

2 Local Infirmaries: A Fruit of the Protestant Revival (1840–1900)

Medical discoveries cannot explain the foundation of local infirmaries in the Canton of Vaud in the years 1840–1880; they were not created with the aim of making new medicine available to the population. On the contrary, a conservative and largely reactionary feeling against the modernisation of society—population explosion, migration, urbanisation and industrialisation—explains the intervention of the traditional local elites in the hospital question. In many respects, the infirmaries in the Canton of Vaud that emerged from

[2] Keir Waddington, *Charity and the London Hospitals, 1850–1898*, Woodbrifge: The Boydell Press, 2000.

[3] Steven Cherry, "Accountability, entitlement, and control issues and voluntary hospital funding c1860–1939", *Social History of Medicine*, 1996, p. 221. See also Steven Cherry, "Before the National Health Service: Financing the voluntary hospitals, 1900–1939", *Economic History Review*, 1997, pp. 305–326.

[4] Germany, where compulsory health insurance was introduced in 1883, served as a model for Austria (1888), Hungary (1891), Norway (1909), Serbia (1910), the Netherlands (1913), etc. Paul Starr, op. cit., pp. 220–245, and Reinhardt Spree, "Krankenhausentwicklung und Sozialpolitik in Deutschland während des 19. Jahrhunderts", *Historische Zeitschrift*, vol. 260(1), 1995, pp. 75–106.

[5] This chapter is based mainly on the annual reports of the hospitals in the Canton of Vaud. In order to avoid a proliferation of footnotes, I do not cite below the source of the accounting data mentioned when they are taken from this source.

the Protestant Revival appear to be the equivalent of provincial philanthropic hospitals founded during the eighteenth century in Great Britain, of which Roy Porter spoke of as "traditional paternalism institutionalized".[6]

The Vaud regional hospitals were a product of the Protestant Revival. This theology, which promoted individual social action as a source of salvation, gave rise to a multitude of social associations and organisations (reading societies, schools, asylums, etc.) in the nineteenth century, among which were the regional infirmaries. Their emergence in the second half of the nineteenth century was the result of a revival of religiosity in a changing society. The founder of the Institution of Deaconesses (1842) and emblematic figure of the Protestant Revival in the Vaud Canton, Pastor Louis Germond declared in the early 1850s, "a hospital administered in a Christian spirit is the best means of evangelisation".[7] This conservative ideology aimed to maintain the old social order through social action among the proletarianising working classes. Thus, the declared cause for the foundation of an infirmary in Yverdon was "the increase in the town's population, especially the working-class population",[8] while Hottinger, a member of the committees of the Vevey-Samaritain Infirmary and the Saint-Loup Institution, declared in 1865: "I hope that, little by little, there will be an infirmary in every town, in every large village in our canton. The ever-increasing number of the floating population makes this absolutely necessary".[9] This is exactly what Pastor Henri Germond, son of Louis, meant when he gave a presentation on the question of local infirmaries in French-speaking Switzerland to the Public utility society of the Canton of Vaud in 1870: "The suffering of the lower classes has often been greater than it is today; but never has their desire been more ardent; never has the heart of the disinherited, as they call themselves, overflowed with more bitterness or more irritated desires. [...] To postpone the shock, and, if possible, to cushion it, let us multiply the cooperative societies, let us fight pauperism hand to hand, let us fraternise with the worker, let us instruct the ignorant, let us care for the sick; let us pay with our own hands; let us not shrink from any sacrifice; let us spare nothing!".[10]

Religion played an important role in the infirmary: the hospitalised patient must accept both his fate in the face of illness and his position of inferiority in society as resulting from divine will, which explains the words attributed to Ambroise Paré, "I bandaged him and God healed him", often mentioned in speeches, commemorative brochures, annual reports and on the walls of the

[6] Porter Roy, "The gift relation: Philanthropy and provincial hospitals in eighteenth century England", in Granshaw Lindsay and Porter Roy (eds), *Hospitals in History*, London/New York, 1989, p. 172.

[7] J. de Mestral Combremont, *Vies données... vies retrouvées. Les diaconesses de Saint-Loup*, Lausanne: Payot, 1932, p. 40.

[8] *Journal de la Société vaudoise d'utilité publique (JSVUP)*, 1858, p. 162.

[9] BGC, 18 January 1865.

[10] JSVUP, 1870, pp. 261–262.

Saint-Loup Hospital in 1928. Similarly, the administrators of the Rolle Infirmary had the following words inscribed on the walls of their establishment: "It is the Eternal One who makes people die and who makes them live, who makes them go down to the grave and who makes them come back up".[11] The paternalistic dimension of the infirmaries is reflected in the admission of patients by a committee that discussed each case. In Yverdon, for example, the minutes of the administrative commission contains the names of the hospitalised patients and the price of the daily pension, decided by the Commission on a case-by-case basis until the 1900s.

The Canton of Vaud was quickly covered with infirmaries: three were founded in the 1850s, four in the 1860s, six in the 1870s, one in the 1880s and one in the 1890s (see Table 1). However, this chronology is more the result of chance than a reflection of diachronic regional socio-economic evolution. Indeed, the dynamics of the foundation of infirmaries only imperfectly reflect the demographic development of the canton. The initiative was left entirely to the private sector, despite a timid intervention by the state in the 1870s. Thus, in the absence of an overall plan, the opening of hospitals depended on the generosity of notables. In many cases, their creation was the result of a bequest or a gift from local dignities: In Vevey, in 1858, the syndic Edouard Couvreu made a house available and offered a plot of land on which the 1877 infirmary was built; in Morges, Henri Monod-Forel made a donation of 18,000 francs in 1869 for the acquisition of a building to be used as an infirmary; in Orbe, the former syndic Georges de Thienne bequeathed a building and 25,000 francs to the town in 1871 for an infirmary; etc. Some of the great names of regional philanthropy, such as the Butini family, were at the origin of several of these establishments. The Genevan doctor Adolphe Butini (1792–1877) was a key figure in the philanthropy of French-speaking Switzerland.[12] Born into a family of magistrates, doctors and bankers, he founded two private infirmaries in Geneva (Infirmerie Butini de Plainpalais 1859; Infirmerie du Prieuré 1876) with the declared aim of competing with the Cantonal Hospital of Geneva opened in 1856 by the radical-democratic government.[13] In the neighbouring Canton of Vaud, Butini was involved in the financing of several philanthropic establishments in the 1850s and 1860s and bought the Hôtel des Bains in Saint-Loup which he made available to his friend, the pastor Louis Germond, to set up his establishment for deaconesses, founded in

[11] Quoted by Henri Germond in JSVUP, 1876, p. 222.

[12] On Adolphe Butini and his family, see Gabriel Mützenberg, op. cit.

[13] See Pierre-Yves Donzé, *Bâtir*..., op. cit., pp. 101–103.

Table 1 Local infirmaries in the Canton of Vaud, 1842–1890

Locality	*Year of foundation*	*Number of beds to the foundation*
Pompaples/Saint-Loup	1842	?
Yverdon	1856	9
Vevey-Samaritain	1858	12
Rolle	1860	17
Payerne	1866	9
Aigle	1867	6
Morges	1869	12
Château-d'Oex	1870	?
Nyon	1874	15
Aubonne	1875	6
Moudon	1876	?
Orbe	1876	?
Montreux	1877	20
Sainte-Croix	1880	?
Bex	1890	12

1842 in Echallens.[14] Butini's descendants remained active in French-speaking Switzerland's philanthropy until the Second World War (see Fig. 1).

The importance of Protestant philanthropic networks on the development of hospitals is perfectly illustrated by the example of the Institution of Deaconesses of Saint-Loup which played a decisive role in the second half of the nineteenth century. During the years 1842–1881, this institution was run by members of the Germond family. The position of director was held by the founder, Louis Germond (1842–1868), and then by his son, Henri Germond (1868–1881), whose wife Louise and daughter Louisa were also members of the administrative commission. During this period, Saint-Loup was at the heart of the Protestant philanthropy. Among the 50 people appointed to the administrative commission between 1842 and 1881, the liberal professions (46%), women (24%) and pastors (18%)—i.e., the social elites traditionally involved in the works of the Revival—largely dominated; doctors were almost absent (6%).[15] Moreover, the Saint-Loup institution was strongly supported by wealthy philanthropists who were not members of the administrative commission, such as the Butini family or the Geneva banker, Jean-Gabriel Eynard-Lullin.

Saint-Loup very quickly sent her deaconesses to social welfare institutions in French-speaking Switzerland and abroad (France and Italy); by 1881, no

[14] J. Vincent, *Aux écoutes de la souffrance. Histoire de l'Institution des diaconesses de Saint-Loup publiée, à l'occasion de son centenaire, par le Conseil général, 1842–1942*, Lausanne: La Concorde, 1942, pp. 109–133; Robert Centlivres and Jean-Jacques Fleury, *De l'Eglise d'Etat à l'Eglise nationale (1839–1863)*, Lausanne: Eglise nationale vaudoise, 1963, pp. 53–56; J. de Mestral Combremont, *Vies données...*, op. cit.

[15] The balance (6%) is accounted for by unidentified persons.

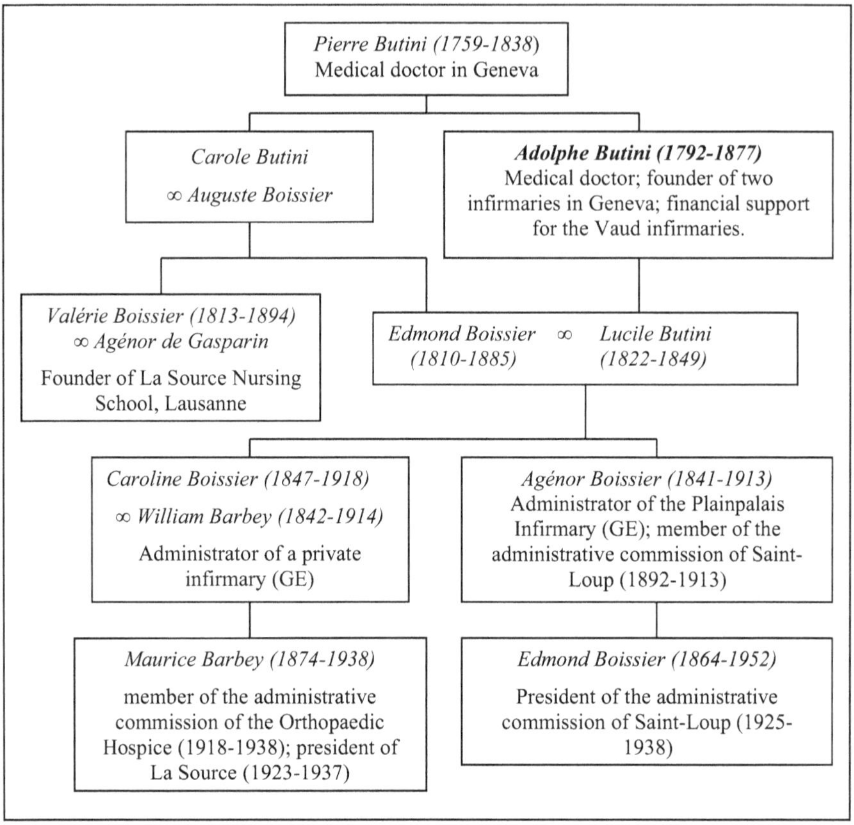

Fig. 1 Simplified genealogy of Dr. Adolphe Butini (*Source* Gabriel Mützenberg, *Une femme de style. Valérie de Gasparin*, Le Mont-sur-Lausanne, Ed. Ouverture, 1995)

fewer than 52 organisations called on them.[16] They were heterogeneous and reflected the general social character of the deaconesses' work in its early days: 24 establishments for the sick, 11 for children (orphanages, schools, etc.) and three for the elderly, as well as five posts of visiting sisters and nine miscellaneous organisations. However, this commitment was very volatile and the deaconesses had already left 38 of these establishments in 1890—including 25 of the 28 non-hospital posts—to refocus their activities on the hospitals. With the death of Henri Germond in 1881, the generalist and purely philanthropic period of Saint-Loup came to an end. The deaconesses then specialised in hospital services, thanks in particular to the support of the medical profession, which needed a disciplined and obedient workforce in its project to modernise hospital medicine.

[16] J. Vincent, op. cit., pp. 295–297.

The First Infirmaries: Homes for the Indigent Sick

Originally, most infirmaries were opened in private residential buildings (Aigle, Aubonne, Morges, Payerne, Vevey-Samaritain) or in the disused Ancien Régime hospital provided by the commune (Moudon, Nyon, Yverdon). Only the infirmaries of Montreux (1877) and Sainte-Croix (1880) were opened in specifically designed new buildings. Buildings generally not intended for medical purposes were used and allowed for installations at low expense. All these infirmaries were financially independent and profitable but were quickly confronted with capacity problems, leading them to build new infirmaries or transform and extend the original buildings. The administrators were generally aware of this reduced capacity but financial considerations kept the founders from building new installations. Thus, they often preferred to open a temporary infirmary in a residential house and hoard donations as much as possible in order to construct a new building when their wealth could ensure a high level of self-financing.

The first phase of (re)construction (1870–1900) did not correspond with the arrival of new medical considerations that would require a reorganisation of the hospital space. The buildings constructed during this period were always small (25 beds in Aigle in 1871; 20 in Yverdon in 1874; 14 in Aubonne in 1896; 28 in Payerne in 1896; 25 in Morges in 1897; 30 in Nyon in 1898; etc.). The architects who carried out the work often had no experience in the construction of hospitals, a field in which there were no experts in the canton. Local personalities, sometimes involved in the administration of the infirmary, were contracted. Philanthropic networks also played an important role in the choice of architect. Several builders of infirmaries were close to the Free Church, for whom they built chapels (François Jacquerod in Aigle; Francis Landry in Yverdon; etc.).[17]

At this time, two new infirmaries were also founded in Lausanne (1907) and Vevey-Providence (1910). The first was opened as part of La Source School to enable student nurses to acquire practical training. An agreement was signed in 1907 with the State to receive indigent patients at the expense of the canton to relieve the Cantonal Hospital. The second, the Providence Infirmary, was opened by the Catholic diaspora of Vevey following a donation of over 110,000 francs.

This generation of buildings was characterised by its "family" style. The infirmaries resembled small houses with bourgeois charm, often of the Swiss traditional *Heimatstil* type, with a balcony, garden, terrace, etc. (see Fig. 2). The administrators of the Infirmary of Moudon celebrated the "chalet-like exterior form"[18] of their hospital building in 1895. Together with its small size, this architectural feature gave the illusion of a family, of a warm home in

[17] Dave Lüthi, *Les chapelles de l'Eglise libre vaudoise, 1847–1965. Histoire architecturale*, Lausanne: Bibliothèque historique vaudoise, 2000.

[18] *Infirmerie de Moudon: Notes historiques*, Mondon, L'Eveil, 1895, p. 8.

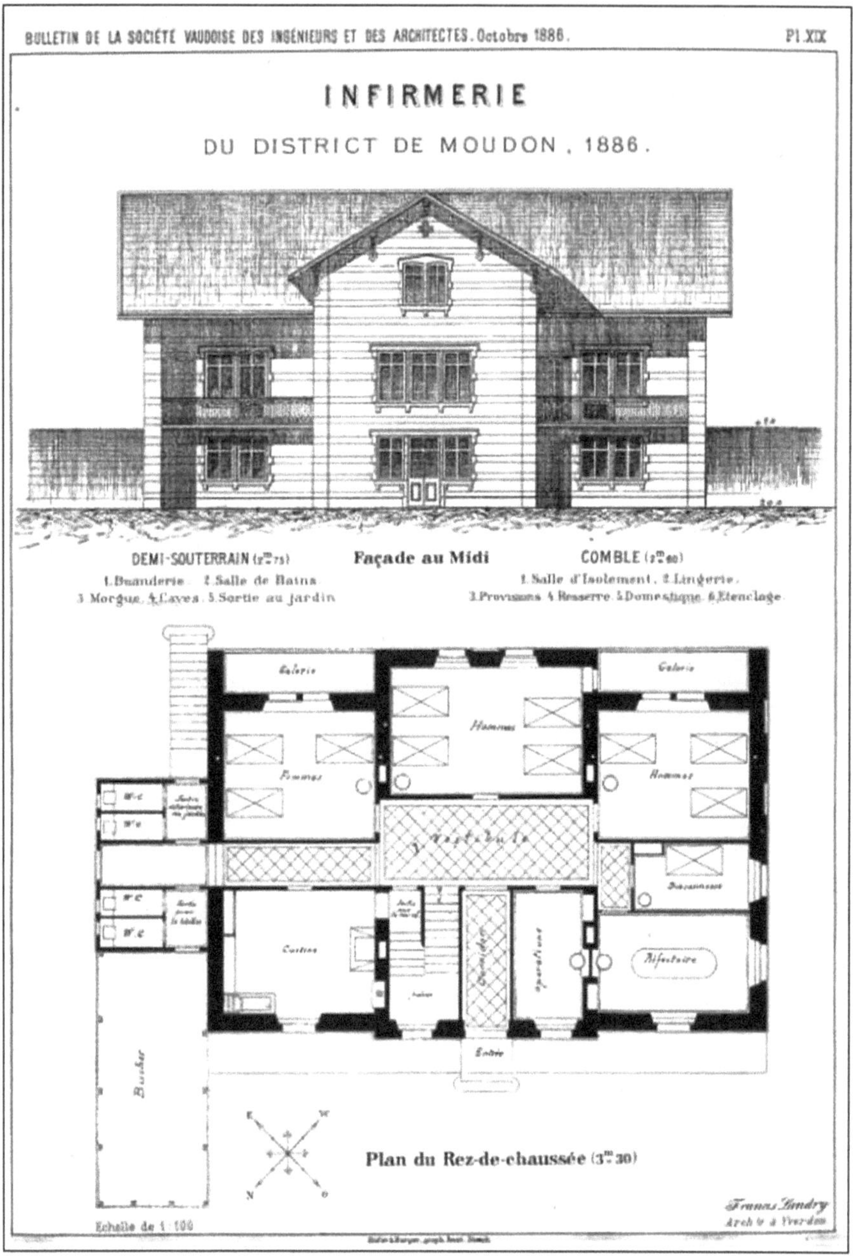

Fig. 2 Moudon Infirmary, 1886 (*Source Bulletin de la Société vaudoise des ingénieurs et des architectes*, 1886, p. 53)

which the philanthropic elites welcome those of the working class experiencing difficulty. The architectural setting of these infirmaries was entirely consistent with their social function.

A Minimal Medical Service

The internal organisation of these infirmaries was very basic because of their small size. The limited number of beds meant that only a limited number of patients could be admitted. In 1880, there were 41 hospitalisations in Aubonne, 67 in Moudon, 112 in Nyon, 92 in Orbe, 87 in Payerne, 90 in Rolle and 139 in Yverdon. Under these conditions, it is obvious that the hospital staff and the internal organisation of the hospital were reduced to their simplest expression. In general, there were one or two lay servants, or even a deaconess of Saint-Loup, the latter being present in Yverdon (1857), Vevey-Samaritain (1858), Rolle (1860), Morges (1869), Montreux (1877), Sainte-Croix (1880), Payerne (1885) and Moudon (1888).

These establishments were open; that is, every doctor in the locality was allowed to come and practice there. However, doing so was not very lucrative as patients were essentially indigent and could not afford to be treated at home. This is why doctors accepted their appointment more than they claimed it. Very often, they practised free of charge during their first years as a doctor; however, this type of voluntary work disappeared during the 1880s because the administrative commissions wanted greater attention from them. The administrators of the Yverdon Infirmary spoke of paying the doctors in 1881 "so that they could not demand, but at least expect a visit every day".[19] Auguste Garin, a doctor in this establishment, refused to submit to a fixed schedule and resigned because he preferred to give priority to his private clientele. Similarly, at the Bex Infirmary which opened in 1890, the three local doctors refused to receive an allowance. While the president of the committee proposed in 1892 to pay them, "doctors refused and want to continue to treat our patients in an absolutely disinterested manner".[20] They accepted compensation in 1894.

The administrative commissions in each locality generally established a rotation among the various practitioners who accepted this responsibility. The length of service varied between three and six months, meaning there was no chief doctor at the head of the infirmaries, with some exceptions. In Aigle, for example, the doctors informed the infirmary administrators in 1867 of the disadvantages inherent in this mode of operation. As a consequence, they appointed Alois Mandrin as the only doctor in charge of the hospital service and he remained at the head of the establishment until 1899, when he was replaced by two colleagues in rotation. These facts illustrate that access to the infirmary was not considered important by doctors for their daily practice.

[19] Yverdon Hospital, minutes of the steering board, 27 April 1881.

[20] ACV, PP 324/1, minutes of the committee, 8 February 1892.

Until the end of the nineteenth century, local infirmaries were not considered as working tools by the medical profession whose main income still came from home visits. Similarly, apart from a few special cases, doctors were hardly ever present in the administrative commissions of the infirmaries and did not get involved in hospital management. From time to time, from the end of the nineteenth century, the commissions called on doctors for their expertise, particularly in the medico-technical field, but the medical profession never claimed to be a member of the commission.

Unstable Balance of Finances

The notables who founded the various local infirmaries also managed and financed them. As these were small establishments with a very limited medical and technical infrastructure, their financial needs were limited and easily covered by a private charity so there was no fundamental difference between the management of infirmaries in small rural towns and those in urban centres. However, material difficulties appeared with the construction of the first generation of hospital buildings, regardless of the size and geographical location of the institution.

Administrative Organisation

The organisational structure of these infirmaries was relatively simple: there was a general assembly of donors—sometimes important donors were appointed for life—who met once a year to approve the management of the hospital. This assembly elected the administrative committee responsible for day-to-day operations. Sometimes, a smaller management committee presided when a large number of people were in the administrative committee (Aigle, Nyon, Payerne, Sainte-Croix, Yverdon). This organisational structure allowed for the potential democratisation of the control of hospitals through the possibility of making a donation, even a small one, and access to the general assembly.[21] In practice, this right was hardly used and the various administrative commissions were composed of traditional notables (pastors, notaries, landlords and merchants), confirming their social power. The functions of bursar, cashier and secretary of the infirmary were not entrusted to salaried employees but carried out by members of the administrative commissions on a voluntary basis. The internal control of the establishment (kitchen, supervision of the sick, etc.) was entrusted to the deaconess superior in the case of infirmaries that called on Saint-Loup or a lay bursar-supervisor in other cases.

Finally, the commission was assisted by a committee of ladies that sometimes depended on the general assembly but in fact functioned on the basis of co-option. The committee was made up of women from dominant families

[21] Thierry Christ, "Du zèle piétiste à l'activisme républicain. Démocratisation de la gestion et du contrôle de l'hôpital à Neuchâtel au 19^{e}siècle", *Revue historique neuchâteloise*, 1999, pp. 19–31.

whose husbands generally sat on the administrative commission. Their role in the infirmary was similar to their household: supplying the house with linen, sheets, pillows, etc., listening to the patients to "hear their complaints about the food or the care of the staff, which were sometimes well-founded, but more often exaggerated", collecting donations in kind, organising sales and Christmas parties, etc. The ladies' committees left few written records of their activities and are hardly visible in the hospital archives. The wives remained in the shadow of their husbands who organised, managed and directed the hospitals, thus producing the documents kept in the archives. The role of the women's committee was that of stewardship, not of speaking out and making decisions.

Original Funding from Private Sources

At the financial level, the same structure of operating income was found in most infirmaries. They can be classified into three main categories: own funds (interest on assets and rental of real estate), private resources (donations and legacies from individuals, sales, etc.) and patients' pensions. Finally, some institutions benefitted from other sources of funding, the amounts of which are almost negligible (municipal fines and various taxes) (Table 2).

Despite the diversity resulting from the specific conditions of each institution, private funding predominated. These resources came mainly from donations and legacies and occasionally from sales organised sporadically, bringing in several thousand, or even tens of thousands, of francs. The importance of these donations explains the infirmaries' reliance on their own resources as operating profits were generally capitalised, sometimes in a special construction fund for a new building. This private funding ensured the independence of local infirmaries but left little room for manoeuvre for administrators who were not in control of their institution's income. Donations or legacies were uncertain which caused problems when the infirmaries developed and were financed by bank loans.

To a large extent, the size of the donations determined the size of the pensions paid by the patients; the administrators had to make up for any shortfall in income and avoid operating deficits. Finally, there was no direct public

Table 2 Financial resources of local infirmaries in Vaud in their first years, in %

Type of resources	*Nyon 1877*	*Moudon 1880*	*Morges 1885*	*Orbe 1880*	*Rolle 1861–1867*	*Vevey-Samaritain 1860*	*Yverdon 1857–1858*
Own	–	3	11	4	–	3	–
Private	95	12	40	46	79	74	85
Pensions	5	85	49	47	20	22	15
Various	–	–	–	3	1	1	–

Source Hospital annual reports, various years

funding, either from the municipalities or the Canton, apart from paying the costs for certain indigent inpatients but this was generally included under the heading "pensions" in the annual reports and was therefore difficult to measure. The state became timidly involved in this financing from the 1870s onwards (see Chapter 5).

An Unstable Financial Balance After the Construction of New Buildings
This donation-based funding structure was suitable for small institutions with very limited needs. However, when infirmaries moved into new buildings, they had to rely on other financial partners. Some relatively wealthy infirmaries developed without taking out any loans (Aubonne, Nyon, Sainte-Croix, Vevey-Samaritain); however, in the majority of cases, recourse to external capital was the only possible solution. Sometimes, the bank loan was only temporary and did not lead to serious financial dependence in the long run; for example, in Moudon, a new building was constructed in 1888 thanks to donations and a loan which was paid off three years later. In other cases, the loan had serious consequences. In Aigle, in order to build an infirmary, the administrators founded a real estate company in 1869 to which the operating profits were paid. This company contracted a debt for the construction of the new buildings which were placed at the disposal of the infirmary in return for the payment of rent and the amortisation of the loan. Until 1885, the infirmary paid a very large part of its annual operating profits to the real estate company. This financial dependence occasionally led to a delay in investments, as in 1877–1878 when it was decided to suspend the construction of a bathing and laundry room that was not completed until 1879. It was not until the second half of the 1880s that the financial burden decreased significantly.

These financial problems show the difficulty of making major investments within the framework of a traditional financing system that was highly dependent on private generosity. However, this method of financing the infirmaries was not fundamentally questioned. Only in Morges were there problems that could not be solved via philanthropic management. The new infirmary, opened in 1897 at a total cost of more than 110,000 francs, was only marginally financially dependent (a loan of 17,000 francs) but swallowed up the institution's assets. The proportion of self-financing in the house's operating income was only 2% in 1900, compared to 11% in 1885, so the total income only covered 65% of operating expenses that year, decreasing to 59% in 1906. In 1908 the directors declared they were "in the situation of a ship that is slowly sinking".[22] This difficult situation was only overcome with new resources generated by an increase in pension prices and private financing, thanks to the regular organisation of sales. In addition, in 1909 the district's municipalities were officially asked to include a contribution to the infirmary in their budgets. Some of them accepted this payment, but only as a voluntary donation.

[22] Morges Hospital, annual report, 1908, p. 6.

Table 3 Financial resources of local infirmaries in the canton of Vaud, around 1900

Type of resource	*Aubonne 1912*	*Montreux 1900*	*Morges 1900*	*Nyon 1900*	*St. Croix 1900*	*Vevey-Samaritan 1895*	*Vevey-Providence 1915*	*Yverdon 1900*
Own	42	–	2	11	26	10	30	14
Private	8	55	55	17	37	67	9	37
Pensions	49	43	38	72	37	23	61	48
Various	1	2	5	–	–	–	–	1

Source Hospital annual reports, 1895–1912

These examples illustrate the difficulties trustees had in finding the resources for heavy investment within a traditional management framework. The means most used by infirmaries to increase their resources was to increase the price of a day's boarding, whose growing importance in the financing of infirmaries is reflected in Table 3. The increase in hospital expenditure was thus passed on to the patients and those who subsidised them. Even though it is difficult to estimate the share of the pensions paid by insurance companies, municipalities and the state, it can be said that the proportion of patients admitted free of charge decreased significantly. Originally, the infirmaries were intended to be medical institutions for the working classes and accepted a large number of free hospitalisations. However, faced with the success of these infirmaries with the public at large, not only the underprivileged, the various administrations restricted this charitable policy and made the hospitalised participate in financing the institution. In Aigle, for example, the number of free hospitalisations fell sharply, from 26.9% of patients in 1878–1882 to 7.4% in 1889–1893.

Although the proportion of free admissions decreased, the administrative commissions did not solely pass the costs of hospitalisation on to the patients themselves. The second half of the nineteenth century saw the signing of numerous agreements with mutual aid societies in order to guarantee the hospitalisation of their members at a price fixed in advance. However, it is very difficult to obtain usable data on these societies before 1900. In the study published in 1888 by the Swiss Statistical Society, Hermann Kinkelin lamented the lack of reliable accounting data, writing, "we have no data of general value concerning the expenses incurred for medical treatment and care in hospitals".[23] Indeed, these various societies insure their members against loss of earnings in the event of illness and accident, sometimes with a contribution to a hospital or outpatient medical costs, but this share is difficult to identify and quantify (Table 4).

[23] Hermannn Kinkelin, *Les Sociétés de secours mutuels en Suisse en 1880*, Berne, 1888, p. 55.

Table 4 Mutual aid societies in the canton of Vaud in 1880 and 1903

	1880		*1903*	
		in % of total		*in % of total*
Total number of societies	31		65	
Societies paying for hospitalisation	6	19.4	7	10.8
Total expenditure (in francs)	175′374		930′836	
Hospital expenditure (in francs)	5′837	3.3	8′050	0.9
Total number of members	12′615		18′542	
Members covered for hospitalisation	3′027	24.0	4′676	25.2

Source Hermann Kinkelin, op. cit., *Les sociétés de secours mutuels en Suisse en l'année 1903*, Berne, Federal Department of Industry, 1907

According to the official data reproduced in Table 4, there was a strong development of mutual aid societies between 1880 and 1903 in the canton of Vaud: the number of funds doubled and the number of insured members increased by 47%, while their expenditure rose by 430%. However, this growth did not lead to an extension of the coverage of hospital costs. Although a quarter of the insured were members of a fund that covered hospital expenses, access to this type of coverage was undoubtedly very restrictive, since it only amounted to 3.3% of fund expenditure in 1880 and 0.9% in 1903. As a proportion of the total population of the canton, members of funds paying hospital costs represented only 1.3% of the population of Vaud in 1880 and 1.7% in 1903.

The primary aim of the mutual aid funds was to help people who had fallen into indigence due to illness, accident or death in the family, all of which were unforeseeable events that no longer allowed an individual or a family to live from their work.[24] It seems that the signing of an agreement between an infirmary and a mutual aid fund did not automatically imply that the latter would pay hospital costs. Above all, it guaranteed a fixed price per day, sometimes at a preferential rate, for members of the mutual funds.

The public authorities also financed all or part of the hospitalisation of their indigents. The municipalities were particularly active; for example, they paid for the hospitalisation of 35.9% of patients in Aigle between 1878 and 1893. Finally, by virtue of the law about infirmaries adopted in 1875, the State subsidised the hospitalisation of indigent patients who could not be admitted to the Cantonal Hospital for lack of space. This state intervention should be seen in the context of the beginning of a comprehensive hospital policy at the cantonal level and the redeployment of the Cantonal Hospital during the

[24] David Muheim, *Le mutualisme contre l'assurance sociale. La Fédération des Sociétés de secours mutuels de la Suisse romande et les premiers projets d'assurance maladie (1893–1912)*, University of Lausanne, unpublished dissertation, 1998, p. 96.

1870s. The State's payment of hospitalisation costs for indigent patients in local infirmaries was a characteristic feature of Vaud's hospital policy for more than a century (see Chapter 5).

Between Philanthropy and Medicine: Lausanne's Specialised Hospitals

The philanthropic hospital establishments in the canton of Vaud were not limited to local infirmaries. Three specialised institutions founded in the city of Lausanne in the mid-nineteenth century should be added: the Blind People's Asylum (1843), the Children's Hospice (1861) and the Orthopaedic Hospice (1876). These institutions originated from the Protestant philanthropic milieu and have many similarities with the local infirmaries. Firstly, in terms of management, these institutions also owed their existence and annual resources to charitable gestures, although the financial commitment was on a completely different scale. The philanthropists of Lausanne invested considerable sums of money in their private hospitals but this had nothing to do with those funds made available to the local infirmaries. The Blind People's Asylum was founded and financed by an English aristocrat living in Lausanne, William Haldimand, who was responsible for the establishment's annual deficits until his death (1862), contributing a total of more than one million francs to the institution.[25] Alongside Haldimand, the liberal families of Lausanne and a few foreign aristocrats, including the Queen of England, provided the bulk of the Asylum's resources, whose fortune rose from some 65,000 francs in 1860 to over 730,000 francs in 1910. As a result, the rate of self-financing was high and constantly increasing (5.1% in 1850 and 44.2% in 1890). Donations and the institution's resources accounted for more than 80% of its income until the 1880s. Although less wealthy, the Children's Hospice and the Orthopaedic Hospice also depended on private generosity.[26] More than 80% of the income of the former depended on private support until around 1900, compared to almost 70% of the latter's income during the 1870s. Another point in common with the local infirmaries was that, in Lausanne, these specialised institutions were managed by administrative commissions in which members of the upper social strata of Lausanne, generally close to the Liberal Party and the Free Church, predominated. The size of these three establishments was also limited at the time of their opening: there were 22 beds at the Children's Hospice and eight beds at the Orthopaedic Hospice, while the Blind People's Asylum had 122 hospitalisations in 1850 and 201 in 1860.

It is mainly at the medical level that these three institutions differed from the local infirmaries. The position they occupied not only filled a niche in the

[25] Jacques Clavel and Jacques David Chausson, *La pérennité d'une vocation: Asile des aveugles, Lausanne: centre d'accueil, d'instruction et d'adaptation pour aveugles et faibles de vue: 1843–1993*, Lausanne: Fondation de l'Asile des aveugles, 1993.

[26] The Children's Hospice had capital assets of 22,550 francs in 1900 and the Orthopaedic Hospice about 40,000 francs in 1911.

philanthropic market but also in the healthcare market. As Lindsay Granshaw pointed out, in England, the existence of a specialised hospital could prove decisive in the recognition of a new specialisation in medicine.[27] The Blind People's Asylum fits perfectly into this model. It was born from a meeting between philanthropists and a young doctor who wanted to specialise in ophthalmology, Frédéric Recordon, but did not have access to a hospital department. After spending a few months as an intern at the Cantonal Hospital in 1837, he had only a private practice in the city. His subsequent position as head doctor of the Asylum made him the first recognised specialist in his field in the Canton of Vaud. The situation is somewhat similar in the case of the Orthopaedic Hospice which offered institutional legitimacy to its founder, Henri Martin (see Chapter 2). Only the Children's Hospice deviates from this model since the doctors at its head did not specialise in paediatrics but remained generalists.

Conclusion

Local infirmaries in the Canton of Vaud were originally a product of the Protestant Revival and, as such, were not part of a medical revolution. They were extremely small institutions with limited therapeutic ambitions. These infirmaries were collective works in which a charitable conception of assistance predominated. The idea of helping one's neighbour while respecting the social order was the basis of these institutions.

Moreover, although the local socio-economic contexts were not the same everywhere, there was a certain homogeneity in these infirmaries. Despite the demographic development of the Canton of Vaud during the period 1870–1900 as its population rose from 229,588 to 281,379, the trend towards urbanisation remained limited, with the exception of the city of Lausanne which alone absorbed almost half of the demographic increase—from 28,545 to 46,732 inhabitants—and the Vevey-Montreux area, which was the second urban centre of the canton. In 1900, the canton included three towns with more than 10,000 inhabitants (Lausanne, Montreux, Vevey) which accounted for 25.6% of the canton's population.[28] However, the growth of the canton was also due to the emergence of small regional centres. Until 1900, the socio-economic development of the canton of Vaud did not fundamentally challenge the balance between the various parts of the territory. This relative stability largely explains the homogeneous character of the local infirmaries and their presence throughout the canton. The operating expenses of these establishments in 1900 show no break between urban centres and rural towns; they all amount to a few tens of thousands of francs. In the canton as a whole, the infirmaries were still small and essentially charitable in nature,

[27] Lindsay Grandshaw, "Fame and fortune...", op. cit.

[28] *Annuaire statistique du canton de Vaud - 1985*, Lausanne: Service cantonal de recherche et d'information statistiques, 1985.

not materially ready for the change in scale that took place with the arrival of the surgeon-modernisers, whose intervention dismantled the philanthropic financial structure.

3 The Development of Hospital Surgery and Its Consequences (1900–1960)

The arrival of a new generation of surgeons in the local infirmaries of Vaud, generally trained at the German school and often pupils of César Roux, had a strong influence on the development of these establishments. Eager to put their new knowledge into practice, they demanded an improvement in the hospital infrastructure (new operating rooms, new buildings, hiring of additional staff, etc.) which necessitated profound managerial and organisational reform. Of course, they were not the only doctors to benefit from the transformation of the hospital infrastructure in the first part of the twentieth century—a phenomenon that affected the entire medical profession. However, surgeons stood out from their colleagues by their early involvement in hospitals. They were the first to demand the profound modernisation of hospitals and often imposed themselves as chief physicians. Other types of doctors, such as radiologists and ENT specialists, followed in their footsteps, mainly in the 1950s.

The Arrival of Modernising Surgeons

Before the arrival of the new generation of surgeon-modernisers, surgery did not occupy a special place in the local infirmaries. Some did not distinguish between *surgery* and *medicine* but spoke in their annual reports of *external* and *internal diseases*. The operations carried out in these establishments were essentially related to external pathology (fractures, wounds, sores, contusions, abscesses, etc.). Invasive surgery was almost non-existent before the arrival of modern surgeons. Surgical cases were mainly the result of injuries and accidents treated by the doctor on duty in the infirmary. In the event of a particularly delicate operation, he could call on a specialist surgeon from Lausanne. The surgical infrastructure was thus reduced to its simplest form; the infirmaries were not the temples of triumphant medicine as found in the university centres.

Young surgeons from the Canton of Vaud, most of whom were trained at the universities of Lausanne and Berne, acquired their technical and organisational know-how in the infirmaries that opened their doors to them. The modernisation of the medico-technical infrastructure (operating theatres, radiology, etc.) they demanded made the infirmaries their main working tool. The directors of the Orbe Infirmary declared, in 1935, "our vast house does not only receive hospitalised patients, but also provides more and more services to the private clientele of our doctors, by placing at their disposal the resources of our equipment (X-rays, quartz lamp, diathermy apparatus, pantostat, etc.) and above all the skills of our devoted deaconesses".[29] The hospital thus became the treatment centre for the private clientele of the doctors who operated on an ever-increasing number of patients. They established themselves as the real heads of the establishments, with young interns—a new function created in the regional hospitals during the inter-war period—under their orders, to the detriment of the deaconess sisters who until then had had the upper hand in these infirmaries.

The arrival of these modernising surgeons had a direct impact on the organisation of the medical service of the local infirmaries. The rotation between the various practitioners in the locality was quickly abandoned and led to a separation between the medical and surgical services. Surgery in these establishments thus became autonomous and was henceforth dependent on "specialists"—often holding the title of FMH specialist after the 1930s. In the Château-d'Oex, for example, Jean-Philibert Exchaquet, a general practitioner who was appointed head of the surgical department in 1940, left his hospital service in 1947–1948 to take courses to obtain the title of FMH specialist in surgery. This postgraduate training enabled him to acquire new knowledge as well as to secure his position as head surgeon against the arrival of a possible competitor. On his return in 1948, he reorganised the surgical department and purchased new equipment. Symbolising this entry into the surgical era, the Schaerer mass-produced de Quervain table made its appearance in the operating theatre (1948) (Table 5).[30]

Infirmaries entered an era of growth that was not solely the result of population increase. During the inter-war period, the canton of Vaud experienced a certain demographic stagnation (with a population of 317,457 in 1910 and 343,398 in 1941). The population increase was mainly in the city of Lausanne, rising from 64,446 to 92,541, and, to a lesser extent, in the towns of Yverdon (from 8634 to 10,865 inhabitants) and Morges (from 4564 to 5689 inhabitants). Apart from these few cases, the territory of Vaud showed extremely low growth, becoming negative in some countryside areas.[31] Rather than demographic pressure, it was the change in the nature of the infirmaries and in the population's attitudes towards the use of hospital care that explained the redeployment of hospitals between the two World Wars.

An Example of Modernisation: The Aigle Hospital

The example of the Aigle Hospital illustrates perfectly the influence of the surgeon-moderniser in the transition from the philanthropic infirmary to the modern hospital.[32] This establishment, opened in 1867 by local philanthropists, is a classic example of the Vaud infirmary at the end of the nineteenth century: of small size (25 beds in 1871), with medical rotation between local

[29] Orbe Hospital, annual report, 1935, p. 3.

[30] Château-d'Oex Hospital, annual reports, 1940–1950.

[31] *Annuaire statistique du canton de Vaud - 1985*, op. cit.

[32] Aigle Hospital, annual reports.

Table 5 Surgeons-modernizers in Vaud regional hospitals

Hospital	*Surgeon*	*Period of office*	*Place of training*
Aigle	William Soutter	1925–c.1970	Lausanne (Roux)
Aubonne	Gustave Piotet	1927–1955	Lausanne (Roux)
Bex	Henri Vuilleumier	1916–?	Lausanne (Roux)
Château-d'Oex	Jean-Philibert Exchaquet	1940–1980	Lausanne (Decker)
Lausanne, Orthopaedic Hospice	Placide Nicod	1905–1948	Lausanne (Roux)
Lausanne, Children's Hospice	Henri Vulliet	1910–1925	Lausanne (Roux)
	Léon Picot	1926–1957	Lausanne (Roux)
Lavaux	Charles Rochat	1950–1976	Lausanne (Vulliet) and Geneva (Jentzer)
Montreux	Charles Perret	1909–1949	Berne (Niehans)
	Georges Chessex	1912–1949	Germany, Krefeld
Morges	Raoul Masson	1923–1938	Geneva (Girard)
Moudon	Alfred Goin	1931–1970	Lausanne (Vulliet)
Nyon	Gustave Piotet	1927–1963	Lausanne (Roux)
Orbe	Walter Moehrlen	1905–1945	Lausanne (Roux)
Payerne	Armand Givel	1883–1918	Berne (Kocher)
	Charles Yersin	1895–1951[33]	Geneva (Julliard)
Rolle	Gustave Piotet	1927–1952	Lausanne (Roux)
Saint-Loup	Henri Curchod	1907–1931	Lausanne (Roux)
Sainte-Croix	Armand Sandoz	1926–1942	Berne (de Quervain)
Le Sentier	Jämes Rochat	1934–1963	Lausanne (Vulliet)
Vevey-Samaritain	Charles Perret	1918–1946	Berne (Niehans)
	Paul Niehans jr	1918–1946	Berne (Niehans)
Yverdon	Georges Pérusset	1891–1937	Lausanne (Roux)
	Samuel Cuendet	1923–1949	Lausanne (Roux)

doctors, the presence of the deaconesses of Saint-Loup (from 1896) and very few surgical cases (an average of 62.3 cases per year in 1875–1890). Patients were mainly men (80.6% in 1875–1890), hospitalised for various wounds and injuries (49.4%). The majority of patients were farmers (39.5% in 1875 and 42.5% in 1880), servants and employees (25.5% in 1875 and 15.6% in 1880) and artisans (22.5% in 1875 and 14.9% in 1880). The "surgical cases" were most likely to be men from the working classes who were hospitalised following an accident.

The Aigle Hospital experienced an important turning point with the arrival in the town of a young graduate of the University of Lausanne, William Soutter, who was integrated into the medical team of the establishment in 1925. Surgical operations described in the annual reports as "special" or "important", that is, most likely invasive, were already being performed before Soutter's arrival, thanks to the collaboration of external consultant surgeons,

[33] Yersin was absent from the Payerne Hospital between 1913 and 1935.

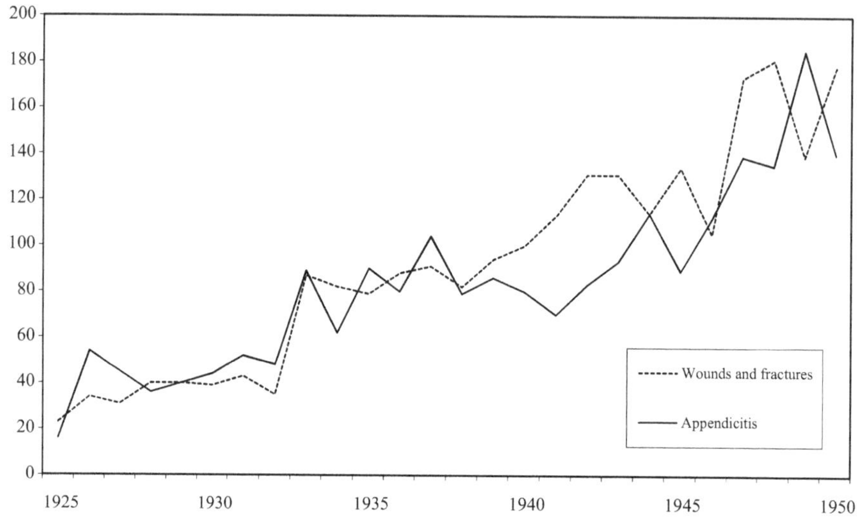

Fig. 3 Hospitalisations in the surgical department of the Aigle Hospital for wounds/fractures and appendicitis, 1925–1950 (*Source* Aigle Hospital, annual reports, 1925–1950)

albeit in very small numbers. Soutter had the knowledge to develop the new surgery on a large scale and thus offered a certain reputation to the local infirmary. The trustees grasped this challenge and stated, in 1927: "Thanks to the presence of a local surgeon, the number of operations performed in our house is constantly increasing and we can dispense with the need to call on outside surgeons for special cases. We are anxious to be able to prove our gratitude to our doctors without too much delay by providing them with a building equipped with medical services meeting modern requirements".[34] A new hospital, equipped with an X-ray facility and designed according to the standard T-shaped model (see pp. 148–149), was inaugurated in 1931.

The appendectomy, exceptional before Soutter's arrival—11 cases in 1923 and 19 in 1924—became symbolic of this new surgery. Between 1925 and 1945, appendicitis operations experienced a very high annual growth rate, amounting to 8.5%, which remained very high in the years 1945–1950 (7.8%). However, the new treatments, such as appendicitis operations, did not replace the more traditional conditions treated in the surgical departments which remained important, as did hospitalisations for "wounds and factures", whose evolution was similar to that of appendicitis operations (see Fig. 3). The new surgical procedures did not replace the older ones but were added to them, also benefitting from the modernisation of the medical and technical infrastructure (X-ray facilities, sterilisers, operating tables, etc.).

[34] Aigle Hospital, annual report, 1927, p. 4.

The new surgery was a highly profitable innovation for the institution. The fees collected from patients for the use of the operating theatre and the X-ray installation amounted to 10,445 francs in 1933 (11.4% of operating resources) and 39,315 francs in 1950 (17.1%). At the same time, the hospital changed gradually in its status. It tended to open up to a wider section of the population, particularly the middle and wealthy classes. This transformation had a welcome financial impact. Pensions for patients rose sharply between 1920 (16,867 francs) and 1950 (214,027 francs). In the 1950s, they became practically the only source of income: their share of operating income rose from 47.1% in 1920 to 94.3% in 1950.

In order to respond to this growth dynamic, the hospital's administrators expanded their services. The medical team was increased: a second surgeon was appointed in 1946 and the radiology department, until then run by a deaconess, was handed over to a doctor in 1951. The commission stated, in 1967, the X-ray installation, paid for by a bank loan, "was very quickly amortised by the very strong and continuous increase in the net output of this department". This was indeed the case as the annual reports show a steadily increasing gross profit for the Radiology Department during the 1950s, rising from 40,245 francs in 1952 to over 95,000 francs in 1960. The surge in the number of hospitalisations perfectly reflects this evolution, from a total of 243 patients in 1920 to 1102 in 1950 and 1278 in 1960.[35]

Internal Reorganisation of Hospitals

When the surgeon-modernisers moved to the regional hospitals, it was not for charitable reasons but for professional motives. The implementation of hospital surgical skillsets acquired at the University required a new organisation of work in the local infirmaries. This was characterised by a clear separation between the internal medicine and the surgery departments, as well as a reorganisation of the hierarchy of nursing staff.

Empowerment of Medical Services

One of the first steps taken by surgeon-modernisers was the separation of internal medicine from the surgery department. This did not usually cause any relational problems with other non-specialist doctors for whom access to the hospital infrastructure was not a professional necessity. Surgeons were often the only ones working permanently in regional hospitals, where they also admitted their private patients, in contrast to other doctors who treated patients at home. In practice, they became the head of the hospital, even if they did not usually have the title of "head doctor". Surgeons were invested with a recognised know-how and the reputation of their masters. It was therefore "natural" that they were entrusted with surgical services.

[35] *1867–1967, Hôpital d'Aigle. Cent années hospitalières*, Aigle, Hôpital, 1967, n.p.

As for the internal medicine departments, they were often organised according to the rotation system between several doctors (Bex, Montreux, Nyon, Payerne, Rolle, etc.), sometimes leading to requests for reorganisation, as in the Montreux Hospital in 1923: "The medical service was provided by three doctors who took turns for three months. In our opinion, this training period is too short, as it does not allow individual doctors to treat patients with sufficient unity. We do not see any possibility of change with the current organisation. As long as doctors have the free medical consultation, where many wealthy people send their employees, the surgical policlinic and the clinical treatment of inpatients, the assistance to surgeons and the tedious but necessary administrative paperwork, they will have to give a lot of their time to the infirmary. Alongside their private professional activities, this is a big job".[36]

This intervention highlights the secondary nature of the hospital service of non-surgical practitioners. As in the nineteenth century, they continued to essentially live off their private practice. However, as was the case at the Cantonal Hospital a century earlier, the growth of the hospital would require a greater commitment—an increased presence of general practitioners which the latter could not concede without risking losing their private and solvent clientele. One of their main requests was the hiring of an intern doctor to carry out subordinate tasks.

Sometimes, the administrative commissions also received another type of demand from non-surgical doctors concerning access to the hospital infrastructure (aseptic operating theatres, radiological facilities, etc.) for their private practice. The case of Yverdon Hospital gives an example of the issues raised by this type of request. During discussions on the organisation of the new hospital, which opened in 1939, the medical profession asked the committee to establish "a permanent medical service, that is, one that was constantly provided by the same doctors".[37] They proposed the creation of four departments (surgery, surgery-medicine, medicine and ENT), each headed by a single doctor. The committee accepted this reorganisation, not without first pointing out "the steering committee remains the sole master of the hospital's internal regulations, including the distribution of medical services".[38] Meanwhile, the question of opening the establishment to external doctors remained delicate. Pache, who was to head the medical service, declared "the door must be open to newcomers without anything automatic being done in their favour".[39] On behalf of the town's doctors, Vodoz, who specialised in pneumology, expressed concern about access to the X-ray facility and operating

[36] Montreux Hospital, annual report, 1923, p. 9.

[37] Yverdon Hospital, letter from the medical corps to the steering committee, 10 March 1939.

[38] Yverdon Hospital, minutes of the steering committee, 20 March 1939.

[39] Yverdon Hospital, minutes of the board of directors, 22 March 1939.

theatre. Bidlingmeyer obtained a guarantee that practitioners from the neighbouring countryside would be put on an equal footing with their colleagues in the town.

A similar organisation was adopted in Sainte-Croix (1940), Aigle (1943) and Payerne (1947). The Lavaux Hospital, which opened in 1940, pushed the logic of the medical profession's work tool the furthest. In 1943, this establishment refused to admit indigent patients, arguing that no doctor had been appointed to head the establishment and so no one could take care of patients who were not solvent.[40] In 1945, this hospital declared that it "worked like a private clinic".[41] The regional hospitals were not, therefore, organisations intended only for surgeon-modernisers. Their medico-technical infrastructure was accessible to external doctors (private surgeons, general practitioners, etc.), even if it was not always at the heart of their professional practice.

Working Alongside the Doctors, the Deaconesses (1880–1930)

With the arrival of Pastor Rau-Vaucher at the head of the Institution of Deaconesses of Saint-Loup in 1881, the latter entered a new phase that could be described as *hospital-based*. Until then, the deaconesses had been active across the private assistance sector (the elderly, orphans, the sick, schools, etc.) but were now refocusing on the hospital sector which was to become their exclusive preserve. Saint-Loup's connections in Lausanne's liberal circles enabled them, through Frédéric Recordon, to be entrusted with the hospital service of the new Cantonal Hospital of Lausanne (1883). Recordon played the role of intermediary between private philanthropic circles and the radical-democratic state. He was the founder and first doctor of the Blind People's Asylum (1843–1880) and, in 1857, was appointed head of the Health Service (Department of the Interior), a position he held until 1885. In this capacity, he supervised the construction and organisation of the new Cantonal Hospital. In this role, he called upon the deaconesses of Saint-Loup.[42] Twelve deaconesses, from a total of about forty in service, entered this establishment in 1883. Access to the Cantonal Hospital, which became a university hospital in 1890, enabled Saint-Loup to train its students and to send them to work in other hospitals. Between 1891 and 1930, no fewer than 194 deaconesses took up their duties at the Cantonal Hospital.[43] Most were at the beginning of their career: 71 were aged between 20 and 25 years (36.6%) and 50 between 26 and 30 years (25.8%). Their length of service was relatively low: 61 stayed for a maximum of two years (34.7%) and 58 between two and five years (33.0%). Only 33 deaconesses (18.8%) remained at the Cantonal Hospital for ten years

[40] ACV, S 73, minutes of the HHC, 1943.

[41] ACV, K VIII D 58, letter from the Lavaux Infirmary to the Department of the Interior, 20 December 1945.

[42] Institution of Deaconesses of Saint-Loup, annual report, 1896–1897, pp. 34–35.

[43] ACV, KVIII E 91–92.

or more. Most only passed through the Cantonal Hospital which confirms the formative role of this institution.

Access to the Cantonal Hospital in 1883 thus represented official recognition by the State for Saint-Loup. However, as the example of Geneva illustrates, recognition by the radical government of a deaconess house was not self-evident. Indeed, the introduction of deaconesses from Berne to the Cantonal Hospital in Geneva in 1891 was the subject of heated political battles in the 1890s between radicals and conservatives.[44] The support of the Canton of Vaud was very welcome in Saint-Loup, as it opened up new prospects for the development of the institution. Its administrators declared, in 1884, "the enlargement of our field of work has brought us friendly relations in that part of the public which previously knew little about us".[45] In the period 1883–1914, deaconesses were employed in 64 institutions, including 27 hospitals. The other posts were part of the tradition of all-out social commitment of the previous years but were not perpetuated; for example, the deaconesses took charge of seven nurseries (six of which were abandoned before 1920), 14 posts of visiting sisters (seven abandoned) and 16 various hospices (three abandoned).[46] The priority given to the growing hospital sector allowed the number of deaconesses in charge to increase. They rose from 41 in 1880 to 68 in 1892, 178 in 1906 and 251 in 1920. The Saint-Loup Hospital was the second training centre for deaconesses. Enlarged, transformed and modernised in 1897, it became a reference establishment in French-speaking Switzerland.

Already present in half of the local infirmaries in the canton of Vaud before 1890, the deaconesses were entrusted with the internal management of the other establishments which were enlarged and modernised (Nyon 1895; Orthopaedic Hospice 1892; Aigle 1896; Aubonne 1897; Orbe 1901; Château-d'Oex 1904; Bex 1911). On the eve of the First World War, the deaconesses were present in all the local infirmaries of the Canton of Vaud. The importance they assumed in these establishments led to a redefinition of their positions—a move that did not always go down well with the lay staff who had previously been highly autonomous. For example, in Montreux, in 1887, the administrators of the institution were obliged to completely change the staff of the house following conflicts between deaconesses and lay employees.[47]

The deaconesses accompanied the doctors in the implementation of the new hospital surgery, thanks to certain professional qualities and values of obedience and self-sacrifice which corresponded to the expectations of the administrators and the doctors. However, the relationship between deaconesses and doctors was ambiguous. For example, in Yverdon in 1905, there were major problems between a former resident of César Roux, Ernest Demiéville, and the

[44] See Joëlle Droux, *L'attraction céleste*..., op. cit., pp. 192–239.

[45] Institution of deaconesses of Saint-Loup, annual report, 1883–1884, p. 8.

[46] J. Vincent, op. cit., pp. 297–299.

[47] Montreux Hospital, minutes of the administrative commission, 1887.

deaconesses who did not follow his prescriptions. The administrative commission had to intervene to "recommend to the sisters and the staff the strict observance of the rules".[48] The young doctor wanted to be obeyed in the infirmary and demanded "that his orders should not be discussed in the presence of the patients".[49] The situation was similar in Morges, where, in 1913, the doctors denounced the excessive authoritarianism of the deaconess superior. They reproached her for being the cause of several early departures of lay nurses and therefore for not having "the collaborators they needed for surgical operations".[50] The administrative commission consequently dismissed the deaconesses and obtained—not without difficulty—new ones.

Appointment of Resident Doctors and Lay Nurses (1930–1950)

The phase of relative harmony with the medical profession lasted until the reorganisation of the hospitals in the 1930s which saw the arrival of resident doctors and lay bursars. The reorganisation of the hospitals involved a redistribution of tasks among the various caregivers. Before the arrival of the surgeon-modernisers, deaconesses ran the infirmaries. They were in charge of both care—as doctors were only temporary—and finances—before the appointment of bursars and salaried accountants. Surgeons fundamentally challenged this organisation. From now on, doctors were the heads of their autonomous departments. They were assisted by interns, appointed in the regional hospitals during the inter-war period and in the 1940s onwards (Children Hospice 1911, Montreux 1928, Vevey-Samaritain 1930, Nyon 1940, Yverdon 1940, Aigle 1943, Payerne 1944, Sainte-Croix 1946, Morges 1959, etc.). It is highly probable that the disorganisation of hospital services caused by mobilisation during World War II reinforced the idea of the need to appoint in-house doctors. For the medical profession, it was a question of ensuring, as at the Cantonal Hospital, a medical permanence and the follow-up of care during their absence. In order to better assert their dominant position in relation to the deaconesses, the doctors could not give up such an important area of autonomy to the latter. Conflicts between deaconesses and the medical profession increased; they reflect the difficulties produced by the redistribution of tasks within the hospitals.

Subsequently, it became necessary to employ more nursing staff to ensure the functioning of these resized hospitals. In Aigle, for example, the number of employees without doctors—rose from 15 in 1931 to 28 in 1945. The rise in the number of lay hospital staff resulted in a sharp growth in the hospitals' wage bills. In Yverdon, the share of salaries in operating costs rose from 11% in 1920 to 39% in 1950. The deaconesses of Saint-Loup still held a very important place in the medical services, particularly in the upper echelons

48 Yverdon Hospital, minutes of the administrative commission, 7 November 1905.

49 Ibid.

50 Morges Hospital, minutes of the administrative commission, 11 March 1913.

of the hierarchy, but they were not enough to meet the demand by themselves. All the hospital administrations regularly asked Saint-Loup to increase the number of sisters available for their establishments. It quickly became difficult for the motherhouse to meet these requests. Facing a lack of availability, the deaconesses were even withdrawn from the Château-d'Oex Hospital in 1945, foreshadowing the great withdrawals of the 1960s.

Qualified lay personnel were called upon from other training courses, such as the La Source Nursing School in Lausanne which, in the 1930s, sent trainees to several establishments (Aigle, Nyon, etc.). Similarly, the opening of analysis laboratories led to the hiring of qualified lay laboratory assistants (Montreux 1934, Château-d'Oex 1943, Payerne 1943, Nyon 1944, Rolle 1946, Sainte-Croix 1950, Morges 1958, etc.). Despite their professional qualifications, these para-medical staff had more than basic working conditions. For example, the laboratory assistant hired in Montreux in 1934 was paid only to cover the meals she received at the hospital, which she left after six months of work.[51] Even if they employed lay professionals, hospital administrators continued to conceive of the work of their employees according to the traditional philanthropic ideal: service to the sick, done in silence, abnegation and sacrifice, forming an integral part of femininity.[52]

Architectural Uniformity of Regional Hospitals

The modernisation of Vaud infirmaries took shape in the construction of new buildings, which were built in two phases (1897–1913 and 1920–1940). Unlike the previous generation, these new hospitals were not built from a local perspective by local architects. Instead, there was standardisation of hospital buildings, both in terms of their medical and technical infrastructure and the organisation of space. This standardisation was favoured by the omnipresence of a few Lausanne architects who had established themselves as true experts in hospital matters. Eager to offer their institution—and the surgeon-modernisers who practised there—a modern infrastructure favourable to the development of scientific medicine, hospital administrators resorted to these experts.

The first of them was the architect Henri Verrey (1852–1928). His reputation in Vaud philanthropic circles preceded his reputation as a builder of hospitals. Indeed, like his father Jules Verrey, he was strongly committed to the Free Church, for which he built many chapels, partly financed by William Barbey.[53] He was also a member of the committees of the Children Hospice and of the real estate association which managed the property of the Free Church of Lausanne. It is therefore no coincidence that his first medical project was the new Saint-Loup Hospital (1897), financed in large part by William Barbey's brother-in-law. This establishment, whose medico-technical

[51] Montreux Hospital, minutes of the administrative commission, 1934.

[52] See Joëlle Droux, *L'attraction…*, op. cit.

[53] Dave Lüthi, op. cit., p. 37.

infrastructure was built on the expertise of prof. Fritz de Quervain,[54] quickly became a model for reference, with its glass rotunda providing optimal lighting in the operating theatre.[55] Verrey also built the new buildings of the Yverdon Hospital (1901), in which there was a modern operating theatre designed on the Saint-Loup model; the private clinic Bois-Cerf, in Lausanne, where his brother, the ophthalmologist Louis Verrey, practised (1902); the Lavigny hospice for epileptics (1907); the Lausanne Infirmary, established as part of the La Source Nursing School (1907); the Monthey Infirmary in the Canton of Valais (1910); the Children Hospice in Lausanne (1910); as well as several alpine sanatoriums.

Not all of these establishments were built according to a uniform model. The diversity of architectural styles is obvious: the Saint-Loup Hospital resembles a mansion, the Yverdon Infirmary a traditional family home, the Bois-Cerf Clinic a hotel in Lake Geneva, etc. It was rather at the level of the medical-technical infrastructure that uniformity was achieved. The operating theatre was equipped with technology produced by Schaerer and with mosaic floors rather than wooden ones, as well as an X-ray installation, which became the symbols of hospital modernity at the turn of the century. Verrey established itself as the leading expert in hospital construction in the canton of Vaud.

The second generation of architects who played a decisive role in the standardisation of hospitals was represented by Georges Epitaux (1873–1957) and Charles Thévenaz (1882–1966).[56] Epitaux made a name for himself as a specialist in hospital matters with the construction of the Maternity Ward of the Cantonal Hospital (1916) and the clinics of Dr. Rollier in Leysin (1927–1928), as well as the transformation of the Hotel Cecil into a private clinic (1931).[57] He reached the peak of his fame with the design of the Athens Maternity Hospital (1933) and the Nestlé Hospital in Lausanne (1935). Although he did not personally design a regional hospital in the canton of Vaud, he was very much involved in the juries that decided on the awarding of works (Montreux 1913; Hospice Sandoz 1928; Aigle 1930; Rolle 1930; etc.), often alongside the state architect Eugène Bron and local personalities who were members of the administrative commissions.[58] As for Thévenaz, he designed the new hospital buildings of the Orthopaedic Hospice (1928)

[54] According to Emile Bonard, op. cit., p. 12.

[55] In its report on the transformations to be made to the establishment, drafted in 1898, the Nyon Infirmary's construction commission asked for "an operating room based on the Saint-Loup model". Quoted by Gustave Piotet, op. cit., p. 31.

[56] Pierre Frey, *Alphonse Laverrière, 1872–1954. Parcours dans les archives d'un architecte*, Lausanne: Presses polytechniques et universitaires romandes, 1999 and *Ingénieurs et architectes vaudois. L'esprit d'entreprise*, Le Mont-sur-Lausanne, SIA, 1987.

[57] Dave Lüthi and Bruno Corthésy, *L'Hôtel Cecil à Lausanne: étude historique*, Lausanne: Bureau de recherche en histoire de l'architecture, 2002.

[58] *Bulletin technique de la Suisse romande*, various years.

and Sainte-Croix Hospital (1947) and built the Germond pavilion of Saint-Loup Hospital (1935). He also sat on the juries for the competitions for the construction of the hospitals in Yverdon (1936) and Lavaux (1939).

These two architects were the main experts used by the hospital administrations in the inter-war period to decide on the awarding of works and, as such, they were essential actors in the standardisation of buildings towards a single T-shaped model (Aigle, Lavaux, Nyon, Rolle, Saint-Loup, Sainte-Croix, etc.). Hugli and Teysseire, architects of the new Rolle Infirmary, representative of this T-shaped model, stated, that in 1934, they had designed their building "following the example of similar constructions carried out in recent years, such as the new Beaujon Hospital in Paris and the Nestlé Hospital in Lausanne [...]".[59] The T-shaped model, as it became established in French-speaking Switzerland in the 1930s, was based on the functional division of hospital space and on the control of internal flows, according to a model imported from the United States.[60] As French architects wrote in the immediate post-war period, "in the United States, there is a growing tendency to abandon the vertical hospital, based on the principle of a pure and simple superposition of pavilions. On the contrary, they try to create, as far as possible, level relationships between the hospitalisation and the diagnostic and therapeutic services. Thus, the operating departments are placed on the same floor as the corresponding hospitalisation departments. Similarly, the laboratory is preferably placed on the same level as the inpatient departments and the general medical consultation departments. This arrangement generally results in a T or H shape, with the wing containing the diagnostic and therapeutic services being perpendicular to the hospital block, which is usually oriented to the south".[61] In Switzerland, establishments designed on this model were built as early as the mid-1920s. One of the first of these was the Lory Hospital, opened in Berne in 1927 and directed from 1929 by a former resident of César Roux, Fritz Dumont, who was also a private doctor of surgery at the University of Berne.[62]

These hospitals were oriented in a north–south direction. The south wing included the hospital block where the patients' rooms were located. The north wing housed the therapeutic services and, in particular, the operating theatre which was ideally located "in a dead end", as recommended by hospital architects to maintain aseptic conditions.[63] The location of the operating theatres to the north met the need for constant natural light, without changing shadows—no longer relevant with the development of artificial light—as well as a temperature that was as stable as possible. Finally, the hotel services

[59] *La Construction moderne*, 1934, p. 130.

[60] Isidore Rosenfield, *Hospitals—Integrated Design*, New York: Progressive Architecture Library, 1947.

[61] «La santé publique», *L'architecture aujourd'hui*, n°15, novembre 1947, p. 34.

[62] See *La construction*..., op. cit., pp. 24–26.

[63] Isidore Rosenfield, op. cit., p. 108.

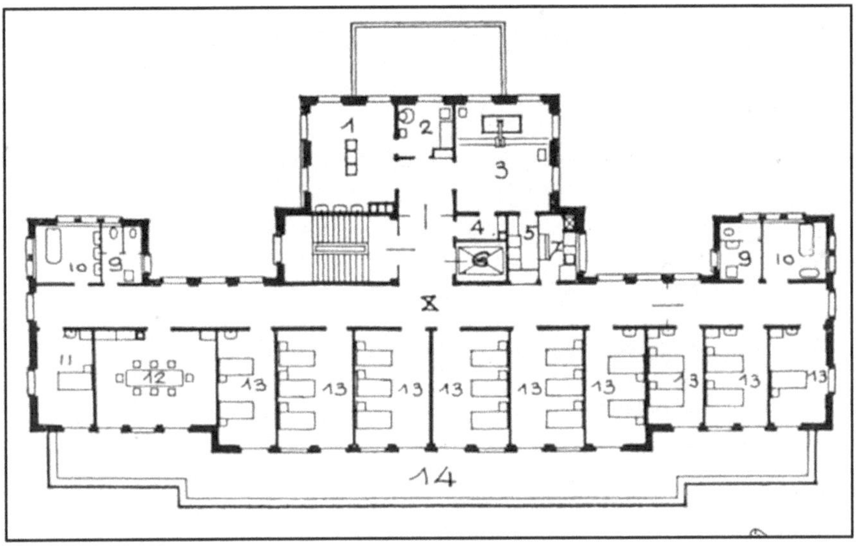

Fig. 4 Plan of Rolle Hospital, 1st floor, 1930 (*Source Bulletin technique de la Suisse romande*, 1938, p. 22)

(kitchens, laundry, etc.) were located in the basement. The straight corridors and the lifts allowed for optimal management of both horizontal and vertical flows within the building. When the new Sainte-Croix Hospital was designed in 1927, the commission explained that the role of the lift was to connect "all the floors and [to facilitate] the transport of patients, who could, if necessary, be taken without a stretcher, in their own bed, to the operating table, to the X-rays or to the baths. It will also be used to take the laundry from the laundry room to the drying room on the second floor".[64]

The Rolle Hospital is an excellent example of the application of this model to the regional hospitals of Vaud (see Fig. 4). The patient rooms (13) are located in the south wing and the operating theatre, with the operating room (1), sterilisation (2) and radiology (3), in the north wing. The lift (6) connects to the hotel services in the basement (laundry and kitchen) and allows quick passage of emergency cases from the main entrance (located under the operating theatre) to the operating theatre.

This new organisation of work was favoured by the systematic use of electrical energy (electric bells on patients' beds, a call control panel in the nurses' room, etc.). Thus, the Vevey-Samaritain Hospital installed an electric kitchen in 1933 which, according to its designer, had many advantages, including

[64] *Feuille d'avis de Sainte-Croix*, 7 September 1927.

Table 6 New hospital buildings and extensions, 1920–1960

	New buildings	*Extensions*
Aigle	1932	–
Aubonne	–	1930
Montreux	1928	
Morges	–	1928; 1936; 1948
Moudon	1954	1925
Nyon	1938	–
Orbe	1933	–
Payerne	–	1939
Rolle	1934	–
Saint-Loup	1952	1928; 1936
Sainte-Croix	1947	–
Le Sentier	1934	1956
Vevey-Samaritain	1956	–
Yverdon	1939	1927

"safety, flexibility, simplicity, cleanliness, hygiene, absence of odours and steam, and above all, its most economical operation".[65]

Ultimately, the management of flows allowed for the care of an increasing number of patients in a rational manner. The hospital building no longer reflects the family atmosphere of the second half of the nineteenth century designed to bring comfort to the patients of the working classes; it became a management tool for hospital medicine (Table 6).

These various efforts made it possible to increase the total number of beds available in the regional hospitals of Vaud from 607 in 1909 to 1340 in 1942.[66] The development of the hospital infrastructure continued in the post-war period. In 1960, the 18 regional hospitals of Vaud had a total capacity of 1527 beds, allowing for the hospitalisation of 22,308 people.[67] Although the internal organisation of these establishments became more complex, with the multiplication of autonomous medical services (radiology, ENT, paediatrics, etc.) and diagnostic tools, they were still designed based on the functional model adopted during the inter-war period and met the same need for organisation and management of the various internal flows.

[65] L. Dénéréaz, "La cuisine électrique de l'Hôpital su Samaritain, à Vevey", *Bulletin technique de la Suisse romande*, 1933, p. 34.

[66] "Statistique des hôpitaux et hospices de la Suisse au 31.12.1909", *Journal de Statistique Suisse*, 1910, pp. 283–318, *Les établissements pour malades en Suisse de 1936 à 1942*, Berne: Federal Statistical Office, 1945.

[67] Yverdon Hospital, statistical tables, 1960.

Improvement of the Medico-Technical Infrastructure

These new buildings were the setting for the very strong development of medical-technical infrastructure. Under the impetus of the surgeon-modernisers, the hospitals were equipped with new operating theatres, radiological facilities, analysis laboratories, etc. From the 1890s onwards, operating rooms were opened or renovated in the regional infirmaries (Nyon 1890/1898, Morges 1893, Vevey-Samaritain 1893, Bex 1899, Payerne 1899/1905, Yverdon 1901, Montreux 1909, etc.), according to modern standards. In Montreux, the administrative commission did not hesitate to call on the advice of Professor César Roux, while Professor de Quervain played a significant role in several hospitals, notably in Saint-Loup and Yverdon. In Payerne, the surgical room was transformed in 1899 "according to the latest known improvements and equipped with all the necessary material and instruments to make it a model operating room".[68] In addition, the new hospital buildings designed in the inter-war period gave great importance to the operating theatre, around which the hospital space was organised.

X-ray installations were introduced and several infirmaries were equipped with them at the end of the 1900s (Vevey-Samaritain 1909, Saint-Loup 1910, Hospice de l'Enfance 1912, Morges 1915, Yverdon 1918, Sainte-Croix 1919, Nyon 1922, Rolle 1924, Montreux 1927, Aigle 1931, Payerne 1931). Separate radiology services were not yet created but, very often, an external doctor, generally from Lausanne, was called in who specialised in this field and regularly visited the regional infirmaries. One of the first radiologists to work in a regional hospital was Marc Ramseyer. He was an assistant at the sanatorium in Leysin and then the first assistant in the Radiology Department of the Cantonal Hospital in Lausanne. In 1946, he moved to the Saint-Loup Hospital and La Source Clinic. The appointment of radiologists to head these departments took place on a massive scale in the 1950s, with the arrival of Paul Anex in Aigle (1951), Robert Kleinert in Rolle (1952) and Nyon (1955), Herzog in Nyon (1958), etc. Alongside the surgeon-modernisers, they were the first specialist doctors to work in regional hospitals. Their arrival was all the more appreciated by the administrative commissions as it generated comfortable financial resources. Indeed, the use of the medical-technical infrastructure for private clients was subject to a tax in favour of the hospital which the patients paid in addition to the medical fees, in principle paid directly to the doctors.

However, the income from operating theatres and radiology departments was often integrated into the patient pensions and therefore difficult to identify over time and from a comparative perspective. A summary document drawn up by the regional hospitals for the year 1960 gives an overview of the phenomenon and makes it possible to measure the extent to which these revenues were generated during the 1940s and 1950s (see Table 7).

[68] Broye Hospital, annual report, 1899, p. 1.

Table 7 Revenues from operating theatres and radiology departments in the regional hospitals of Vaud, 1960

Hospital	*Operating expenses*	*Income from the operating room*	*As a % of expenditure*	*Radiology revenues*	*As a % of expenditure*
Aigle	443′302	28′188	6.4	95′068	21.4
Aubonne	201′433	13′705	6.8	15′773	7.8
Bex	58′799	233	0.4	–	–
Ch. d'Oex	234′804	15′816	6.7	23′480	10.0
Cully	252′827	19′221	7.6	20′083	7.9
Montreux	515′187	7′146	1.4	25′997	5.0
Morges	502′256	39′625	7.9	62′340	12.4
Moudon	271′496	22′713	8.4	31′131	11.5
Nyon	637′603	24′287	3.8	95′027	14.9
Orbe	436′712	29′938	6.9	–	–
Payerne	507′235	54′491	10.7	75′761	14.9
Rolle	299′992	25′517	8.5	41′875	14.0
Saint-Loup	1′295′474	40′503	3.1	100′606	7.8
Sainte-Croix	273′231	31′023	11.4	33′258	12.2
Le Sentier	329′507	21′537	6.5	17′541	5.3
Vevey Prov	402′307	41′125	10.2	61′588	15.3
Vevey Sat	885′443	84′815	9.6	195′371[69]	22.1
Yverdon	1′019′159	100′114	9.8	131′113	12.9

Source Yverdon Hospital, statistical tables, 1960

On average, income from operating theatres covered 7.0% of operating expenses and income from radiology 12.2%. Together, these revenues accounted for almost 20% of expenditure; however, the situation varied considerably from one hospital to another. In some institutions, the medical-technical infrastructure covered more than a quarter of the operating expenses, as in Vevey-Samaritain (31.7%), Aigle (27.8%), Payerne (25.6%) and Vevey-Providence (25.5%). The hospitals that received most of this revenue were those located in urban centres where private doctors and their clients used the hospital infrastructure. Apart from the special case of Montreux, where there were many private clinics and so the doctors' use of the regional hospital infrastructure was less frequent, the establishments that generated the least revenue of this type were located in secondary centres. These included Bex (0.4%), Saint-Loup (10.9%), Le Sentier (11.9%), Aubonne (14.6%), Cully (15.5%) and Château-d'Oex (16.7%), where the market for care (wealthy clientele + independent surgeons) was more restricted.

[69] This figure includes ambulatory radiology revenues, which are not included for other hospitals.

4 Administrative and Financial Reorganisation (1900–1960)

The modernisation of the local infirmaries in the Canton of Vaud and their transformation into regional hospitals was not only due to the implementation of various medical advances. The administrative and financial structure was itself the object of a profound transformation that made the transition to the modern regional hospital possible. The change of scale that took place with the arrival of the surgeon-modernisers required the use of new management methods and new sources of funding. First of all, it was necessary to reorganise the management of flows (patients, money, medical equipment, food, etc.) within the establishment, which the deaconesses and the voluntary management committee could no longer do, but also, new sources of financing had to be found to ensure growth.

Hospital management was modernised on the basis of models imported from the private sector (salaried manager, cost accounting, etc.). The rationalisation process was strongly supported by the Association of Vaud Infirmaries (*Association des Infirmeries Vaudoises*, AIV), which grouped together the private hospitals of the canton. Founded in 1930, this association lobbied the state exclusively until the end of the 1940s. Things changed during this period, as the conflicts between the state and the infirmaries calmed down. To become a credible partner of the state they had to reform and unify their management methods. Those infirmaries that had not yet done so took the name of *hospital* in 1947, while the AIV was transformed into the Group of Vaud Regional Hospitals (*Groupement des Hôpitaux régionaux Vaudois*, GHRV), having a five-member committee with defined attributions: "the research and study, in a spirit of solidarity, of common measures useful to the good functioning and development of the regional hospitals of Vaud".[70] Eugène Zwahlen, director of the Lavaux Hospital and secretary of the GHRV since the end of the 1940s, played a key role in this process. He became president of the GHRV in 1957, director in 1974 and remained its linchpin until his departure in 1980. Authoritarian, dynamic and omnipresent, he transformed the GHRV into an association that intervened in the organisation, management and standardisation of regional hospitals. He was the man who introduced the ideas of rationalisation and scientific organisation of work in philanthropic hospitals.

Professionalisation and Secularisation of Administrative Departments

Until the 1910s, the administrative management of the infirmaries was carried out by the senior deaconess (bursar's office) and the management committee (finances). The transition to a regional hospital no longer allowed this type of operation. The increasing complexity of the pension system as a result of the upsurge in the number of private clients and insured persons, as well as the

[70] GHRV archives, statutes of 9 July 1948, art. 2.

need to control the rise in expenditure caused by both the general growth of the system and the increase in inflation, were all factors that played in favour of restructuring the administrative management of the infirmaries.

At first, the management committees hired lay bursars (Montreux 1923; Yverdon 1932; Nyon 1943; Asile des aveugles 1946; Rolle 1948; Sainte-Croix 1950; etc.) to take care of administrative tasks that, until then, had been carried out mainly by the president, the secretary and the cashier of the administrative commission. As salaried employees dependent on the administrative commissions, these bursars had little power. They implemented the decisions of the administrators and ensured that the hospital was supplied with food, fuel, medical equipment, etc. They also took charge of the emerging hospital bureaucracy (correspondence, cost accounting, patient files, etc.). Alongside them appeared the first lay secretaries and bookkeepers, such as the office workers hired in 1955 in the establishments of Aubonne, Montreux and Sainte-Croix, following the adoption of a new accounting plan. These new administrative staff were mainly from the working classes.

Moreover, whether or not the function of bursar existed, key positions in the governing bodies were taken over by people with a background in financial management. In Payerne, for example, the position of chairman of the committee was taken by the mayor in 1913, whereas it had previously been held by pastors. In Nyon, at the end of the 1950s, the president of the administrative commission was "a very competent industrialist, an organiser and a financier who had proved his worth by adapting his metallurgical factory to the needs of the time".[71] As for the Children Hospice, it was chaired between 1928 and 1948 by Max de Cérenville, director of an insurance company and member of the board of directors of a bank.

There was a real horizontal division of labour between the administrative management (bursar), the nursing management (deaconesses) and the medical management (doctors and interns). Such organisation required a clear definition of the responsibilities between different departments in order to function with minimum conflicts of competence. The arrival of lay directors challenged the domination of the deaconesses and led to sometimes violent conflicts. In Nyon, in 1937, the mother house of Saint-Loup threatened to withdraw its deaconesses if the administrative commission appointed a lay bursar, even though this was part of the reorganisation of the new hospital and the adoption of cost accounting (1943). This downgrading of the deaconess superior was coupled with a conflict between her and the medical profession that shook the establishment in the 1940s. The following position taken by the sister superior of Rolle Hospital in 1948 illustrates these opposing conceptions of hospital management: "[...] addressing herself more directly to Mr Chêne [member of the administrative commission], whose objectivity and constant desire to consider the financial aspect of our institution willingly, she asks us all to see the spiritual side as well. Sister Marie-Madeleine says that she has

[71] Gustave Piotet, op. cit., p. 102.

been so often miraculously granted gifts at Christmas that she was able to prepare the beautiful feast she had dreamed of, that she firmly believes that it will be the same for the purchase of the vegetable garden. [...] She expressed the wish that the annual sale should no longer take place on a Sunday, even if the profit were to be reduced, as God must find a way to meet our needs in another way. Such a conviction made a deep impression. Mr. Chêne thanked Sister Marie-Madeleine for what she had just said: "You have touched my weak point", he said; 'I know that we must trust in the One who directs everything, but I cannot help remembering that financial needs must be resolved for themselves'".[72]

The rationalisation of hospital management took a further and decisive step with the development by Eugène Zwahlen in 1950 of an accounting plan whose stated aim was to unify and make transparent the various management methods used in regional hospitals. The adoption of cost accounting should enable "the administrators of our hospitals to detect the weak point of their organisation"[73] and to remedy it. It's adoption would also make it possible to make comparisons between institutions, in particular with a view to negotiating with the state the reimbursement of the actual costs of hospitalisation of the indigent. This new accounting system provided for the separation of financial accounts (profit and loss), medical operations and hotel operations. Since the 1930s, medical care had accounted for an increasing share of hospital costs. Hospitals needed to know more about the financial effects of this medical modernisation. The 1950 accounting plan, adopted by the GHRV in 1951, was a decisive step in the application of scientific working methods to hospital management. This standardisation of accounting greatly reduced the managerial autonomy that had prevailed until then, possibly explaining the reluctance, or even opposition, of some to implement it. Thus, in 1956, the GHRV explained to the recalcitrants the need for this unified plan: "It is always difficult to defend just claims if the very bases of our expenditure are false or do not correspond to the provisions of the accounting plan".[74] The hospitals benefited financially from this innovation as it favoured the reimbursement of the real cost of hospitalisation of indigents by the state from 1955 (see Chapter 5). This plan remained in force until 1972 when the GHRV decided to adopt a new accounting system developed by Veska at the federal level.

The second area in which the GHRV was involved in the administrative modernisation of hospitals was the professionalisation of their management. The new accounting plan, the growth of hospitals and the various agreements signed during the 1950s required the presence of people with specific administrative skills at the head of hospitals. As Eugène Zwahlen explained in 1959,

[72] Rolle Hospital, minutes of the administrative commission, 13 April 1948. Emphasis added.

[73] Eugène Zwahlen, "De la nécessité d'utiliser le même plan comptable dans les Hôpitaux Régionaux", *Veska-Zeitschrift - Revue Veska*, 1951, p. 372.

[74] GHRV archives, committee activity report, 21 June 1956.

"[...] goodwill is no longer enough. Despite all the dedication and competence of the members of the various committees and councils, it is essential that each hospital benefits from the collaboration of a perfectly qualified and normally paid secretary-accountant or treasurer. The responsibility for very important matters such as purchasing, invoicing, accounting, to name but a few, falls to these 'civil servants'. It is abnormal that deaconess superiors, not prepared for these tasks, are entrusted with them. Their time, so precious, would be better spent, it seems to us, with the patients, in the operating room or in the X-ray room".[75] However, it was not until the deaconesses left in the 1960s that the administrative authorities were given free rein. Administrative directors were successively appointed at the Orthopaedic Hospice (1957), Nyon (1959), Montreux (1960), Aigle (1961), Morges (1964), Château-d'Oex (1971), Vevey-Providence (1972) and Aubonne (1975). The main aim of the reorganisations of the 1960s was to strengthen the administrative power in the hospital and to subjugate the medical profession.

Here, too, the intervention of the GHRV was decisive, directed by André Golaz, the first hospital manager to come out of a specific professionalisation programme, who was appointed director of the Morges Hospital in 1967.[76] Son of a radical-democratic notable from Morges, himself strongly involved in communal political affairs, he attended the French National School of Public Health in Rennes in 1968. This institution, founded in 1960 by the French political authorities wishing to set up professional training for public health executives, enabled Golaz to acquire technical skills (organisation of a hospital within the framework of hospital policy) and to develop a network of knowledge, both of which were to play a decisive role in the realisation of the Vaud Hospital Plan (see Chapter 5). Finally, André Golaz played an important role in setting up a professional training programme for hospital directors in French-speaking Switzerland.[77] Golaz's graduation thesis, carried out on the occasion of the conceptualisation of a new hospital building in Morges (1969), consecrates the ideal of the bureaucratisation of the medical profession. Inspired by Marvin Bower's book *The Will to Manage*, which celebrates "the success of companies through systematized management",[78] Golaz foresaw, "doctors are hired full time"[79] and that "paid extra-hospital medical activity should be exceptional and limited to consultations requested by colleagues".[80] The transition from a non-interventionist and relatively liberal administrative power with regard to the medical profession to a more

[75] GHRV archives, minutes of general meetings, 5 June 1959.

[76] *André Golaz, 11 May 1989*, Morges, Hôpital, 1989.

[77] *ADEHR. Association des directeurs des établissements hospitaliers de Suisse romande. 20th^e anniversary*, Saignelégier: ADEHR, 1993.

[78] André Golaz, *Hôpital de zone - Réalisation et organisation*, Rennes: ENSP, 1968, p. 101.

[79] Ibidem, p. 56.

[80] Ibid.

authoritarian and centralising power was not a smooth one. The question of the status of the medical profession was at the heart of the debate on hospital organisation from the 1960s onwards.

The Limits of the Philanthropic Financial System

The modernisation of hospitals required a financial commitment that went beyond the traditional system of funding. The unstable equilibrium that allowed the infirmaries to function until the 1890s-1900s was broken with the arrival of the surgeon-modernisers. The philanthropic system did not, with a few exceptions, cover the high investment costs of new hospital buildings and the modernisation of the medical-technical infrastructure. Recourse to bank loans was often the only solution. However, this hospital transformation also implied a change in scale: regional hospitals took care of an ever-increasing number of patients for whom they needed more and more nursing staff, as well as increasing maintenance costs (food, medication, heating, etc.). To cope with this situation, regional hospitals had to find new resources.

The Financial Impact of New Construction

The construction of new hospitals in the inter-war period caused difficulties and raised the problem of their financing. Indeed, even though the State intervened in a significant way to support new infrastructure until 1936 when it decided to suspend construction subsidies (see Chapter 5), its participation was not enough to cover all the expenses which exceeded the capacity of self-financing and private financing (donations). Everywhere, recourse was made to external capital (bank loans) which led hospitals to financial dependence. Several establishments took out loans to finance the development of their facilities: Montreux borrowed 400,000 francs in 1927; Aigle 300,000 francs in 1932; Orbe 200,000 francs in 1932; Le Sentier 60,000 francs in 1934; Nyon 230,000 francs in 1938; and Payerne 120,000 francs in 1940.

The financial burden (interest and depreciation) generally represented between five and 15% of the operating expenses—a difficult weight for many establishments to bear. In Nyon, for example, the hospital opened in 1938 was very costly and swallowed up revenue, profits and assets. In 1940, its financial charges amounted to 79,000 francs out of a total expenditure of 202,150 francs; that is, 39%. The administrators of the Sainte-Croix Hospital wrote in 1950: "[…] from 1951 onwards, we will have to find the necessary funds each year to pay the interest on the loan and the amortisation, a total of nearly 38,000 francs. It is therefore a considerable sum that will have to be found in addition to the funds necessary for the operation of the hospital".[81]

It was not only the cost of investment that posed a problem for the various hospitals but also the rapidly increasing operating expenses. For example, the

[81] Saint-Croix Hospital, annual report, 1950, p. 4.

opening of the new hospital in Yverdon in 1939 caused serious financial difficulties in the 1940s. The pensions were not enough to pay for the hotel and medical costs. In 1945, its total income amounted to 383,678 francs, made up of pensions (98%) and private income (2%), while expenditure amounted to 429,676 francs, of which 422,505 francs were for the upkeep of the patients (a 98% share, of which 29% was salary costs) and 7171 francs for financial costs (2%). To remedy this situation, a sale was organised in 1946 but such difficulties remained.[82] The sharp increase in the resources needed to run the Yverdon Hospital was not a reflection of inflation but of the quantitative and qualitative development of the establishment. The number of patients treated rose from 511 in 1910 to 791 in 1930 and 2186 in 1950. In parallel with this growth in capacity, the modernisation of the medical and technical environment (radiology, laboratories, etc.), as well as the professionalisation and densification of the nursing staff, resulted in a sharp increase in the cost of treating patients. In 1910, a day of hospitalisation required 2.78 francs; in 1930 it was 4.12 francs and in 1950 it was 13.45 francs. This phenomenon is extremely important because the cantonal subsidy to regional hospitals was calculated on the basis of the number of days of hospitalisation of indigent patients. The indexation of the subsidy was therefore not sufficient to cover the constantly rising costs and regional hospitals did not cease to demand an increase in state aid and full coverage of hospitalisation costs.

The Crisis of Philanthropy

Hospital philanthropy was in crisis during the inter-war period. The qualitative leap that took place in hospitals during the 1920s and 1930s broke with the paternalistic model established in the nineteenth century, while at the same time making financial needs more extensive. Indeed, the adoption of rational and standardised management methods greatly anonymised the relationship between philanthropists and hospitalised patients that had been the basis of nineteenth-century infirmaries. Henceforth, patients were taken care of by doctors and salaried bursars in a standardised manner as soon as they entered the hospital. Cases were no longer discussed by the hospitalisation committee. There was no longer any direct confrontation between the philanthropists and "their" patients. This was a strong disincentive for the financial commitment of traditional patrons, although they continued to support hospitals only in a more sporadic and less demonstrative way.

The specialised hospitals in Lausanne are a good illustration of this phenomenon. There was an identical downward trend in donations offset by strong growth in pensions. Despite the large differences between these three institutions, pensions became their main source of income by 1940 (see Table 8).

[82] Yverdon Hospital, annual reports, 1910–1950.

Table 8 Structure of income in Lausanne's philanthropic hospitals, in %, 1910–1940

	Children's Hospice				*Orthopaedic Hospice*				*Blind People's Asylum*			
	1910	*1920*	*1930*	*1940*	*1911*	*1921*	*1930*	*1940*	*1910*	*1920*	*1930*	*1940*
Own	9	4	3	1	4	16	1	0	21	37	25	22
Pensions	29	68	65	75	84	75	93	95	15	30	33	44
Donations	60	25	29	22	11	7	6	5	59	25	27	26
Various	2	3	3	2	0	1	0	0	5	8	15	16

Source Annual reports, 1910–1940

Donations were already falling during the 1900s at the Orthopaedic Hospice, perhaps because of the attempts to modernise the medical treatment of patients by Drs Perret and Nicod which, in the eyes of some, betrayed the philanthropic spirit of the institution (see Chapter 2). Donations still accounted for 41% of income in 1902 but only 11% in 1911. Thereafter, the early rapprochement of the Orthopaedic Hospice with state institutions (Cantonal Hospital, Faculty of Medicine) militated against a resumption of donations. As for the Blind People's Asylum, this was characterised by the importance of its own assets, whose interests alone represented almost a quarter of its resources, and by the growing participation of school fees from the Institute for Young Blind People (under the heading "Various") in the institution. Finally, the Children's Hospice followed the classic model observed in the case of regional hospitals. It underwent widespread development in the new building opened in 1910, including a doubled medical service. The number of children hospitalised, which had fluctuated around 220–230 per year since the end of the 1870s, rose to 429 in 1920, 544 in 1930 and 801 in 1940. As a consequence of this growth, operating expenses rose sharply from 22,451 francs in 1910 to more than 115,000 francs in 1940. This change in scale was unfavourable to private participation. The limited resources of this Hospice did not allow it to meet the needs of an ever-growing establishment so deficit years followed one after another: between 1910 and 1955, only 13 out of 46 years were profitable.

In regional hospitals, the situation was identical. In 1920, the administrators of the Montreux Hospital stated they were "entirely dependent on private charity".[83] That year, donations amounted to 40% of their resources. After the opening of the new hospital (1927), donations dropped sharply and their share did not reach 2% of their revenue in 1930. In these conditions, the hospital administration had to find resources other than the traditional contribution from philanthropists. Dr. Gustave Piotet declared, in 1961, "a hospital must be able to run on its own resources and that it must no longer rely on charity

[83] Montreux Hospital, annual report, 1920, p. 7.

[...]".[84] He was thinking of a stronger intervention of hitherto secondary actors (the state, insurance companies, patients themselves) in favour of the reimbursement of hospitalisations.

Pensions for the Sick: The State, Insurance and Private Clients

In this financing structure, increasing the price per day of hospitalisation appeared to be an easily achievable solution that did not fundamentally call the system into question. The new costs were passed on to the inpatients or, indirectly, to the public authorities (state and municipalities) and the insurance companies that subsidised them. Generally speaking, hospitals no longer admitted patients free of charge. Thus, pensions quickly became their main source of income. In 1930, they represented 70% of the operating revenue in Bex, 76% in Montreux, 63% in Morges, 81% in Nyon, 63% in Vevey-Samaritain and 80% in Yverdon. The trend became more pronounced in the 1940s and 1950s.

The state, which legally covered the hospitalisation of indigent patients, remained an essential financial partner although its subsidies did not keep pace with the growth of regional hospitals (see Chapter 5). The state contribution was still calculated based on a specific price per day of hospitalisation paid by the state in regional hospitals. However, the value of the day as reimbursed by the state changed slowly during the inter-war period and covered less and less of the real cost. From the 1920s to the 1940s, the regional hospitals constantly demanded an increase in the state's contribution. This position led them to form a well-structured lobby in 1930, the Association of Vaud Infirmaries.

Although health insurance was almost non-existent in 1900, it became more important during the inter-war period. For the whole of Switzerland, the mutual aid funds recognised and subsidised by the state spent a total of 9.3 million francs in 1933 on the hospital costs of their members—that is, 11.7% of their expenditure—whereas in 1895, this proportion was only 0.3% for French-speaking cantons.[85] The health insurance companies subsequently devoted more and more of their money to hospital costs, allowing the middle and working classes to have greater access to hospital care and, at the same time, guaranteeing the modernised hospitals a part of their income. The entry into force of the Swiss National Accident Insurance Fund (*Caisse Nationale Suisse d'Assurance en Cas d'Accidents*, CNA) in 1918 favoured the development of hospitalisation of accident victims and ensured an income for the Vaud hospitals which signed an agreement with the CNA. In Montreux, the various insurance companies paid for 9% of hospital days in 1920 and 8% in 1930; in 1938, they financed the hospitalisation of 155 patients out of 868 (17%).

Finally, the patients themselves were increasingly responsible for their own hospitalisation costs. The progress of hospital medicine, especially in the

[84] GHRV archives, minutes of general meetings, 28 September 1961.

[85] *Bulletin de la Fédération des Sociétés de secours mutuels de Suisse romande*, 1897, pp. 308–309 and 1936, p. 126.

surgical field, brought a whole non-indigent population to the hospital who paid for their own care. Hospitals built in the first part of the twentieth century generally had one- or two-bedrooms for wealthy patients. During the discussion on the financing of the general reorganisation of the Rolle Hospital in 1945–1946, an administrator stated that "most of the costs can be recovered from the patients' bills".[86] In Montreux, 56% of the patients paid their own pensions in 1950. However, after 1945, the development of health insurance and the increase in the population covered encouraged the transfer of the burden from the patients themselves to the insurance companies. In the 1950s, the state, in collaboration with the GHRV, intervened to guarantee the hospitalisation of the entire population in a context of rising costs. Dr. Piotet stated, in this respect, "as a result of the price of medicine [...] the majority of those hospitalised become 'indigent', more or less at the expense of the state".[87]

Late Intervention by Municipalities

As important as these increases in pension prices were, they were not enough to make up for the shortcomings of the philanthropic funding system. It was, therefore, necessary to call on the direct contribution of new partners: the municipalities. Until then, they had not been involved in the financing of the operating budget through annual subsidies, but they did participate indirectly by paying the hospitalisation costs of their patients—a burden that traditionally fell to the municipalities. The management of a hospital was one of the new sectors of public intervention at the end of the nineteenth century where there was a tendency for the central state to take charge of expenditure, with local authorities assuming the development of older responsibilities (assistance, schools, etc.).[88] However, this mode of operation, as far as the management of regional hospitals was concerned, was called into question by the redeployment of these establishments at the end of the inter-war period.

It was often the construction of new buildings which, by upsetting the precarious balance of finances, raised the question of public funding. However, the participation of the municipalities did not come without difficulty. Very often, they accepted a voluntary contribution in favour of the hospital but refused to formalise these donations (Aubonne, Morges, Orbe, Payerne, Sainte-Croix, Vevey-Providence, Vevey-Samaritain, Yverdon). In this case, communal aid remained very limited. For example, the financial support of the commune of Vevey to the Providence Hospital amounted to 300 francs in 1940, then 500 francs in 1950 and 1000 francs in 1960. As for the communes of the Aubonne district, their subsidies represented 4–5% of the hospital's

[86] Rolle Hospital, minutes of the board, 8 February 1946.

[87] Nyon Hospital, minutes of the administrative commission, 26 June 1954.

[88] André Lasserre, *Finances publiques et développement. Le canton de Vaud, 1831–1913*, Lausanne: Bibliothèque historique vaudoise, 1980, pp. 389–390.

resources in the years 1930–1950. Overall, the local authorities were not promoters of hospital development in the canton of Vaud.

It was during the expansion and construction of new buildings in the 1950s and 1960s that the communes began to intervene massively in hospital financing, particularly with the aim of guaranteeing the necessary bank loans. Most of the hospitals built during this period required assistance from the municipalities (the districts of Yverdon and Grandson in 1955, Vevey in 1956, Payerne in 1957, Aigle in 1959, Aubonne in 1960, Orbe in 1962, Nyon in 1962 and Morges in 1968).

In the canton of Vaud, therefore, the regional hospitals remained strongly independent of local public authorities until the 1950s. When cash flow difficulties arose, the regional hospitals turned first to the cantonal government and not to the communes.

Some Examples of Hospital Management

While local infirmaries had a relatively homogeneous model of organisation, management and financing until the inter-war period, this was no longer the case thereafter. The contrasting evolution of the Vaud in the 1950s and 1960s—strong growth in the urban areas of the Lake Geneva region and industrialised regions while the peripheral regions stagnated—directly affected the management of the infirmaries. The various restructurings of these establishments and their transformation into hospitals led to a marked differentiation between certain small peripheral establishments (Aubonne, Bex, Château-d'Oex, etc.) and others located in rural towns (Aigle, Payerne, Orbe, etc.) or urban centres (Montreux, Vevey, Yverdon, etc.). The economic and demographic dynamics specific to these different regions, in particular, the structure of the medical market, largely explain the type of regional hospitals that emerged.

The Financial Difficulties of Peripheral Establishments Following the Modernisation of Their Equipment: The Case of Aubonne Hospital

The redeployment of the Aubonne Hospital at the end of the 1920s corresponded to the arrival of Gustave Piotet as a consultant surgeon. Until then, this small establishment which hospitalised fewer than 300 people per year worked on a traditional philanthropic basis, relying on the internal management of the deaconesses, a medical service organised on a rotating basis and financing that depended to a large extent on donations and income from a small real estate fortune.

Shortly after Piotet's arrival (1927), the management committee decided on a new extension that would increase the capacity to 55 beds but which required a bank loan of 150,000 francs.[89] The transformed hospital opened

[89] ACV, K VIII D 4, Memorandum presented by the Committee of the Aubonne Infirmary on the financial situation of this establishment, 7 June 1934.

in 1930 and was quickly criticised by the Department of the Interior which considered the establishment to be overdeveloped for local needs.[90] However, it experienced significant growth and saw the number of patients increase to 350 in 1940, 433 in 1950 and 560 in 1960, with a decreasing average length of stay (30.4 days in 1915 and 23.1 days in 1960).

From a management point of view, the establishment experienced difficult financial years until 1950. For the whole of the period 1938–1950, the gross operating finance was too little to cover the necessary depreciation and repayment of the mortgage debt. The infirmary's assets thus lost more than a quarter of their value between 1940 (190,663 francs) and 1950 (136,807 francs). There was a chronic deficit in the institution that can be explained by a general lack of resources to cover expenses. The structure of its income was similar to that observed elsewhere: for the years 1938–1950, patient pensions dominated with an average of 79.6% of income, followed by donations (14.5%), municipal subsidies (4.8%) and its own income (1.1%). These revenues did not cover all the expenses and were difficult to extend. First of all, patient pensions depended largely on agreements signed with external partners (the state, municipalities, insurance companies, etc.) which defined the amount paid for a day's hospitalisation and could not be extended indefinitely. While in many regional hospitals the modernisation of equipment was financed by the arrival of new, profitable hospital clients, this seems to be lacking in Aubonne. The income from the radiology service, which is a good indicator of the profitability of the clientele, was not as important as in other regional hospitals: in 1950, it reached a maximum of 3.6% of total income. The new hospital in Aubonne, which opened in 1930, was not financially in line with the local medical market. This fact largely explains the deficits seen in its accounts. It was primarily a response to a social demand on the part of the local notables who wanted to have an establishment similar to those in neighbouring towns. However, this local elite did not have the means to fulfil its ambitions. On the one hand, private income alone could not ensure the institution's development. The general context of a crisis in philanthropy, linked to the limited resources of a local elite that was essentially winegrowers and remained on the fringes of industrialisation, proved unfavourable to the extension of this type of resource. On the other hand, the municipalities of the district were already participating in the voluntary financing of the establishment, with an average annual subsidy of 4066 francs from 1938 to 1950.

In the end, Aubonne Hospital owed a large part of its survival to its participation in the regional hospital union (GHRV). Since the early 1950s, the GHRV had negotiated hospitalisation agreements with the State and then with insurance companies, to cover the operating costs of the various establishments in the canton (see Chapter 5). In Aubonne, this resulted in a substantial increase in resources from pensions (89.6% of the average income for the years 1950–1960), despite the lack of access to profitable private clients. The 1950s

[90] ACV, S 73, minutes of the HHC, 1933.

brought comfortable profits. In 1960, its assets amounted to 194,626 francs and the board of directors planned a new extension in 1961, which brought the capacity to 65 beds.

The Transformation of Rural Town Hospitals: The Case of Broye Hospital

Broye Hospital is a good example of the financial dimension of modernisations affecting hospitals in rural towns. The medical market was relatively large and not very competitive—often the regional hospital was the only establishment in the region. Its capacity doubled between 1902 (55 beds) and 1940 (100 beds). The establishment was saturated in the 1920s and 1930s, with a ceiling on hospitalisations of around 600 patients per year. The opening of the new hospital in 1940 doubled the number of people treated annually (1415 in 1950). At the same time, the equipment was modernised (with X-rays in 1931 and a new operating theatre in 1934).

The new hospital inaugurated in 1940 represented a qualitative and quantitative leap that had to be financed. Until then, the Broye Hospital was in a good financial situation. Before the construction of the new hospital, it only had two years of deficits which allowed an increase in its assets (11,224 francs in 1921 and 145,005 francs in 1935). Interest on these assets became an important element of its operating resources, representing 2% of its income in 1921 and 8% in 1938. The construction of new buildings from 1938 to 1939 was made without too many financial difficulties. The hospital limited itself to a loan of 120,000 francs but most of its assets were spent on the construction. While capital expenditure in 1938–1939 was not a problem for the Broye Hospital, the same could not be said for operating expenditure. The change in scale broke the unstable balance of the philanthropic financial system. The care of a growing number of patients logically implied a sharp increase in operating expenses.

This growth in financial needs implied a trend towards increased resources which the traditional philanthropic channels did not meet. In absolute figures, the private share (donations) remained broadly the same, with an annual average of almost 25,000 francs for the period 1921–1948. However, this participation, which amounted to 27.4% of income in 1921, fell sharply and continuously in the context of the growth of resources so it was only 12.5% in 1948. Despite the strong downward trend in donations from the 1930s onwards, private charity was mobilised for specific actions. The sale organised in 1939 for the new hospital, as well as the donations of that year, brought in 39,090 francs which were included in the operating income but were used to pay for the new buildings.

In the end, the absorption of wealth into capital expenditure and the crisis of philanthropy left the institution's administrators with little choice but to pass on the bulk of the cost of growth to the patients. Pensions, which on average accounted for 63.1% of income in 1921–1930, rose to 76.8% in 1940 and 86.9% in 1948. At the same time, there was a very strong declining trend of state-funded pensions. During the period 1923–1935, the state's share was relatively stable, hovering around an average of 33.0% of total pensions. A breakthrough came in the mid-1930s, corresponding exactly to the opening of the new operating theatre (1934) and the appointment of the surgeon Charles Yersin (1935). The share of state pensions fell sharply (34.4% in 1935; 15.7% in 1940; 7.5% in 1947) and revealed the arrival of a new clientele; from then on, patients from the middle and upper classes, whose hospitalisation was not covered by the state, came to be treated in the reorganised and modernised local hospital, to whose financing they thus contributed directly.

Modernisation of an Urban Hospital: The Case of the Montreux Hospital

Finally, let us take the example of a hospital located in an urban centre, that of Montreux. At the beginning of the twentieth century, this establishment, which experienced difficulties due to insufficient resources, found solutions in the 1920s to ensure not only the financing of its operations but also its development within the framework of profound transformation. Indeed, the abandonment of the philanthropic model and the inauguration in 1927 of a new hospital with a hundred beds, demanded in particular by the doctors, allowed the adoption of a highly profitable management model.

Two main sources of funding were used: patient pensions and municipal subsidies. The opening of the new hospital was clearly aimed at the middle classes who could afford the costs of their care. Priority was no longer given to the needy, which led to the intervention in 1933 by a representative of the commune of Le Châtelard who "found the price of 5.50 francs too high compared to what was charged at the Cantonal Hospital for people with limited means".[91] The pensions paid by the patients appear to be an essential source of financing, amounting to an average of 84.7% of its income for the period 1938–1960. Information on the type of patients published in annual reports shows that the hospital was not primarily intended for indigent patients. When free hospitalisation disappeared completely in 1941, indigent patients covered by the State represented only 17.3% of hospitalisations in 1938–1960 and those dependent on insurance, 20.0%. The remainder were patients who paid for their own hospitalisation (62.7%). Within this category, patients in private rooms increased constantly, representing 4.4% of hospitalised patients in 1940, 13.1% in 1950 and 19.7% in 1960.

The second strong aspect of the hospital's management was the very early participation of the communes in financing the operation of the hospital. In view of the financial difficulties at the beginning of the century and wishing to build a new establishment, in 1924, the administrators obtained from the Grand Council the authorisation to collect a local hospitalisation tax. This public participation amounted each year to a sum varying between 20 and 30,000 francs; that is, 10.1% of operating revenue for the period 1940–1960.

[91] Montreux Hospital, minutes of the administrative commission, 21 December 1933.

Opening up to a profitable clientele and the massive intervention of the public authorities was to the detriment of the philanthropic character of the institution, which tended to fade away. Donations represented only 4.3% of its income for the years 1940–1960 and the local economic elite deserted the board of directors. Among the 16 people on the board in 1950 were four doctors working at the hospital and three representatives of the public authorities; thus, it was now people who had a direct interest in the hospital who became involved in its management.

The management organisation set up in Montreux during the inter-war period led to financial success. The operating profits accumulated during the years 1938–1960 amounted to more than one million francs. These financial resources allowed the Montreux Hospital to serenely tackle its growth in equipment—with a new extension in 1961 which brought the capacity to 125 beds—and to assert itself as one of the main hospitals of the canton within the framework of the new hospital policy of the 1960s.

Conclusion

The growth and development of the philanthropic infirmaries in the Canton of Vaud very soon raised the question of their financing. The provisional solutions established in the years 1880–1900 led to an unstable equilibrium suggestive of the difficulties a redeployment of the infirmaries would bring.

Their transformation into generalist hospitals equipped with high-tech equipment which took place at the beginning of the twentieth century, more particularly during the inter-war period, appears to have been a breakthrough, manifested by the adoption of the name of *hospital* by most establishments (Montreux in 1926, Aigle in 1933, Château-d'Oex in 1934, Yverdon in 1937, Payerne in 1940, Rolle in 1948, etc.). First of all, as far as the structure of the establishments themselves was concerned, there was a real homogenisation following the changes brought about by the surgeon-modernisers. The same model of a general hospital built according to a T-shaped plan and centred on the operating theatre was imposed on all the infirmaries. However, although there was a movement towards standardisation of the hospital infrastructure, this transformation did not take place at the same pace, to the same extent or with the same financial resources available, so heterogeneity emerged in terms of their management and financing. At the end of the 1950s, the GHRV emerged as a lobby that included both large regional hospitals, which had nearly one million francs at their disposal and admitted more than a thousand patients a year, and small establishments, whose infrastructure was less developed and which were generally located in regions where the medical market was smaller and less profitable. The participation of the latter in the GHRV was ultimately beneficial in that the hospital union entered into bilateral negotiations with the state to take into account all member institutions and thus enable the less viable to survive.

Despite differences in size and profitability, all regional hospitals faced similar organisational problems. As in the case of the Cantonal Hospital, they needed to create a new material framework for the modernisation of their infrastructure. Indeed, there were insufficient philanthropic resources to guarantee their redeployment towards a new hospital medicine focused on surgery. In the end, the regional hospitals had to pass on the costs of hospital growth to the patients whose pensions became the main source of income during the first decades of the twentieth century, as was the case in similar institutions in other countries (Great Britain, Spain, Germany, etc.). However, in the Canton of Vaud, the modernisation of local infirmaries implied a particular type of relationship with the state. Originally set up by men close to the Free Church and the Liberal Party who were strongly opposed to state intervention, these establishments retained a very pronounced private and local character until at least the 1950s, their philanthropic nature taking on an identity-based, even regionalist dimension, despite their modernisation. The budget of regional hospitals was largely based on the pensions of the patients who came to be treated there and a large part depended on state funds (for indigent patients). From the 1890s onwards, the administrative commissions of the regional hospitals constantly demanded an increase in state subsidies for indigent patients while refusing to allow the state to intervene in the internal affairs of the regional hospitals. This paradoxical demand led to a consensual agreement with the state that was representative of the cantonal hospital policy established after 1945. This issue is discussed in Chapter 5.

CHAPTER 5

Building a Hospital Policy

1 Introduction

The hospital system does not operate in a perfectly liberal economic environment based solely on the law of supply and demand. The imperatives of public health and the training of medical professionals make the State an important player in the hospital system.

Despite the State's involvement, it is difficult to speak of any statewide *hospital policy* enacted throughout the nineteenth century. The various establishments in the hospital system were operating in a complementary fashion that was quite favourable to a certain non-interventionism and the State authorities let the establishments develop "naturally". Neither the cantonal administration, whose Department of the Interior was very small before 1945, nor the medical profession, nor the representatives of the regional hospitals, nor any other actor attempted to intervene at the level of the hospital system to influence its evolution. There was only a timid intervention by the State in favour of the hospitalisation of indigent patients in the local infirmaries, although this measure was more a question of assistance than a desire to coordinate the hospital system.

The unrestrained growth of hospitals in the first part of the twentieth century highlighted the limits of this laissez-faire approach. The competitiveness within the hospital system, a direct consequence of the development of hospital facilities, led to fears and demands on the part of many actors: the Cantonal Hospital and the professors of the Faculty were not happy about the questioning of the dominant position of their institution, as much for professional reasons as for financing and prestige; the philanthropic hospitals did not have the material means of their policy (developing hospitals without

P.-Y. Donzé, *The Formation of the Swiss Hospital System (1840–1960)*,
https://doi.org/10.1007/978-981-19-3911-2_5

state support); the doctors denounced a healthcare market that was more and more competitive and therefore less and less profitable; the health insurance providers wanted to limit the increase of their contributions; etc. In the end, all these actors turned to the State demanding public intervention in their favour.

The new economic and political situation that emerged after 1945 was particularly favourable to tackling these various expectations. The State intervened more and more in the hospital system and entered into discussions with the various players in order to meet their expectations, becoming one of the main financial backers of the system. In the 1950s and 1960s, it asserted itself as the manager of the hospital system as a whole. This change in the scale of health management was largely due to the arrival of new actors—the planning specialists, mainly architects and sociologists. The emergence of these experts expresses the advent of a statewide hospital policy conducted at the system level.

2 The Beginnings of a Statewide Hospital Policy: The 1875 Law on Infirmaries and Its Consequences

Until the beginning of the 1870s, the Vaud authorities' hospital policy was limited to the management and organisation of the Cantonal Hospital. This did not mean they were not interested in the hospitalisation of the population but rather, they considered the public institution in Lausanne could meet the needs of the indigent patients. This explains the general tendency between 1810 and 1860 to focus on the curable sick while other types of people who had previously been hospitalised at the Cantonal Hospital were admitted to new specialised institutions (for lunatics, prisoners and abandoned children). The policy of this period was characterised by the extension of the population cared for by the Cantonal Hospital (non-Vaud Swiss, foreigners, etc.). For the political authorities of the Canton of Vaud, this establishment was sufficient to regulate the issue of hospitalisation; therefore, the concept of hospitalisation was centralised which explains why the Public Relief Commission did not intervene elsewhere in the territory. However, during the 1860s, the Cantonal Hospital proved too small to fulfil its function. This was an opportunity for the Department of the Interior to redeploy its hospitalisation policy throughout the canton, taking into account the local infirmaries founded by philanthropists.

The Department of the Interior

The Department of the Interior was not considered an important and prestigious department until the mid-1870s. The strong men of the Council of State preferred to deal with departments such as Public Education or Justice and Police, leaving the Interior to less charismatic men. For example, the Department of the Interior was left to the sole liberal councillor of State after the radical victory in the 1866 elections. This relative lack of interest explains to a large extent the non-interventionist policy of the State in hospital matters before the mid-1870s. In the view of the State Council, the Cantonal Hospital, whose modernisation was approved, was sufficient to ensure the hospitalisation of the indigent. The political situation was completely different from the second half of the 1870s when the Radical-Democratic Party showed a desire for social modernisation, of which the Department of the Interior became an integral part. The political authorities wanted to give the entire population general access to hospital medicine which was undergoing profound changes—Dr. Dupont adopted the antiseptic method around 1876 and César Roux settled in Lausanne in 1883.

Hospital medicine and public health were incorporated into the project to modernise society and thus became decisive political issues. The State of Vaud entered a phase of redeployment in the years 1870–1880 which resulted in an increase in operating expenses in certain sectors, such as schools and social welfare, as well as significant capital expenditure following the construction of the railways, mainly in the context of hydraulic works and roads.[1] State intervention in the hospital sector was part of both social welfare policy and major capital works.

This political context explains, to a large extent, the presence after 1875 of influential radicals—often strongmen of the government—at the head of the Department of the Interior for periods of more than ten years. It should also be added that welfare spending and social policy became more important in the management of the State in the 1870s and 1880s. The Department of the Interior thus lost its secondary status. The arrival of State Councillor Charles Estoppey as its head in 1875 marked a time of strong politicisation of the Cantonal Hospital, along with the appointment of Samuel Cuénoud as its director (1876). The administrative power was strengthened and became more interventionist. This new interest in public health led to the extension of hospital policy to local infirmaries and the construction of a new cantonal hospital.

Organisation of the Department of the Interior (1845–1914)

During the years 1845–1862, the Department of the Interior included a Public Relief Commission, appointed by the Council of State, which was responsible for administering the property and controlling the operation of the establishments attached to this service (Cantonal Hospital, Lunatic Asylum, Detention House, etc.). This commission had six civil servants under its command, including the director of the Cantonal Hospital. Its main focus was on questions of order and discipline: it monitored the various cases of hospital patients, decided on the dismissal of disobedient employees and discussed the amount of pensions.[2] Neither the commission nor the civil servants appear as

[1] André Lasserre, *Finances publiques...*, op. cit.

[2] ACV, K VIIIa 42/1–5, Hospice protocol, 1849–1864.

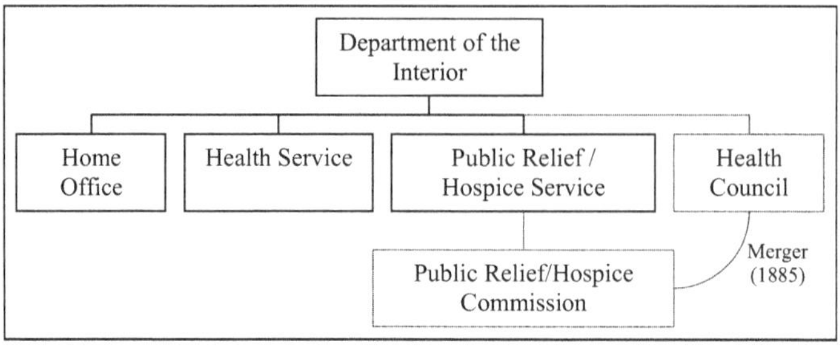

Fig. 1 Organisation chart of the Department of the Interior, 1863–1957

modernising elements. Their intervention was limited to ensuring the efficient functioning of the establishments for which they were responsible.

The reorganisation of the cantonal administration in 1862–1863 led to a strengthening of administrative power in hospital matters. At this time, the commission was dissolved and its functions were attributed to a Public Relief Service, consisting of five officials, with whom "the chief secretary exercised, under the authority of the department, the supervision of the incorporated, the accounting, the economy and the police of the hospices".[3] Therefore, civil servants were responsible for the supervision of the Hospital, with no other control than that of the State Council. There is, however, little trace of the administrative decisions taken during the period 1862–1875, in the absence of minutes from their meetings (Fig. 1).

The Department of the Interior was given two other services, the Home Office (three civil servants in 1863), which dealt with the day-to-day and general affairs of the Department, and the Health Service, responsible for supervising the practice of medicine and public health. The latter consisted of only two civil servants: the cantonal doctor and a secretary. The Health Service developed considerably in the 1880s, notably with the opening of a bacteriology laboratory, directed by Louis Roux, nephew of César Roux, from 1905 to 1941. Finally, the Department of the Interior could rely on the Health Council which had existed since the 1800s but was not a service of the administration but a consultative commission appointed by the government.

The reform of 1862–1863 thus enabled the Department of the Interior to set up the first organisation to supervise the administration of public health. This basic structure was reinforced in 1875 with the intervention of the radical modernising elites. State Councillor Estoppey strengthened the administrative power of the Department with the reintroduction, in 1875, of a Hospices Commission; however, it was not very interventionist. This is mainly because the management of the hospital was strengthened at the same time. For example, the power to dismiss disobedient employees was given to the hospital director in May 1875 whereas, until 1862, the Public Relief Commission had

[3] Ibidem, art. 22.

been responsible.[4] The members of the new commission were often men who, essentially, kept a distant eye on the management of the institution. Most of the power was passed on to the management of the hospital which, in 1876, was entrusted to a man from the radical ranks: Samuel Cuénoud (see Chapter 3).

The size of the Public Relief Service remained limited (five civil servants until 1938) which did not allow it to assert itself as a major player in hospital policy formation. In practice, his head worked in close collaboration with the hospital management and the Health and Hospices Council, created in 1885, of which Cuénoud was a member until 1892. The Public Relief Service lost the decision-making power it had between 1862 and 1875; from then on, it simply implemented the policy decided by the Health and Hospices Council—the real heart of Vaud's hospital policy-making from 1885 onwards.

The Health and Hospices Council Between 1885 and 1914

In 1885, the State Council decided to combine the Health Council, an advisory body on the practice of medicine, and the Hospices Commission, responsible for the administrative supervision of the Public Relief Service, into a single commission: the Health and Hospices Council (HHC). This centralised power within a single commission was responsible for supervising the private practice of medicine in the canton, public health problems (epidemics, sanitation, etc.), the treatment of tuberculosis patients and the management of public hospitals.

The socio-political profiles of the 18 people who sat on the HHC during the years 1885–1914 clearly illustrate the connection between the medical community and the cantonal administration.[5] The most represented group (seven) were civil servants from the Department of the Interior (heads of service and secretaries). This was followed by radical career politicians (five), professors of medicine (four), a veterinarian and a cantonal judge. There were only three liberals on the commission, two of whom were professors of medicine. This council was made up of men with recognised administrative and managerial skills. Several held seats on the boards of directors of large public companies. The experience they had acquired in these companies was put to good use in the management of establishments dependent on the Department of the Interior and in the organisation of a cantonal-scale hospital policy.

The HHC intervened in hospital affairs at several levels. First of all, there was a general policy for monitoring the proper functioning of the Cantonal Hospital. In the 1880s and 1890s, the members of the HHC made numerous personal visits to the establishment and issued reports in which problems of employee discipline and building maintenance dominated.[6] From the 1900s

[4] ACV, K VIII B 61, Hospice protocol, 20 May 1875.

[5] ODCV, 1885–1914.

[6] ACV, K VIII B 8, Board of Health, individual reports, 1887–1899.

onwards, these tasks were left to the director of the hospital and the HHC concentrated on financial management and organisational problems. This was indeed its main function. In the case of the Cantonal Hospital, the HHC implemented, in collaboration with the director, new management methods and a new organisational structure that allowed for the growth of the institution (e.g., financial autonomy, rapprochement with the private sector, etc.). As for medical concerns, they were little present in the minutes of the HHC, despite the presence of several doctors and professors of medicine. A large degree of autonomy was left to the doctors in charge of the hospital's departments.

The Public Relief Service: Financial Aspects

The Public Relief Service was not profitable and had a permanent operating deficit. Its revenue, mainly from the income of its landed assets, notably the former rich Villeneuve Hospital acquired by the State in the 1800s, could not cover its expenses; however, until 1872, the situation remained under control. The average annual deficit was about 46,500 francs for the period 1856–1872. This was a negligible expense for the Canton of Vaud, representing 1.4% of the State's operating expenses. The Cantonal Hospital played an important role in this service. It accounted for no less than 59.2% of its expenditure for the period 1856–1872, but only 10.2% of its income. The Hospital had no assets of its own and its self-financing rate was almost zero which explains its dependence on public relief.

The situation changed in 1873 with the opening of a psychiatric asylum for 300 patients, making it the largest hospital in the canton.[7] In addition, the Public Relief Service granted subsidies to private infirmaries in the canton from 1875 onwards. As for the Cantonal Hospital, it was also growing, with a deficit that rose to nearly 163,000 francs in 1880. The number of patients taken in by the Service multiplied during the 1870s, explaining the sharp increase in its operating expenses and the growth of its deficit which reached more than 214,000 francs in 1880. The increasing burden of this service was felt heavily, representing 3.4% of the State's expenditure in 1875 and 4.8% in 1880.[8]

The Cantonal Hospital Becomes Too Small: The Beginnings of a Statewide Hospital Policy

Although the political authorities had been discussing the need to renovate and enlarge the Cantonal Hospital since the mid-1860s, it was not until 1873 that a hospital policy was developed for the whole of the canton. In fact, the decision to build a new cantonal hospital was taken that year, as was

[7] Catherine Fussinger and Deodaat Tevaearai, op. cit, Claude Secrétan, *L'hôpital de Cery, 1873–1973*, Lausanne, Payot, 1973.

[8] RSC, Department of Finance, 1875–1880.

the decision to encourage the foundation and development of local private infirmaries.

For the first time, the State Council adopted a global vision of hospitalisation and sought to make the local private infirmaries and the Cantonal Hospital complementary, thus laying the foundations for coordination within the Vaud hospital system. Since 1871 at least, the former had been petitioning the State for recognition as legal entities in order to benefit fully from the donations and legacies allocated to them which constituted an essential part of their income. The Grand Council granted their request in 1873. Meanwhile, the State Council knew that its Cantonal Hospital was too small to meet the needs of a growing population and the construction of new buildings would not solve the problem. By approaching private infirmaries, it sought to supplement the public hospital offers. In 1873, the State Council wrote to its prefects asking them to study the question of setting up a private infirmary in their district, in collaboration with local notabilities. This led directly to the foundation of establishments in Montreux and Nyon in 1874. The State Councillor Ruchonnet went further than this policy of encouragement and suggested to the Grand Council "to make them branches of the Cantonal Hospital [...], the State Council [being] very much in favour of the decentralisation of our hospital assistance".[9]

This position was opposed by philanthropists who wanted to keep their establishments private while accepting collaboration with the State. The law on infirmaries, accepted in 1875, thus adopted a consensual position. It aimed to make the philanthropic establishments complementary to the Cantonal Hospital and contributed to their development through the introduction of two types of subsidies. On the one hand, the State intervened by means of construction and transformation subsidies (10% of the total cost of the work), in order to encourage the development of private infrastructure. On the other hand, the principle of a public contribution was adopted "for the maintenance of patients who, being in the conditions required to enter the Cantonal Hospital, and not having been able to be received there for lack of space or for any other reason, have been admitted to an infirmary at the request of the cantonal administration".[10] This participation was based on the payment of hospitalisation days for indigent patients. The calculation of the price of the reimbursed hospitalisation day quickly became a fundamental issue in the relations between local infirmaries and the State.

By securing the collaboration of local infirmaries, the State hoped to have 17 private infirmaries in the canton with an average of 12 beds; that is, a total of 204 beds which, added to the 200 beds of the Cantonal Hospital, should have corresponded to the estimated needs of the time.[11] This policy of complementarity lasted until the end of the 1910s but the first warnings

[9] BGC, 20 February 1874.

[10] Law on infirmaries of 15 May 1875, art. 3.

[11] Catherine Lehmann-Jomini, op. cit., pp. 14–15.

Table 1 Patients treated by the State in some local infirmaries, in %, 1880–1910

	Montreux	*Morges*	*Nyon*	*Payerne*	*St. Croix*	*Yverdon*
1880	5.9	–	13.4	–	–	36.0
1890	–	19.3	29.6	40.3	14.8	53.4
1900	0.3	18.4	32.7	42.1	7.6	38.6
1910	13.3	41.9	63.0	43.2	54.0	52.3

Source RSC, Department of the Interior; annual reports of individual institutions

against the generalised and uncontrolled development of the system appeared at the end of the 1890s. Jean-Marc Morax, head of the Health Service, declared at the inauguration of the new Saint-Loup Infirmary in 1897 that "the decentralisation of hospital services is most welcome. However, it has its limits, because we cannot have doctors or surgeons everywhere who are as experienced as those who practice in a large hospital".[12] These words met with little response at the time but were truly premonitory. The new Saint-Loup Infirmary inaugurated an era of transformation and modernisation of local infirmaries which made them competitors of the Cantonal Hospital in the inter-war period and led to the questioning of the hospital policy adopted in the 1870s (see Chapter 4).

The Financial Importance of Public Support for Local Infirmaries

At first, State subsidies remained limited: before 1900, they fluctuated around an annual sum of 32,000 francs. Their growth in the twentieth century was mainly due to the development of local infirmaries, whose increased capacity and constantly improving medical and technical infrastructure (X-ray facilities, aseptic operating theatres, wards for contagious patients, laboratories, etc.) allowed for a steady increase in hospitalisations. The amount of subsidies reached 130,400 francs in 1910 and 193,503 francs in 1920. This phase of growth did not cease throughout the twentieth century.[13] The State subsidy was granted according to a daily reference price set at two francs in 1875.

For the infirmaries, this State participation soon became a financial resource they could no longer do without as their development and operation were strongly dependent on the increased financial participation of patients and increased pensions. Despite the varying situations of the infirmaries, a general trend towards an increase in the number of patients whose hospitalisation was paid for by the State can be observed during the period 1880–1910. In 1910, almost half of the patients in most establishments received cantonal aid, as shown in Table 1. The infirmaries' financial dependence on public subsidies increased with their development.

[12] Institution of deaconesses of Saint-Loup, annual report 1896–1897, p. 34.

[13] RSC, Department of the Interior, 1875–1920.

The situation was different for the State. Subsidies to infirmaries became an increasingly important part of the Public Relief Service. There was a general upward trend between the mid-1880s (around 6–7% of the public relief budget) and 1914 (16.6%).[14] However, these amounts remained of almost negligible importance in the general State budget. They represented an average of 0.53% of ordinary expenditure over the whole period 1875–1914, with a slight upward trend in the years 1900–1914 (0.49% in 1880; 0.45% in 1900; 0.85% in 1910; and 0.97% in 1914).[15]

Even though subsidies to the infirmaries grew relatively slowly, they were called into question from the 1880s onwards. Indeed, the opening of the new Cantonal Hospital forced the State to make budgetary savings, particularly within the framework of the Department of the Interior. The government proposed to reduce the price of a day's hospitalisation reimbursed to the infirmaries for indigents to 1.2 francs, a reduction of 40%. This proposal led to a collective reaction from the private infirmaries, marking their first structuring into a lobby.

The Formation of a Private Hospital Lobby

At the instigation of the Moudon Infirmary, representatives of each private infirmary met in Lausanne in April 1883 in order to present a united opposition to the attempt to reduce public subsidies.[16] They succeeded in negotiating a limited reduction in the daily rate of reimbursement to 1.80 francs. This first confrontation between the two partners revealed the fragility of a mode of hospital development based on resources over which the infirmary administrators had no control. The infirmary delegates subsequently met on several occasions, to defend the subsidies they had acquired and demand they be increased to the real cost of a day's hospitalisation.

The State would not discuss a possible increase in subsidies; instead, it planned to reduce them to a rate of 1.50 francs a day by 1904, leading to the strong mobilisation of the infirmaries.[17] Their delegates met again in December 1903 in Lausanne and decided to improve the structure of the lobby by appointing a committee of three people "who will serve as a link and will convene delegates to a conference once a year to discuss all questions that may be of interest to the infirmaries in general".[18] In addition, at the instigation of the Nyon Infirmary, a petition was sent to the State Council while the liberal deputy Armand Piguet, a member of the Yverdon Infirmary's steering committee, intervened in the Grand Council and succeeded in restoring the subsidy to 1.80 francs. Despite this success and an initial structuring of the lobby, the delegates of the infirmaries rarely met before the end

14 RSC, Department of the Interior, 1875–1914.

15 RSC, Department of Finance, State Accounts, 1875–1914.

16 Yverdon Hospital, minutes of the administrative commission, 4–10 April 1883.

17 Ibidem, 27 January 1904.

18 Gustave Piotet, op. cit. p. 41.

of the 1920s. The State's contribution increased, thanks in particular to "pressure from the infirmaries"[19] (2.10 francs in 1917; 3.00 francs in 1922; etc.), and thus helped to settle disputes, even if it still did not cover the real cost of a day's hospitalisation. It was not until the 1930s that the movement became more assertive within the context of relative State withdrawal and increased competition between establishments within the hospital system.

3 Attempts to Reorganise the Hospital System During the Inter-War Period

The inter-war period was a time of rebalancing power within the hospital system. At the beginning of the twentieth century, the power was in favour of the local infirmaries, although the socio-economic evolution of the Vaud territory was clearly favourable to the city of Lausanne. While the cantonal policy of austerity and privatisation of the Cantonal Hospital did not allow for the planned growth of this establishment, local infirmaries were the object of profound transformation following the arrival of the surgeon-modernisers. The infirmaries' transformation into modern hospitals made them competitors to the Cantonal Hospital, mainly in the field of surgery, which led some professors to call for the adoption of a new policy based on organising the hospital network and the distribution of tasks between the various care institutions in the canton—a real division of labour applied at the level of the hospital system.

The Demand for the Centralisation of Investments in Lausanne

The modernisation of the local infirmaries had resulted in an increasingly competitive environment in the hospital system. This was to the detriment of the Cantonal Hospital which demanded the centralisation of investments in its clinics and the sharing of tasks between the various institutions in the hospital system. The division of medical work that was beginning to take place (for example, in Decker's surgical department) required increased financial resources and a critical mass of patients. Both of these resources suffered from the increased competitiveness of the hospital system. The question of the hospitalisation of chronically ill patients—who the modernised infirmaries no longer wanted to accommodate in large numbers—provided the first opportunity for the HHC and doctors close to the Faculty to demand State intervention in the 1920s.

Warnings About the Hospitalisation of the Chronically Ill in the 1920s

Gustave Delay, head of the Health Service and then chief doctor of the University Polyclinic, was a major player in hospital rationalisation. He intervened on numerous occasions at the HHC to request changes to the Cantonal Hospital that would allow savings to be made (limiting the number of employees,

[19] Ibidem.

combating the misuse of pharmaceutical specialities, etc.) and was an active promoter of the privatisation of certain hospital services. Delay was also one of the first to denounce the widespread development of local infirmaries which resulted in the poor distribution of chronic patients in the canton's establishments. Already in 1922, Delay declared, "there is a tendency to transform small infirmaries into large hospitals",[20] which revealed the desire of the surgeons in charge to concentrate on acute cases, which were more profitable for the infirmary, and to refuse the hospitalisation of the elderly and chronically ill. This habit led to an increasing number of chronically ill patients being admitted to the Cantonal Hospital, which led to a reaction from the medical profession and the administrative management of the establishment, denouncing the overcrowding of hospital beds by this type of patient. The evolution of the average length of stay—generally a decreasing trend in hospitals that are modernising—is a good indicator of the presence of chronic patients. The average length of stay at the Cantonal Hospital increased significantly between 1914 and 1935, from 29.5 days to 34.4 days.[21] In collaboration with the management of the Cantonal Hospital, Delay proposed to reverse the trend by offering special conditions to infirmaries that hospitalised chronic and incurable patients; however, his proposal did not meet the expected interest. The HHC itself intervened in the matter and decided, in 1923, to transform the Romainmôtier Infirmary, the only local healthcare establishment in the possession of the State, into an asylum for the elderly and incurable. However, it was a very small establishment and could not solve the problem of the centralisation of chronic cases in Lausanne—in 1915, it only had 18 beds that could accommodate 170 patients per year.[22]

Delay intervened at the HHC again in 1924 to denounce the refusal of infirmaries to accept tuberculosis patients and incurables, even though they tended to fill the beds of the Cantonal Hospital. He also stated their "surgical facilities [...] are in no way necessary; he cited the case of the Montreux Infirmary, which proposed to create a similar facility, estimated at 150,000 Swiss francs, and which did not meet a need".[23] Delay demanded the State stop subsidising the development of the hospital infrastructure outside of Lausanne. In January 1926, the chief doctors of the Cantonal Hospital intervened alongside Delay to complain about the modernisation of the local infirmaries. Taillens stated, in particular, that "the new spirit of the infirmaries comes from an improvement of the medical corps; the medical plethora also intervenes, and the doctors want to keep the interesting cases with them".[24] Three years later, Demiéville asked that hernia operations, which were technically very simple, no longer be performed at the Cantonal Hospital: "there

[20] ACV, S 73, minutes of the HHC, 29 March 1922.

[21] RSC, Department of the Interior, 1914–1935.

[22] ACV, K VIII B 113, report from Comtesse Infirmary, 1915.

[23] ACV, S 73, minutes of the HHC, 15 October 1924.

[24] Ibidem, 20 January 1926.

are enough young surgeons in the canton, who have been to the school of Prof. César Roux and who are perfectly qualified to operate on hernias in the infirmaries, without it being necessary to bring them all to the Cantonal Hospital".[25]

These demands began to bear fruit and the subsidy of 10,000 francs granted in 1927 to the Sainte-Croix Infirmary for its enlargement was only made in return for the provision of some beds for tuberculosis patients in the region. However, the transformation of this establishment served, above all, to turn it into a hospital equipped with modern materials and so it was more competitive than complementary to the Cantonal Hospital. The creation, by the Vaud Tuberculosis League and philanthropic circles, of pavilions for tuberculosis patients and the chronically ill in the districts was an essential step in resolving the issues with hospitalisation for these types of patients. The creation of new ad hoc establishments made it possible to satisfy both the local infirmaries and the Cantonal Hospital. In 1931, the State granted construction subsidies to the hospitals of Aigle, Orbe and La Vallée without requesting any compensation for the care of chronic patients. Similarly, in 1932, the opening of the Sandoz Hospice as a special unit of the Cantonal Hospital allowed the latter to be relieved of its chronic patients and to settle the controversy over the hospitalisation of these types of patients. Another, more specific problem arose with the appointment of Pierre Decker to the chair of surgery in 1932—that of the hospitalisation of surgical cases and competition between the surgical departments of the Cantonal Hospital and local hospitals.

Prof. Decker's Questioning of the Cantonal Hospital

Shortly after taking office (1932), Pierre Decker, head of the Department of Surgery, distinguished himself by his active opposition to the cantonal hospital policy which allowed the development of local infirmaries in all directions. He called for a concentration of financial resources in Lausanne and for the networking and prioritisation of the various healthcare establishments in the canton. The difficulties encountered with the creation of a new surgical clinic, requested since the beginning of the 1930s but only opened in 1947, largely explain Decker's vehement opposition to the generalised development of the regional hospitals of Vaud. In the 1930s, the surgical department of the Cantonal Hospital was too small and poorly equipped with medical and technical infrastructure to allow the development of team surgery and the affirmation of surgical specialities. Moreover, the improvement of the surgical equipment of the regional hospitals made these institutions serious competitors for the Cantonal Hospital. According to Prof. Michaud, "if the infirmaries also want to keep these patients [acute cases], this is because the country doctor likes to operate, because the public sees an immediate success. It is therefore easy for him to make a good reputation for himself by this means, and this quickly. Internal medicine cases, on the other hand, are boring. Often

[25] Ibidem, 9 March 1929.

these cases are unclear, it is difficult to make a diagnosis, so they prefer to send them to the university medical clinic".[26]

Decker needed a considerable number of patients, not only for the purposes of university teaching, but also to enable surgical research to take place. Behind the demand for a new surgical clinic was the desire to centralise the State's financial investments and to turn the regional hospitals into second-rate establishments for the care of chronic patients, tuberculosis patients, convalescents, etc.; that is, cases less interesting to the State. Decker's demands were supported by the HHC which saw two possible ways to combat the excessive decentralisation of infrastructure. In the short term, the State was to use its subsidies given to regional hospitals to implement a real spatial planning policy for hospital infrastructure. In 1935, Prof. Delay stated, "there can be no question of demolishing existing infirmaries, but the building of new ones can be prevented. The budget for the infirmaries is essentially based on the cost of boarding patients in the State"[27] but also, in the longer term, "we need to train fewer surgeons at the Cantonal Hospital".[28] The hospital system had become competitive and Decker was concerned about the place of his surgical department in the healthcare market, especially as there would be a decline in surgical hospitalisations in the early 1930s.

This question was debated within the HHC throughout the 1930s. The State Council was very sensitive to the professor's arguments, especially as centralising investments in Lausanne would allow budgetary savings. Indeed, under the 1875 law on infirmaries, the State granted subsidies for the construction of hospital buildings—a windfall that proved decisive for several of them: in the mid-1930s, Montreux received 16,270 francs as cantonal aid for the construction of a new hospital (1934); Saint-Loup 44,876 francs (1935); Rolle 48,150 francs (1936); and Nyon 44,000 francs (1938).[29] On the advice of the HHC, the Vaud government decided, in 1936, to stop granting construction subsidies to regional hospitals.[30] The financial interests of the State were perfectly in line with the HHC's desire to rationalise.

Decker was not satisfied with this decision. In January 1939, he wrote a report for the HHC and the Department of Public Education in which he wondered whether it was "justified to create, as has just been done in a very short time, hospitals that are expensive to set up every 15 or even 10 kms".[31] Decker thought in terms of the spatial organisation of the hospital system and was considering the negative effects for the Cantonal Hospital of the competition brought by the modernisation of the infirmaries. He denounced

[26] ACV, K VIII D 68, annual conference, 25 June 1946.

[27] ACV, minutes of the HHC, 8 November 1935.

[28] Ibid.

[29] RSC, Department of the Interior, 1930–1940.

[30] Decree of 24 March 1936.

[31] ALS, report by Professor Decker to the Department of Public Education, 14 January 1939, unlisted.

the excessive density of surgical facilities, and the high cost of amortising new infrastructure in small general hospitals and demanded, in the context of a public financial crisis, the centralisation of investments in Lausanne. In conclusion, Decker called for a reorganisation of the Vaud hospital system on the basis of sectoral complementarity between establishments: "What we need is a central hospital that is normally equipped, with a normal budget that allows us to treat our patients in the same way as those from other Swiss cantons or other countries. What we need, on the other hand, is to find a way of hospitalising with sufficient comfort, but as economically as possible, the indigent who cannot be treated at home, the elderly, the chronically ill, the incurable".[32] He was supported by La Source, who stated, "the present boom has been largely caused by the remarkable preparation of young surgeons at the Cantonal Hospital"[33] and "our Infirmaries will [...] certainly have broad enough views to understand that it is in their own interest to take account of the general and distant concerns of Professor Decker"[34]; however, the report caused an outcry in the canton.

After the opening of the new Surgical Clinic (1947), Decker became less insistent and less determined. The post-war situation favoured the general development of the hospital system and the growth of regional hospitals occurred without detriment to the Cantonal Hospital. Decker was nonetheless aware of the problems posed by this phenomenon. In a letter written, in 1953, to the Fribourg State Councillor, Paul Torche, he supported the project of a Cantonal Hospital in the neighbouring canton of Fribourg and warned him of the difficulties he could expect: "What seems likely to me is that the spirit which already prevails in the canton of Vaud of dispersion of means, of extremely advanced decentralisation, will also develop in the canton of Fribourg in the more or less distant future. There is nothing to be done about it, I think: it is the inevitable consequence of the medical plethora".[35] Decker's resignation is largely explained by the success of the lobbying of the local infirmaries, against which he had been unable to do anything during the previous two decades.

Regional Hospitals' Opposition to the Cantonal Policy

The modernised regional hospitals were strongly opposed to the policy of centralisation and the disengagement of the State. First of all, they rejected the restructuring plans of the Department of the Interior and those of Prof. Decker. The doctors working in the regional hospitals, mainly surgeons, had made these establishments into working tools they used for their private practice. There was, therefore, no question of them reorganising the hospital

[32] Ibid.

[33] ALS, letter from the management of La Source to AIV, 24 February 1939, unlisted.

[34] Ibid.

[35] ACF, DSPa 229, letter from Pierre Decker to Paul Torche, 31 January 1953.

Table 2 Patients treated by the State in selected regional hospitals, as a % of the total, 1920–1940

	Aigle	*Montreux*	*Morges*	*Nyon*	*Payerne*	*Vevey-Samaritain*	*Children's Hospice*
1920	59.3	22.9	45.1	45.7	46.8	34.5	5.1
1930	33.9	15.9	34.2	36.6	33.2	23.2	6.3
1940	36.0	15.3	32.2	23.7	16.5	16.1	3.3

Source Annual reports of the various regional hospitals; CRCE, Department of the Interior, 1920–1940

system in the sense of sharing care between the Cantonal Hospital (acute care, particularly in the surgical field) and their hospitals (minor surgery and chronic patients). At the Lavaux Infirmary, Charles Rochat, a surgeon, was opposed to accepting chronic patients from the Sandoz Hospice for essentially economic reasons. In 1943, he wrote to the board of directors of his establishment, "the chronic patients evacuated from the Sandoz Hospice will increase the operating deficit of the Lavaux Infirmary. In fact, a doctor on duty is needed to treat them, and this costs the Infirmary Fr. 1200 per year. These patients require much more assiduous care from the staff of the house. Most of them are elderly and dirty their beds, hence the need to wash and change their bedding and linen very often, which is very expensive in these times. [...] It is a bad business for the Lavaux Infirmary to want to relieve the Sandoz Hospice. I think we have enough chronically ill patients in our Lavaux clientele, and I see the day coming when we will no longer be able to accept these acute and profitable cases (accidents, small operations) because all the places will be taken by chronically ill patients who cannot be evacuated. The Lavaux Infirmary will be, in a way, a dead end" (Table 2).[36]

This financial argument went to the heart of the matter. By modernising, the regional hospitals opened up to a non-indigent and profitable clientele that did not depend on aid from the State. During the 1920s and 1930s, the proportion of indigent patients, whose stay was paid for by the Hospices Service, fell sharply in all regional hospitals (see Table 2). Establishments such as Morges, Payerne or Vevey-Samaritain, for example, had only 15–16% indigent patients among their clientele. The proportion of non-indigent patients became dominant yet it was precisely with the pensions and various taxes of this new clientele that the regional hospitals financed their operations. Under these conditions, it was unthinkable to accept a restructuring of the hospital system in the sense of the centralisation of acute and profitable cases in Lausanne.

The surgeon-modernisers of the local infirmaries had important political connections which they used to organise resistance against the policy led by Decker and the HHC. This struggle to save the regional hospitals took place

[36] Lavaux Hospital, letter from Dr Rochat to the Board of Directors, 3 March 1943.

in a particular socio-economic context which, during the inter-war period, saw the city of Lausanne assert its demographic and economic predominance while the rest of the canton was stagnating. Opposition to the centralisation of hospital medicine in the city of Lausanne thus depended as much on regional and political factors as on strictly medical reasons.

Even though few surgeons personally sat on the Grand Council—only Alfred Goin, surgeon of the Moudon Hospital and liberal deputy, was a member—they were strongly inserted in local political networks. A good number of these surgeons were municipal councillors (e.g., Chessex in Les Planches, Curchod in La Sarraz, Goin in Moudon, Moehrlen in Orbe, Piotet in Nyon, Vuilleumier in Bex). Association networks also played an important role, such as alumni societies and service clubs, like the Rotary Club, which enabled links to be established with the political world. Mario Guex, a surgeon at the Morges Hospital since 1944, is a fine example of this commitment: he was a town councillor, president of the local Liberal Party and governor of the Rotary for Western Switzerland. Finally, these surgeons were fully supported by the management committees of the various hospitals which generally included local MPs. Decker and the Department of the Interior were faced with a strong and structured political opposition. Payot, head of the Health Service, was well aware of this and warned his fellow professors, in 1946: "If we insist any further, we will be exposed to a barrage of interventions in the Grand Council".[37] Some deputies began to express their opposition to the development of the Cantonal Hospital towards the end of the 1930s, such as the liberal deputy from Montreux, Marius Léderrey, who, in 1937, unsuccessfully requested that the matter not be discussed when credit for the expansion of the ENT department of the Cantonal Hospital was being debated. He intervened a second time in 1946, again in vain, on the occasion of credit of more than 700,000 francs for the Cantonal Hospital, demanding greater attention from the State to regional hospitals.

The Structuring of the Lobby: The Association of Vaud Infirmaries (1930–1947)

In order to better defend their interests, contest government policy and fight for an increase in state subsidies, the infirmaries grouped to form the Association of Vaud Infirmaries (*Association des Infirmeries Vaudoises*, AIV), founded on 12 February 1930. The will to adopt a united line of demands against the State was taken up from the start. It was, therefore, no coincidence that the State-owned Romainmôtier Infirmary was excluded from the AIV at this meeting.[38] One of the major actions of this lobby was their intervention with

[37] ACV, K VIII D 68, annual conference, 25 June 1946.

[38] ALS, minutes of the IAC meeting of 12 February 1930.

the State to demand an increase in the price of a reimbursed day of hospitalisation for the indigent (1931, 1932, 1938, 1941)[39] which it finally obtained in 1942.

Although the various demands of the AIV might lead one to believe otherwise, the State continued to support the hospitalisation of the indigent. The total annual public contribution even increased slightly during the inter-war period, from 193,503 francs in 1920 to 372,686 francs in 1945.[40] For the State, these contributions represented an increasingly important part of the expenses of the Public Relief Service (5.2% in 1920; 7.2% in 1930; and 8.0% in 1940) due to the policy of austerity adopted in other areas.

The AIV also intervened in the question of the reorganisation of the cantonal hospital system and responded strongly to the report by Prof. Decker.[41] The local infirmaries were in favour of collaboration with the State but on a voluntary basis. They categorically rejected any intervention by the State in their organisation and management, recalling that they are private companies. As a structured, determined and effective lobby, the AIV was able to maintain the status quo of its establishments from the years 1930–1945. This relative position of strength thus favoured the affirmation of the hospital union as an inevitable interlocutor in post-war hospital policy.

4 The Implementation of a New Hospital Plan (1945–1966)

The financial difficulties of the State during the inter-war period undoubtedly explain the absence of reform within the hospital system and the lack of coordination in the hospitalisation of patients between the various establishments. The situation was quite different after 1945. Public finances were no longer an obstacle to State intervention in the coordinated development of the hospital system. In addition, the socio-economic evolution of the canton after 1945 was characterised by urbanisation and reorganisation of the territory which required the redeployment of the hospital system. The aim was to eliminate competition between hospitals and replace it with geographical and sectoral complementarity, offering equal treatment to the various inhabitants of the canton, regardless of their status (indigent, insured, etc.) and their place of residence. In order to achieve this system-wide rationalisation, the cantonal authorities called on external experts to draw up a hospital plan.

[39] ACV, K VIII B 213/15, letter from the AIV to the Department of the Interior, 11 February 1938.

[40] RSC, Department of the Interior, various years.

[41] ACV, K VIII B 213/15, AIV report on Decker's requests of January 1939, 27 April 1939.

The Affirmation of the State in Public Health

In 1946, the arrival of Gabriel Despland as the head of the Department of the Interior marked an important turning point in cantonal hospital policy. The wait-and-see position adopted during the inter-war period was abandoned in favour of a consensual interventionist approach with the aim of ensuring a functioning hospital system and responding to the demands of the main actors involved (institutions, doctors and insurance companies).

The number of civil servants responsible for monitoring the cantonal hospital policy increased for the first time since the 1860s, from a total of five people before 1945 to eight in 1950 and eleven in 1960. Above all, the 1950s and 1960s saw the emergence of experts in the field of hospital policy from outside public administration, as mandated by the Council of State to conceive a homogeneous hospital system organised and managed as a whole. The restructuring of the Department of the Interior from 1957 to 1958 is a good expression of this desire for reform. This reorganisation was characterised by the separation of management and assistance tasks in hospital policy. Until then, the Hospice Service had been responsible for all these functions. This service was dissolved in 1957 and replaced by two new departments with clearly defined responsibilities. Firstly, the Social Welfare and Public Assistance Service included various offices (assistance, hospitalisation, accounting and litigation) and was involved in hospital policy concerning the conditions of hospitalisation at the Cantonal Hospital and the agreements negotiated with insurance companies, doctors and regional hospitals. Secondly, the Public Health Service replaced and took over the responsibilities of the former Health Service and was also given the onerous task of coordinating the development of the hospital system, including drawing up a hospital plan.

As for the HHC, it continued to include, in addition to the State Councillor at the head of the Department of the Interior and the head of the Health Service, representatives of the medical professions and personalities with specific skills. Among the twelve people appointed to the HHC during the years 1946–1955, there were five doctors and seven experts, including a lawyer and businessman, a professor of psychology, and a company director. In 1958, however, the HHC was reorganised to focus on medical rather than managerial skills. Bringing together the cantonal doctor, the head of the Public Health Service, the cantonal veterinarian and the public prosecutor, along with the State Councillor in charge of the Interior, the HHC concentrated on questions of medical practice, leaving managerial and organisational issues to the officials of the Department of Interior.

This new organisational structure corresponds to the affirmation of the State as an essential player in the reorganisation of the hospital system. Its intervention took place in two stages. Firstly, during the 1950s, it was a question of guaranteeing the hospitalisation of patients in a uniform manner, in the context of rising costs and of harmonising the conditions of access to the various establishments. Secondly, the question of the standardisation of hospitalisation conditions raised the issue of relations between establishments within the hospital system and the transition from a situation of competition to one of complementarity. These problems were discussed in the early 1960s and led to the adoption of a hospital plan in 1966.

Guaranteeing the Hospitalisation of Patients

The rising cost of hospitalisation caused by changes in hospital medicine was at the heart of the political debate in the 1950s. It posed a double problem. First was the question of ensuring the material viability of hospitals whose main resources came from patients' pensions. The second problem was also a social one: guaranteeing wider access to hospital medicine as an integral part of the State's tasks. The agreement signed in 1953 between the State and the regional hospitals solved the problem of the hospitalisation of the indigent. The problem of the hospitalisation of patients covered by health insurance and the "economically weak"—i.e., people with average incomes, not considered indigent and without a health insurance fund who risked falling into poverty in the event of illness—remained unsolved. Several interventions in the Grand Council raised the problem of these categories of people.

The 1953 Convention for the Hospitalisation of Indigents

The main cause of conflict between the State and the regional hospitals since the end of the nineteenth century, the question of reimbursement for the days of indigent patients, found a satisfactory answer in the early 1950s under pressure from the GHRV. A report sent to the Department of the Interior in 1947, highlighted the importance of regional hospitals in hospitalising patients and the little financial support they received from the State.[42] It compared regional hospitals and the Cantonal Hospital, showing that in 1944 the former had 1466 beds and 473,779 patient days, while the Cantonal Hospital had only 1077 beds and 356,419 patient days. In 1946, the financial burden for the State amounted to 2.5 million francs for the Cantonal Hospital and only 343,000 francs for the regional hospitals. This report was an opportunity for the GHRV to demand the State pay the real cost of a patient's day of hospitalisation.

At the beginning of the 1950s, the regional hospitals pushed for the creation of a hospital plan which would organise the hospitalisation of patients throughout the canton. This would be a recognition by the State of its role and, therefore, of its participation in the management costs. Around 1951, a study commission was founded with the aim of defining the relationship between the State and regional hospitals. In the same year, a unified chart of accounts was imposed by the GHRV on its members and came into force. It

[42] ACV, PP 324/9, report on the financial situation of the regional hospitals of the canton of Vaud, 18 November 1947.

was intended not only as a management tool but also as an information and communication tool. By having a streamlined and unified accounting system in all its institutions, the GHRV could present itself to the Department of the Interior as a credible partner with scientifically established figures (see Chapter 4).

The State Council finally agreed to the GHRV's requests and signed an agreement with it to cover the actual costs of the hospitalisation of indigent patients (in 1953). In addition, this agreement led to the creation of a joint commission for the rationalisation of hospitalisation, bringing together representatives of the State, the Cantonal Hospital and the regional hospitals to discuss the reorganisation of the hospital system.

The Forel Motion on Hospital Conditions (1953)

In 1953, the communist deputy Armand Forel submitted a motion to the Grand Council requesting a study of the general revision of the conditions of hospitalisation throughout the canton. In fact, the agreement signed with the regional hospitals only regulated the question of indigent patients and left aside those who were members of a health insurance fund, as well as those without support. For these categories of patients, there were still major disparities depending on the institution in which they were hospitalised and/or the insurance company to which they were affiliated. Furthermore, the indigent status was treated differently depending on whether one was cared for in a GHRV facility or in the Cantonal Hospital. In the latter, there was a sliding scale between the completely indigent, who paid nothing, and the non-indigent; it was the hospital management team who decided the amount of a hospitalised person's contribution according to his or her material conditions. In regional hospitals, by virtue of an agreement with the State, the latter reimbursed the entire cost for the completely indigent and nothing for others. The Forel motion thus called for "the standardisation of hospitalisation conditions between all the establishments in our canton, as well as the extension of the agreements signed with the health insurance companies to the regional hospitals".[43]

This intervention had no other aim than to establish true equality of treatment between all the inhabitants of the canton; however, it raised the question of the status of the Cantonal Hospital, whose privileged conditions of hospitalisation ensured the presence of a large number of patients. The faculty's leading figures feared the perverse effects of the Forel motion on the Cantonal Hospital in terms of the number of hospitalisations. This was an opportunity for Prof. Decker to reaffirm his point of view. Together with Prof. Rochat, he wrote a report defending the Cantonal Hospital, approved by the Faculty Council. In the report, Prof. Vannotti "expresses his gratitude to Messrs Decker and Rochat. The Nestlé Hospital became an asylum for the elderly. Some regional hospitals, for example, the one in Yverdon, never send him

[43] BCG, 9 December 1953.

interesting cases, but only old arteriosclerotic patients. He had the impression that the Vaud doctor had much less pride in his faculty than the doctors in Berne or Zurich".[44] As for Prof. Rochat, he "says he is surprised that some hospital doctors have joined forces with the Forel deputy to organise an offensive against the Cantonal Hospital. He is convinced that most of the doctors in the regional hospitals are enemies of the Faculty and are completely uninterested in the teaching mission of the Faculty".[45]

The only member of the Faculty Council who defended the regional hospitals was Prof. Urech, who was personally involved in the problem, as he was then the head physician of the Saint-Loup Hospital in addition to his teaching practice. He fought against the idea of a medical plethora and found another explanation that did not question the medical power: "What has greatly increased the overheads of the regional hospitals are above all the salaries of the nurses, which have been greatly increased, which is fair enough".[46] In the end, the fact that the Faculty Council and the Cantonal Hospital rejected the Forel motion meant that it was referred to the State Council for study. The latter instructed the newly created Joint Commission for the Rationalisation of Hospitalisation to take into account the problems raised by the communist deputy in its reflections.

The Joint Commission for the Rationalisation of Hospitalisation (1954–1960)

Desiring to perpetuate the dynamic resulting from the tripartite meetings between the State, the Cantonal Hospital and the GHRV that led to the signing of the 1953 agreement, State Councillor Gabriel Despland set up a Commission for the Rationalisation of Hospitalisation, chaired by a Cantonal judge and with representatives of the three partners. This commission was a discussion forum for actors who had been in latent conflict for more than fifty years and proved to be a decisive step in the construction of a policy based on complementarity between the various elements of the hospital system. The GHRV recognised the regional hospitals could no longer afford their individualistic policy and only State support would enable them to develop their infrastructure and remain modern general hospitals in the near future. For the first time, in 1954, the GHRV accepted the need to discuss a new distribution of patients between the two partners and the principle of centralising "all serious cases and cases of scientific interest" in Lausanne.[47] It was also within this commission that the representatives of the GHRV demanded, in 1959, the adoption of a cantonal hospitalisation plan. They stated, "the various hospitals must all be integrated into a co-ordination plan in order to play the role

[44] Archives of the University of Lausanne, minutes of the meetings of the Council of the Faculty of Medicine, 30 October 1953.

[45] Ibid.

[46] Ibid.

[47] AFHCV, minutes of the meeting of 29 June 1964.

assigned to them. No hospital can or should go it alone. It is, among other things, essential that any innovation, any new construction be submitted to the Joint Rationalisation Commission to study how it fits into the hospitalisation plan".[48] This desire to coordinate the development of the canton's hospital infrastructure was reinforced by the motion of the liberal deputy François Cuénoud on hospital status (1957) which "had the effect of a bomb in the Grand Council".[49]

Since the inauguration of its new surgical clinic, the development of the Cantonal Hospital had led to new fears on the part of surgeons and administrators of regional hospitals. The agreement signed with the State in 1953 for indigent patients was not sufficient to guarantee them the resources needed to ensure their modernisation. The small Lavaux Hospital, some fifteen kilometres from the Cantonal Hospital, felt directly threatened by the expansion of its powerful neighbour. Charles Rochat, a surgeon in Cully, intervened with the president of the board of directors of the Lavaux Hospital, the deputy Cuénoud, and suggested he "set up a political hospitalisation programme"[50] more favourable to regional establishments. Hostile, in principle, to the development of the State and the Faculty of Medicine, Cuénoud tabled a motion in 1957 calling for "the modification of the Vaud hospital statute",[51] supported by the GHRV and the Vaud employers' associations. The discussion of nine million francs in credit that the State Council proposed to grant to the Nestlé Hospital (the medical clinic of the Cantonal Hospital) was an opportunity to demand the decentralisation of hospital facilities as well as collaboration between the Cantonal Hospital and regional hospitals. Cuénoud said, "We know that after the Nestlé Hospital and its nine million, it will be the turn of the Sandoz Hospital, then other pavilions, other services and so on. This is why it seems logical and necessary to us to ask the State Council to define a clear and precise hospital policy".[52]

This motion was referred twice to a commission for further study (in 1957 and 1958). A second commission was then appointed by the State Council in 1959 to examine the issue with the aim of defining a new statewide hospital policy. The Vaud government was all the more sensitive to this problem as some departments of the Cantonal Hospital were experiencing serious overcrowding problems in the mid-1950s. In February 1955, the State Council replied to Fernand Petit, a socialist deputy who was concerned about the overcrowding of the Cantonal Hospital in an interpellation to the Grand Council, that "the first remedy for the permanent overcrowding of certain departments of the Cantonal Hospital lies in a more judicious distribution of patients

[48] AFHCV, hospitalisation plan, undated [1959].

[49] AFHCV, letter from Zwahlen to Bel, bursar of the Payerne Hospital, 2 December 1957.

[50] AFHCV, note from François Cuénoud to Charles Rochat, undated.

[51] BGC, 27 November 1957.

[52] Ibid.

among the various hospitals in the canton"[53] and that the Commission for the Rationalisation of Hospitalisation had been entrusted with this issue.

Despite these various interventions carried out by the Grand Council, the Rationalisation Commission did not address the problem of reorganising hospital policy in its entirety. Its work focused on the introduction of a hospitalisation agreement for patients insured by a health insurance fund in all the canton's hospitals, except for private clinics. The principles that led to the adoption, in 1960, of a hospital agreement for patients insured by the State, regional hospitals, insurance companies and doctors were the standardisation of hospital conditions and the abandonment of competitiveness within the hospital system. Negotiations within the commission for the rationalisation of the hospital system lasted throughout the period 1954–1960 and aimed to meet the expectations of all parties in a consensual manner.

For the regional hospitals, the challenge was to obtain identical hospitalisation conditions compared to those practised at the Cantonal Hospital which they accused of "a kind of unfair competition or rather intolerable dumping".[54] Indeed, the State's coverage of its budget deficit allowed it to charge hospitalisation rates for insured patients that were below the institution's profitability threshold—a policy that was not feasible in regional hospitals. The GHRV's position vis-à-vis the State and the insurance companies was unequivocal: "Insured inpatients must pay the same price in all public or semipublic hospitals".[55] Moreover, this hospital tariff should not be lower than the average cost price.

The Cantonal Hospital and the Department of the Interior agreed to the GHRV's request—a necessary condition for the desired standardisation. The agreement signed in 1952 between the Cantonal Hospital and the Vaud Federation of Mutual Aid Societies (*Fédération vaudoise des sociétés de secours mutuels*, FVSSM) was thus denounced by the State in 1958 to add the regional hospitals which required a sharp increase in the agreed tariffs for the insurance companies. However, the latter had serious difficulties due to the rise in prices (inflation + hospitalisation costs) being much higher than the increase in federal subsidies. The most important health insurance companies in the canton had large operating deficits; for example, the *Société vaudoise des secours mutuels* (approx. 60,000 members) lost 544,000 francs in 1957 and *Helvetia* (approx. 27,500 members) more than 320,000 francs in 1958.[56] Increasing the agreed tariffs could only lead to an increase in membership fees.[57] This situation led to several interventions in the Grand Council in 1958–1959

[53] BGC, 3 May 1955.

[54] AFHCV, presentation by Eugène Zwahlen to the Vaud Medical Society, 16 January 1958.

[55] Ibid.

[56] BGC, 27 May 1959.

[57] The FVSSM registered, in 1958, an increase in monthly contributions of almost 10%. AFHCV, presentation by Eugène Zwahlen to the Vaud Medical Society, 16 January 1958.

by left-wing deputies, who advocated easier access to hospital care for the entire population, and representatives of the health insurance companies who demanded negotiations with the State. In order to guarantee a single agreed tariff in the canton's establishments and to encourage the population to join a health insurance scheme despite the increase in contributions, the State Council adopted a law on the encouragement of insurance, which came into force in 1957 and provided support for disadvantaged social categories.[58]

After the question of insurance had been resolved, the question of doctors working in regional hospitals and the reimbursement of their fees remained. Here, too, the diversity between institutions was extreme. In order to rationalise the system and control the growth of costs, the GHRV, the insurance companies and the State demanded a switch to flat-rate fees but they were opposed by the Vaud Medical Society (*Société vaudoise de médecine*, SVM) which defended the principle of fee-for-service for its members. After negotiations, the SVM accepted the principle of fixed fees (1.5 francs per day per patient in 1958), except for the surgeons who demanded to be paid on a fee-for-service basis. In order to overcome this opposition, the GHRV proposed the creation of an organisation responsible for collecting lump sums from patients and insurance companies—calculated on the basis of the average fees paid the previous year—and paying surgeons on a fee-for-service basis.[59] While this measure met the requirement of the surgeons, it entailed bureaucratic red tape in the regional hospitals and the hiring of administrative staff (see Chapter 4).

The agreement signed between the various partners in 1960 led to the opening of a Central Collection Office responsible for its financial operation (see Fig. 2). Its aim was to guarantee the insurance companies an identical price of hospitalisation in all the hospitals in the canton which, added to State aid, covered the actual expenditure of the hospitals as well as the medical fees. After a reserve—in the guarantee funds—to cover a possible deficit of one or other of the compensation funds, the money collected by the Central Office was given to the hospitals and doctors. After the adoption of this method of financing, the renewal of the agreement was discussed on the basis of the indexation of hospital costs and medical fees. This agreement remained in force until 1980 when the principle of a budgetary envelope for each hospital came into force.

As Eugène Zwahlen explained in 1958, the real challenge of the 1960 agreement lay in the fact that "with the application of this system, the famous competition from the Cantonal Hospital would be purely and simply eliminated".[60] The elimination of competition within the hospital system, as well as the consideration of the demands of its various actors (insurance companies,

[58] Law of 3 September 1956 on the promotion of health insurance.

[59] AFHCV, presentation by Eugène Zwahlen to the Vaud Medical Society, 16 January 1958.

[60] Ibidem.

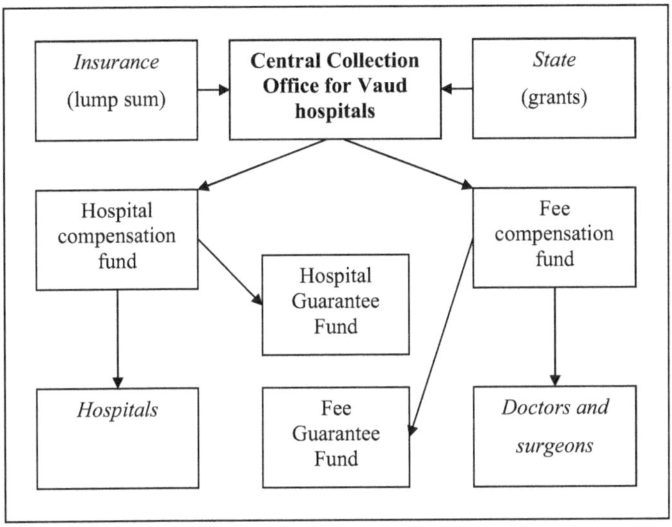

Fig. 2 The operation of the hospital convention, 1960–1980

doctors, hospitals), made it possible to construct, during the 1960s, a new hospital policy based on complementarity between hospitals. This new stage was achieved through the intervention of a new category of experts which will be discussed in the next section.

The 1966 Hospital Plan: A Guarantee for the Widespread Development of the System

Negotiations leading to the signing of agreements for indigent patients (1953) and insured patients (1960) showed that rationalisation of hospitalisation was feasible provided the expectations of the various partners were taken into account. On the basis of these consensual experiences, rationalisation was extended to hospital equipment in the 1960s.

The Hospital Advisory Commission (1959–1961)

In 1959, the State Council decided to set up a new consultative commission on hospital issues to bring together the main players in the field of hospitalisation in the canton. Chaired by a cantonal judge, it included representatives of the medical profession, insurance companies, regional hospitals and the State. Its official mandate was to make "proposals for the establishment of normal relations between health insurance companies, regional hospitals and cantonal hospitals, in the best interests of patients and other interested parties".[61] However, in an informal way, this commission played a decisive role in the

[61] AFHCV, Council of State order, 21 April 1959.

construction of the new cantonal hospital policy. It brought together representatives of the various actors in the hospital system to discuss a solution that satisfied them all on issues that went beyond the 1960 agreement which only regulated the problem of hospitalisation of insured patients. This new commission continued the consultative work carried out during the period 1954–1960 by the rationalisation commission which was dissolved in 1961. In September 1960, the State Council mandated it to take up the whole issue of hospitalisation, which had been raised by various motions and petitions since 1953 and to which no formal response had ever been given, and to provide guidelines that would satisfy the various partners.

Under pressure from a petition submitted to the Grand Council in February 1960, the commission asked the State Council to continue the policy of encouraging health insurance with the aim of increasing the proportion of the population covered by insurance which, in 1960, was only about 50%.[62] This proposal was taken into consideration and the State budget for health insurance promotion was increased from 450,000 francs in 1960 to 750,000 francs the following year.[63] Several members of the commission, led by the director of the Cantonal Hospital, even called for the adoption of compulsory health insurance subsidised by the State, Piotet arguing, "the assisted, like the economically weak [i.e. the middle classes], are far from all having the capacity for discernment that would allow them to conceive of the obligation to be provident".[64] However, this proposal was opposed by State Councillor Despland, who was more in favour of the private initiative and the status quo in this area; he stated, "the term 'assistance' no longer exists and that the left-wing parties use it for their political propaganda".[65] He asked the commission to abandon its reflections on health insurance and to concentrate on the problems of coordination of hospital policy.

In the report sent to the State Council in March 1961, the commission drew up an inventory of the existing hospital infrastructure in the canton. Dividing the various establishments according to the type of patients treated (acute, chronic or other), it stated, "the patients were not rationally distributed among the hospitals"[66] and the 8910 hospital beds available in the canton were insufficient, particularly for chronic patients. The functional complementarity of the various components of the hospital system became a new challenge for hospital policy, in line with the abandonment of competition.

[62] This proportion would then be 90% in the canton of Zurich and 70–80% in the canton of Berne. AFHCV, minutes of the Consultative Commission on Hospitalisation, 2 November 1960.

[63] AFHCV, minutes of the Hospitalisation Advisory Committee, 14 December 1960.

[64] Ibidem, 11 January 1961.

[65] AFHCV, summary of the meeting held on 31 January 1961 between Mr. State Councillor Despland, Head of the Department of the Interior and Mr. Cantonal Judge André Rossel, President of the Hospitalisation Advisory Commission.

[66] AFHCV, report to State Councillor Despland, 13 March 1961.

The Working Group for the Establishment of the Hospital Building Programme (1959–1966)

Originally, this working group, founded in 1959 by the State Council, had the task of setting up the extension of the Cantonal Hospital, particularly in terms of property. At its request, the working group was assisted by a Design office for Vaud Hospital City (*Bureau d'études pour la Cité hospitalière vaudoise*), founded by the State Council in 1960 and headed by a Lausanne architect, William Vetter. The appointment of Vetter as director of this office corresponded to the desire of the cantonal authorities to have recourse to an internationally recognised expert in hospital development. The design of the new surgical clinic at the Cantonal Hospital (1947), in collaboration with Jean-Pierre Vouga, enabled him to be noticed by the World Health Organisation (WHO) and be entrusted with numerous missions in developing countries (Jordan, Syria, Turkey, Vietnam, etc.) during the 1950s where he supervised the construction of large hospital units. The work carried out in Lausanne by Vetter's office was directly responsible for the design of the Vaud University Hospital Centre (*Centre hospitalier universitaire vaudois*, CHUV).[67]

Freed from the problem of extending the Cantonal Hospital, the working group was given a new task, in 1961, of "promoting a real cantonal hospital plan"[68] and coordinating the development of the Cantonal Hospital with other hospital buildings. To this end, in 1961, it brought together representatives of the medical profession, insurance companies and regional hospitals. Noting "the canton's hospital facilities had developed without any overall vision",[69] the working group wanted to plan for future needs, taking into account the existing hospital system and its development possibilities. Here, too, the working group proposed the use of experts who could assess the situation in a scientific manner. The State Council accepted the principle of a hospital plan in 1962 and entrusted its implementation to the Design office directed by Vetter. Sociologists were called in to support the working group and the Public Health Service. Hospital planning thus left the realm of advisory commissions and was placed in the hands of experts. In 1964, the sociologist Pierre Gilliand explained to representatives of the medical profession and regional hospitals that "planning [...] is the effort to organise, coordinate and forecast in order to increase the capacity to control events".[70] In the 1960s, he carried out a prospective socio-demographic study in which he assessed the need for hospital infrastructure in the early 1980s. Highlighting the ageing

[67] Anne-Marie Clavel and Louis-Samuel Prod'hom, *Historique de la mutation de l'Hôpital cantonal de Lausanne en Centre hospitalier universitaire vaudois de 1959 à 1990*, s.l., 1993, Véronique Dreyfuss, *Le Bloc hospitalier du CHUV: Essai de géographie urbaine*, Lausanne, L'Aire, 1979.

[68] AFHCV, minutes of the discussions of the Working Group for the establishment of the hospital building programme, 27 November and 18 December 1961.

[69] Ibid.

[70] AFHCV, minutes of the meeting of 29 June 1964.

of the population as the main feature of future demographic change, he concluded this "profoundly modifies the structure of hospital needs expressed in terms of the number of beds per age group, per admission department and per diagnostic group. As a result, geriatrics is taking on an increasing role in existing general hospitals. This directly raises the question of the structure of the general hospital and even the general hospital network".[71] Gilliand's studies for the development of the hospital plan were defended in the form of a doctoral thesis, supervised by Pierre Jaccard, professor of sociology and member of the HHC, Armand Delachaux, professor of social and preventive medicine, and a French WHO official, Robert Frédéric Bridgman, who had been one of the promoters of hospital planning on the European continent since the 1940s. Gilliand became the main expert on hospital planning in French-speaking Switzerland in the second half of the twentieth century.[72]

Vetter's team developed multilateral collaborations with regional hospitals, doctors and insurance companies, whose demands remained the same (absence of competition, a flat rate for hospitalisation, fee-for-service surgery, etc.). After two years of work, the Public Health Department presented the status of its work to the doctors and regional hospitals. The functional complementarity between the establishments of the hospital system was based on a double movement of centralisation at the Cantonal Hospital of "complicated medical and surgical techniques" and decentralisation in the districts of "medicine and general surgery, maternity and geriatrics".[73] In order to evaluate the developing needs as well as possible, economic and demographic projections for the year 1980 were carried out, as well as a survey of "the clientele of our various hospitals".[74] These studies showed the need to avoid too much decentralisation of equipment. The Canton of Vaud was thus divided into health zones and the construction of new general hospitals with 150–250 beds (called "zone hospitals") was planned for each. Within each zone, other regional hospitals that focused on the care of chronically ill patients and geriatric patients were retained.

This hierarchical structure between hospitals was a consensual position that made it possible to obtain the agreement of the GHRV, whose political weight was important, on the limited centralisation of the hospital system and the maintenance of all its member establishments—one of the group's primary objectives. In June 1964, Eugène Zwahlen, president of GHRV, informed the administrators of the Lavaux Hospital "confidentially, that certain hospitals would only be maintained by tradition and that they were already more than sufficient to meet the needs of their districts, in particular Château-d'Oex, La

[71] Pierre Gilliand, *Vieillissement démographique et planification hospitalière. Etude fondée sur les données de la Suisse et du canton de Vaud*, Lausanne, Department of the Interior, 1969, p. 165.

[72] Pierre-Yves Donzé, *Bâtir...*, op. cit., pp. 302–303.

[73] AFHCV, minutes of the meeting of 29 June 1964.

[74] Ibid.

Vallée and Orbe, which would only be maintained thanks to the reputation of its surgeon".[75] For the regional hospitals, the hospital plan was necessary to obtain construction subsidies from the State for new hospital buildings as philanthropic resources could no longer finance these.

Now that the GHRV had gained support for the hospital plan, it was necessary to obtain the support of the medical profession. Its representative informed the working group, in December 1964, "the climate within the SVM was not very favourable, partly because of the fear of State control and partly because of the concern of general practitioners about their future activity".[76] The surgeons and other specialists feared a move to a flat-rate remuneration or even a full-time contract with a fixed monthly salary. General practitioners were afraid that the appointment of full-time doctors in regional hospitals would restrict access to the infrastructure of these institutions (radiology, laboratories, etc.). This issue was hotly debated with regard to the new zone hospitals and the status of surgeons whose fee-for-service principle led to "a disproportion between the sums allocated to surgeons and those received by other practitioners".[77] Some surgeons defended the principle of fee-for-service, arguing that medicine was "a liberal profession [which] must retain the minimum of freedom conferred by its dignity" and that "to a certain extent, the hospital doctor fulfils the functions of a boss, since he is the only one who can understand in their complexity and achieve the goals of the institution where he works".[78] The surgeons thus defended the idea of a double remuneration for the medical profession, with a fixed annual base salary plus a variable income depending on the total amount of fees collected by the hospital during the year. This method made it possible to reconcile the requirements of the medical profession and those of the hospital administrations. Finally, after discussion, the principle of closing zone hospitals, except for assistant doctors with specific skills accepted as external consultants, and appointing full-time doctors, with the possibility of having beds for their private clientele, was adopted. The smaller hospitals remained open to the entire licensed medical profession.

The 1966 Hospital Plan

The Vaud Hospital Plan adopted by the Grand Council in 1966 was the result of a new way of thinking about the territory and its organisation, influenced by theoretical models such as those of Walter Christaller on central squares (1933) and Auguste Lösch on spatial balance and market areas (1940). These analyses asserted the principle of a hierarchy between urban centres based on

[75] Lavaux Hospital, report by Eugène Zwahlen to the Board of Directors, 30 June 1964.

[76] AFHCV, minutes of the Working Group, 3 December 1964.

[77] Ibidem, 28 December 1964.

[78] AFHCV, letter from Dr Piotet to Eugène Zwahlen, 29 November 1965.

the differentiation of services provided to their hinterland, that is, a functional division of space. They appeared to be the theoretical foundations of the spatial planning policies that emerged in the Western world in the immediate post-war period, with the aim of reducing regional disparities in development and facilities.[79] After 1945, the first health planners who worked on the spatial reorganisation of hospital systems set up a new territorialisation of public health, also based on the same logic.

In the Canton of Vaud, the architect Jean-Pierre Vouga played a decisive role in the affirmation of spatial planning.[80] Appointed State architect in 1960, Vouga was particularly concerned with mitigating the negative effects of economic growth in terms of spatial organisation, based on the observation of "the catastrophic state in which our cities and regions find themselves, both in terms of their anarchic expansion and in terms of pollution and the gradual disappearance of the natural or built heritage".[81] As soon as he was appointed, he began to carry out theoretical and methodological studies with the aim of setting up a master plan on a cantonal scale. In 1961, he was approached in this capacity by the Public Health Service's working group.[82] Vouga's experience in the hospital sector, alongside William Vetter, in the construction of the Decker surgical clinic (1947) and in numerous projects carried out on behalf of the WHO, played a role in the consideration of the health dimension of spatial planning. This concern was not new; in 1948, shortly after the opening of the surgical clinic at the Cantonal Hospital, Vetter and Vouga had presented the various hospitals in the Canton of Vaud in the professional journal of French-speaking engineers and architects, emphasising the strong decentralisation of hospital facilities.[83] Favourable of the achievement of functional complementarity between the various hospitals, they advocated the implementation of an "organic health plan"[84] and declared "the charm of small-scale solutions should not cause us to lose sight of the fact that the enhancement of existing buildings can only be achieved through an overall plan, abandoning the administrative fragmentation so dear to our traditions".[85]

[79] Joseph Lajugie and others, *Espace régional et aménagement du territoire*, Paris Dalloz, 1979.

[80] Bruno Marchand (ed.), *Jean-Pierre Vouga, architecte de l'Etat*, Lausanne, Payot, 2000.

[81] Ibid, p. 97.

[82] AFHCV, minutes of the discussions of the Working Group for the establishment of the hospital building programme, 27 November and 18 December 1961.

[83] William Vetter and Jean-Pierre Vouga, "Hôpitaux et cliniques du Canton de Vaud. Bases d'un plan de santé", in *Bulletin technique de la Suisse romande*, 26 June 1948, pp. 176–182.

[84] Ibidem, p. 180.

[85] Ibidem, p. 182.

These two architects were inspired, in particular, by the French example. Very close to the Christaller model, the French hospital reorganisation plan was based on the idea of a hierarchy and the sharing of functions between the various health establishments (see Fig. 3). The result was a hospital system based on the functional complementarity of its various components. According to one of the promoters of this model, Robert Bridgman, the realisation of this "coherent and efficient health organisation [...] requires considerable technical and financial efforts, but it is important, in order to avoid their dispersal, that rigorous coordination be foreseen and that the different parts of our health arsenal be closely harmonised and no longer work in dispersed order".[86] As a doctor attached to the WHO, Bridgman played an essential role in the implementation of hospital planning in several European countries and was directly involved in hospital planning in Vaud in the early 1960s. He was not only one of the directors of the thesis of the sociologist Pierre Gilliand, which appears to be the main theoretical basis of the Vaud hospital plan but he was also consulted by the working group on various issues.[87] Bridgman promoted the idea of classifying the various establishments according to the functions they performed in the hospital system to plan the long-term expenditure on equipment necessary to perfect the system "where any idea of competition is excluded".[88] The State became highly interventionist and became a territorial organiser, whose aim was "to ensure the transition of the hospital from a market economy to a managed economy".[89] Lastly, the French influence was reinforced by a mandate to assess the hospital plan entrusted in 1965 by the Council of State to Dr. Jean-Simon Cayla, Director of the National School of Public Health in Rennes and France's representative at the WHO, whose report sanctioned the hospital policy implemented.[90]

The Vaud hospital plan had the same spatial organisation characteristics as those mentioned above (see Fig. 4). Its aim was to define a structure for the hospital system that could serve as a basis for the modernisation of hospital facilities. The canton was divided into eight zones corresponding to socio-economic areas requiring a general hospital with 150–300 beds. These "zone hospitals" offered care in acute surgery, gynaecology-obstetrics, internal medicine and paediatrics which were complementary to the Cantonal Hospital and thus avoided its congestion. The latter played the role of a university research and training centre, a zone hospital for the Lausanne region, and a hospital for the treatment of specialised cases. Each health zone also included "regional hospitals" which were not structured as closed services and which

[86] Ibidem.

[87] *Planification hospitalière 1966*, Lausanne, Département de l'Intérieur, 1966, p. 4.

[88] Robert-Frédéric Bridgman, "Problèmes de gestion hospitalière du point de vue administratif", *Revue économique et sociale*, 1965, p. 79.

[89] Ibidem.

[90] AFHCV, *L'organisation et la gestion hospitalière dans le canton de Vaud—Suisse. Report on a Mission Carried Out Between 15 October and 3 December 1965*, Geneva: WHO, 1965.

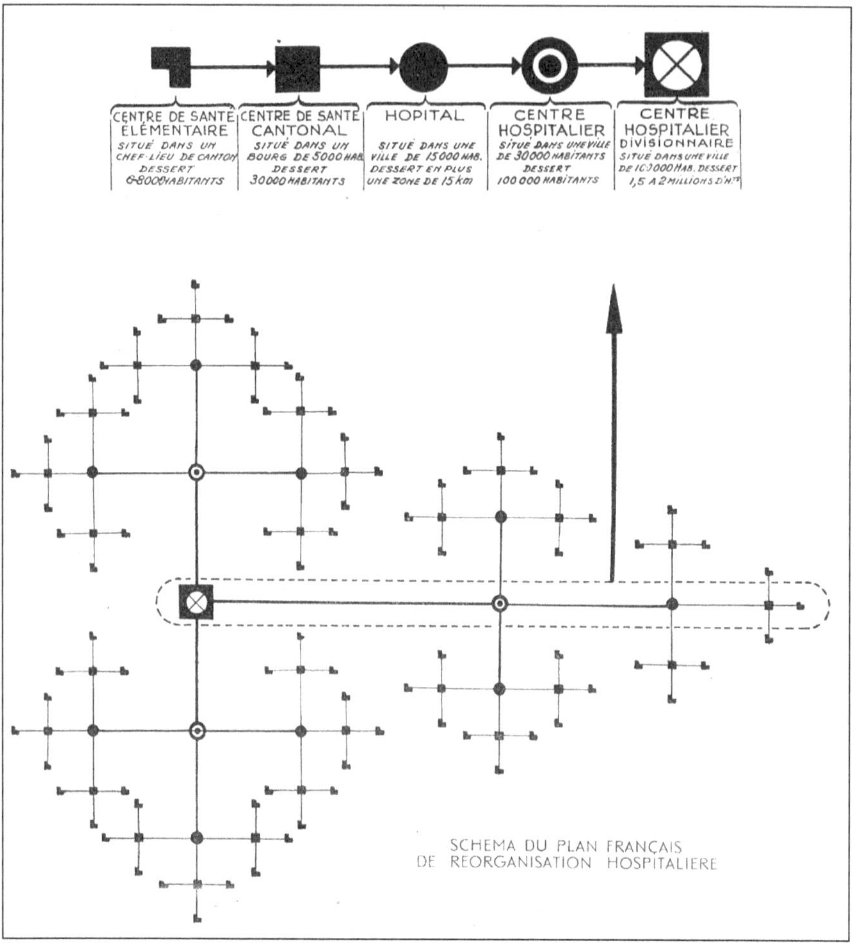

Fig. 3 French plan for hospital reorganisation, 1947 (*Source* "La santé publique", *L'architecture aujourd'hui*, no. 15, November 1947, p. 6)

functioned as medical hotlines as well as facilities for the care of chronic and convalescent patients. Finally, the hospital system was completed by a few institutions that specialised in the care of particular types of patients (e.g., psychiatry, geriatrics, etc.).

This plan made it possible to assess the existing infrastructure and the needs of each zone by 1980–1985, the idea being to plan the construction of the various missing facilities in a rational and economic manner, taking into account the demographic growth and ageing of the population. The evaluations revealed the inadequacy of the 5260 beds existing in 1962 and the need for nearly 8300 beds in 1985, especially "for functional rehabilitation and [...] for the chronically ill and disabled elderly, thus filling a major gap

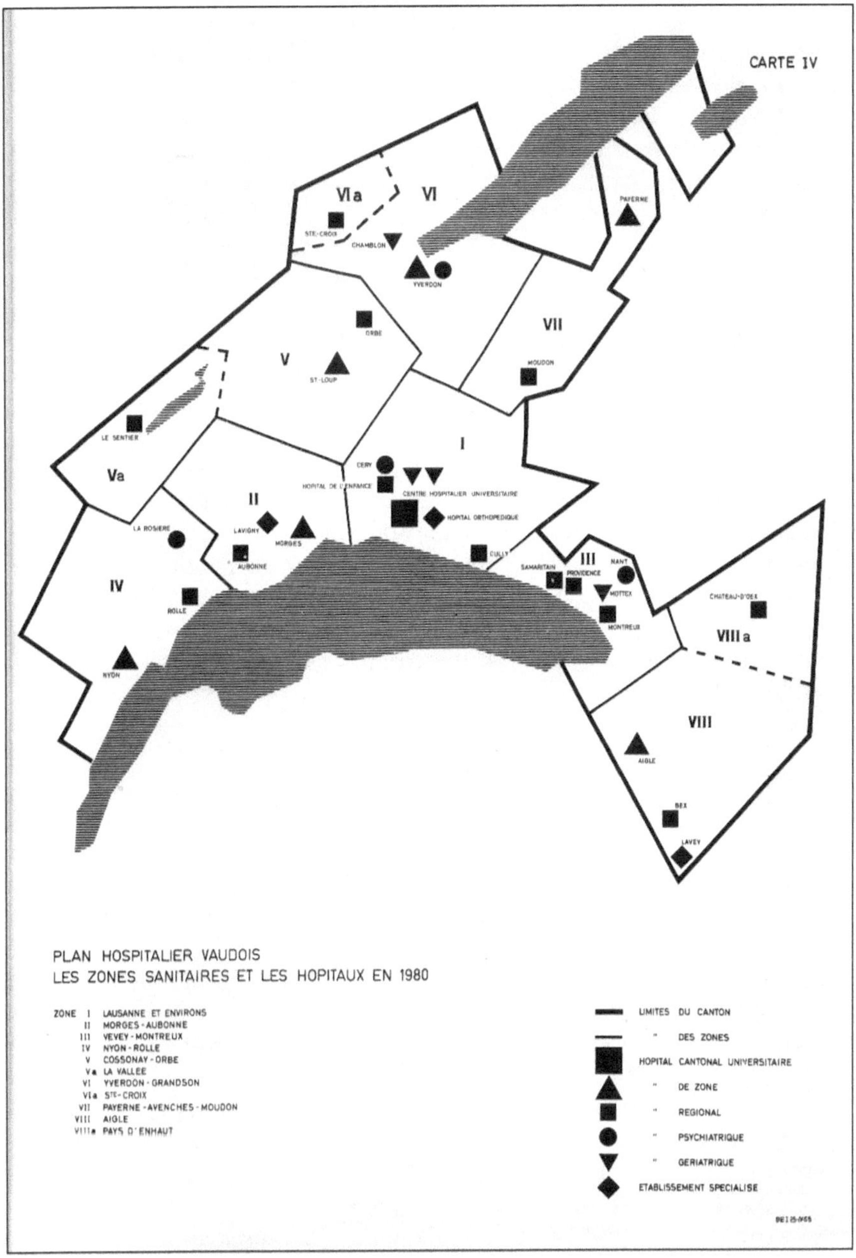

Fig. 4 Hospital organisation in Vaud according to the 1966 hospital plan (*Source Planification hospitalière 1966*, Lausanne, Département de l'Intérieur, 1966, Map IV)

in the Vaud equipment".[91] However, this ambitious policy had a high cost. Investment expenditure was estimated at a total of over 570 million francs for the period 1966–1984. The operating costs for 1985 were estimated at more than 267 million francs. In order to solve the financial problems, the State Council appointed a study commission in 1968 and the following year created a banking pool led by the Cantonal Bank and Crédit Foncier.

The State Council adopted the hospital plan in December 1966 and submitted it to the Grand Council for its opinion, the Grand Council issued its own report in May 1967. The scale and duration of the financial commitment gave rise to numerous interventions, generally on specific points that did not call into question the principle of having a hospital plan. The only issues that remained concerned health zone I (Lausanne region) and the question of the construction of the Vaud University Hospital (CHUV) which would fulfil "the mission of a teaching centre, a highly specialised establishment and a public hospital for the Lausanne conurbation".[92] This project was opposed by a large part of the medical profession, who feared the affirmation of a medical elite based at the CHUV working against doctors practising in regional hospitals or on an outpatient basis, as well as by several non-Lausanne deputies who did not accept that the State should make available to the capital a CHUV playing the role of an area hospital when these establishments were private elsewhere in the canton. However, these remarks did not lead to the rejection of the hospital plan.

5 Conclusion

The 1966 hospital plan was based on a consensus and the consideration of the demands of the various actors involved in the hospital system, which largely explains its success at the Grand Council. The economic situation and the growth of public resources made it possible to take the various demands into consideration.

The State played a decisive role in the construction of this consensual hospital planning because it was able to meet everyone's expectations. First of all, there was the problem of maintaining existing institutions. The GHRV was in favour of health planning but defended and obtained the survival of all its members. Regions in which the density of hospitals could lead to a rationalisation of facilities were guaranteed the existence of their institutions. At the same time, the State acceded to the request of the Faculty of Medicine and set up a Design office to conceive a new University hospital (CHUV). Then came the question of the standardisation of hospitalisation conditions between the regional hospitals and the Cantonal Hospital, an issue that was settled by the adoption of agreements based on the principle of an identical cost per day of hospitalisation: the levelling of prices was carried out from

[91] Ibidem, p. 18.

[92] BGC, 10 May 1967.

the top, so as not to harm any establishment. The resulting increase in health insurance contributions was a perverse effect in terms of guaranteeing access to healthcare for the middle classes but, since 1957, the State paid subsidies to people of modest means to help them join an insurance scheme. As for the medical professionals—especially surgeons—who rejected the principle of fixed fees, they obtained satisfaction through attachment to the compensation fund provided for in the 1960 agreement which collected fixed fees from patients and distributed fee-for-service income to the medical profession. Here, too, the State was a guarantor of the proper functioning of the fund and covered part of the deficit.

Regional hospitals, the Faculty of Medicine, insurance companies and doctors thus had their main concerns taken into account. The construction of the hospital plan did not prejudice any of the actors, thanks to the intervention and the money of the State for whom the expected rise in costs was not considered problematic. The 1966 plan was largely consensual and thus formed the basis for the general growth of the Vaud hospital system until the 1990s.

CHAPTER 6

Conclusion

The example of hospital medicine in the Canton of Vaud during the nineteenth and twentieth centuries shows that the history of medicine approached from the angle of hospital systems makes it possible to highlight a certain number of elements that have been little understood until now. Indeed, the economic history of hospitals, as it has developed into an autonomous field of research in Anglo-Saxon countries, has essentially been carried out within a monographic framework, around a hospital establishment or a town. It has thus shown that the transition from a charitable to an entrepreneurial model was largely based on the intervention of various actors within the hospital (doctors, administrators, municipal authorities, and the middle classes). These various studies emphasised that the technical modernisation of medicine took place in hospitals, mainly because they allowed a rationalisation of medical work (centralisation, standardisation of infrastructure, economies of scale). The financing of a more complex medico-technical infrastructure required an increase in the number of profitable clients, which was achieved through the intervention of insurance companies (for the indigent and the middle classes) and wealthy patients, as well as the affirmation of a new bureaucracy intended to ensure the functioning of these institutions. The Vaud example presented here corroborates this typical pattern of hospital transformation. However, the interplay of actors within hospitals alone does not appear to be a sufficient explanatory factor. Indeed, the hospital system approach makes it possible to introduce the notion of territory into the explanation of developments in hospital medicine and to better highlight the influences of the market.

P.-Y. Donzé, *The Formation of the Swiss Hospital System (1840–1960)*, https://doi.org/10.1007/978-981-19-3911-2_6

This dual importance of the territory and the market as explanatory factors in the development of hospital medicine has so far received little attention in the historiography, which makes it difficult to compare the case of Vaud with other hospital systems, whether in Switzerland or abroad. It is highly probable that the organisation of public health at a national level in most Western countries has worked against historical research conducted at the system level and taken into consideration all the hospitals concerned, because of the extensive size of these systems. Thus, historians have often preferred to focus on individual hospitals. Although this approach has led to some excellent work, it prevents any attempt to highlight the reciprocal impact of the territory and the market on the evolution of hospital medicine. It is true that the market is an omnipresent factor in the American historiography of hospitals, but the latter does not place a territorial limit on this market and does not really take its structure into consideration. Thus, the conditions of inter-hospital competition within the system, which impact the nature of the supply of care, are rarely taken into account. The economic aspect is often reduced to the sole extension of demand, which distorts the analysis in terms of the market.

The situation is somewhat different in Switzerland, where public health is the responsibility of the cantonal states. Geographical scales are, hence, small enough to easily allow the study of a territorialised hospital system and a coherent approach to the healthcare market. The Vaud hospital system thus appears to be an exemplary case of the evolution of Western hospital systems during the nineteenth and twentieth centuries. The territorialisation of hospital systems can be explained by the fact that they are not without limits. They are built within a coherent and autonomous geographical framework, which gives them a certain homogeneity shaped to certain structuring axes that directly affect the transformation of the various hospital establishments. Oppositions such as those between the centre and the periphery, the public and private sectors, or the acute and chronically ill, which in the case of the canton of Vaud are formed between the Cantonal Hospital of Lausanne and the regional hospitals, strongly structure the configuration of the hospital system and the internal organisation of its various establishments. However, the territory is not an immutable substrate on which the hospital system is built. Its internal structure and the balance between its various socio-economic regions are, on the contrary, strongly evolving over time. The dynamics of the territory, therefore, influence those of the hospital system. The widespread development of the hospital system in the second half of the nineteenth century corresponded to a socio-economic context in which the whole of the canton experienced demographic growth and the emergence of urban centres, even if this was more marked in the Lausanne and Vevey-Montreux regions. As for the questioning of the cantonal hospital policy by the professors of the Faculty of Medicine, who demanded during the interwar period that the infrastructures be centralised in the capital, this can be explained by the contrasting evolution of the Vaud territory during these years—growth in the city of Lausanne and stagnation in the rest of the canton. In this context, the struggle of the local infirmaries against the centralising tendencies of the faculty appears as a claim to identity and politics of the hinterland in the process of marginalisation, and not only as a protectionist reaction of the doctors running these establishments. Finally, the generalised growth of the canton after 1945 and the territorial recomposition in the direction of strong urbanisation shed light on the intervention of the state and the adoption in 1966 of a hospital plan aiming at resizing the hospital system according to this spatial reorganisation.

The study of the Vaud hospital system also highlights the importance of the hospital care market as a structuring element, within which the various establishments must position themselves in relation to each other. The dimension of the market arises from the interpenetration of the medical technical system and the hospital system that took place during the nineteenth and twentieth centuries. At first, until the end of the nineteenth century, these two systems did not interfere much with each other and functioned relatively autonomously. Surgery can then be seen as a technical craft system, based on ingenious and evolving technical knowledge, but not standardised, and on a decentralised way of working. The surgeon usually worked in the patients' homes and undertook each case individually. The hospital, whether cantonal and public or local and private, was not a central place of work in this technical system. The hospital system did not primarily respond to a medical needs. It was set up in the canton of Vaud mainly during the years 1840–1880 and can be explained first and foremost by the importance of the social question in the context of a society undergoing a process of demographic growth, industrialisation and modernisation: it was clearly a question of providing assistance and support to members of the disadvantaged social classes. The hospital system was organised according to the principle of complementarity between its various components, a complementarity that took several forms. Firstly, it was geographical. The Cantonal Hospital of Lausanne and the local infirmaries catered for the same category of people—the indigent who were ill or injured—but in different areas. The fact that the Canton of Vaud is crisscrossed by twenty or so general hospitals is a sign of a territory that experienced widespread growth. Secondly, the complementarity between institutions was also social. Some institutions, such as the private clinics in Lausanne and on the Lake Geneva Riviera, catered to the wealthy and developed in line with the growth of tourism. However, they were not in any way in competition with the other establishments in the hospital system because they took care of a particular type of patient which was not taken into account by the latter. Finally, there was complementarity at a functional level. The few specialised establishments in the system, intended for the indigent classes and located in Lausanne (Blind People's Asylum, Children's Hospice, and Orthopaedic Hospice), responded to a marketing type of logic, both on the philanthropic and the care markets. The multiplication of philanthropic works in the city of Lausanne led to a diversification and specialisation of charitable financial commitments. This desire met the interest of certain doctors in positioning themselves in a medical niche that would enable them to establish themselves as specialists in the field. Here again, the specialised establishments remained complementary to the general hospitals which were not interested in these various specialities.

The interaction between the medical technical system and the hospital system began to develop at the end of the nineteenth century. The transformation of the medical technical system towards a new model led to a profound reorganisation of the hospital system which put an end to the complementarity between the various establishments. Under the influence of César Roux, who joined the surgical department of the Cantonal Hospital in 1887 and was appointed Professor of Surgery in 1890, and other surgeons mainly trained in the German-speaking world, surgical work underwent a double movement of concentration and mechanisation similar to that observed in other economic sectors. Working methods and the medico-technical infrastructure (operating tables, X-ray equipment, sterilisers) tended to become standardised. Finally, the work environment became highly hierarchical and saw the first division of labour at a vertical level, with the surgeon at the head, who essentially abandoned home visits. Surgery was now performed in hospitals, where new equipment and patients were concentrated, thus facilitating the care of a growing number of patients.

The intervention of the surgeon-modernisers in the hospital system disrupted its internal organisation. Hospitals were modernised and transformed with the integration of a new medico-technical infrastructure and the construction of new hospital buildings, a redeployment that began at the end of the 1890s and lasted until the interwar period. It was then a question of releasing the resources necessary for the amortisation of this equipment and the operation of establishments that had become more expensive. The growth of hospital admissions, and therefore income, was a necessary condition for the perpetual modernisation of technical equipment. This growth was essentially ensured by the arrival en masse of the middle classes, and even the wealthy in certain cases, in hospitals, which were now at the heart of the medical market. The various hospital administrations sought to attract as many profitable patients as possible, to increase their market share and to position their establishments in relation to each other. The hospital system lost its complementarity and tended to become much more competitive. The only area in which complementarity remained was in the functional relationship between the private specialised hospitals, in which some university clinics were decentralised, and the Cantonal Hospital, which did not compete with these institutions as it did with the regional hospitals and private clinics. While complementarity remained at a functional level, this was no longer the case at the geographical and social levels. The modernised regional hospitals attracted a whole category of patients, especially acute surgical cases, who used to come to the Cantonal Hospital for treatment. Similarly, the hospitalisation of wealthy patients was no longer the prerogative of the private clinics but became an object of struggle with the Cantonal Hospital and the regional hospitals, all of which sought to hospitalise this type of profitable patient. The hospital system had thus moved from a situation of complementarity to one of competition.

This competitive situation proved unfavourable, however, to the transition to a new medical technical system. In fact, surgical work methods and techniques evolved during the 1930s in the direction of a horizontal division of labour, favoured in particular by the emergence of medical specialities. The introduction of this medical technique from the United States into the Cantonal Hospital would require a larger number of patients and new equipment. Thus, Pierre Decker, who had been the head of the University Surgical Service since 1932, constantly called for a reorganisation of the hospital system based on the abandonment of competition between institutions and a division of tasks between them. The obstacle to the realisation of a new surgery was economic: it required the centralisation in Lausanne of public financial investments along with acute surgical cases, and the decentralisation of chronic patients and classic surgical cases—scientifically less interesting—among regional hospitals. Only a return to a complementary hospital system—but one whose complementarity would be of a purely functional nature—would seem to allow a transition to team-based surgery.

The faculty's desire for reform was very poorly received by the other agents in the hospital system, especially as the territory of the Canton of Vaud was being reorganised in favour of the city of Lausanne in the interwar period. Decker's projects provoked a strong reaction from the regional hospitals and the surgeon-modernisers, who could not imagine abandoning scientifically interesting and financially profitable patients for the benefit of the Cantonal Hospital. Their authority as local notables and their reputation as surgeons were at stake. The surgeons' modernism thus showed its limits. However, this opposition in principle came up against the harsh reality of the financing of these institutions. The regional hospitals experienced serious difficulties due to insufficient financial resources, which were essentially based on the pensions paid by the patients or those who supported them (state, insurance). In order to balance their accounts, the regional hospitals demanded an increase in these contributions and thus greater state support, while the insurance companies also turned to the state to guarantee services accessible to a large part of the population. After 1945, most of the actors in the hospital system, with the exception of the modernising surgeons who demanded that the status quo be maintained, turned to the main funder of the system, the state, and undertook a whole series of discussions and negotiations. These negotiations led in the 1950s and 1960s to the signing of agreements and the adoption of a hospital plan which had the effect of eliminating competition within the hospital system in favour of its cartelisation: the care market was no longer governed by the law of supply and demand but was shared between the various establishments of the hospital system. A new complementarity, which was not geographical but functional, was established through the hospital plan. The existence of the various hospitals was guaranteed—a minimum condition required by the GHRV—and they were given functions within the hospital plan, with medical research and the treatment of acute surgical cases being centralised at the Cantonal Hospital. With the adoption of the 1966 hospital plan, hospital management was thus approached at the system level and no longer at the level of each institution. Although the latter retained a certain amount of autonomy in their internal organisation and the implementation of choices made at the cantonal level, the real decisions were henceforth taken at the level of the hospital system as a whole. A total change of perspective, which made Gustave Piotet, former head of clinic at César Roux and surgeon at Nyon Hospital, say in 1966 to certain rather cautious regional hospital administrators: "You are linked to a hospital system, you are all a cell of this system".[1] The development of the various hospitals in the canton no longer depended solely on the will of local councillors and the surgeons at their head, but on a hospital plan negotiated between various partners in a cantonal perspective and organised by new public health managers (sociologists, architects). It was therefore a reorganisation of the hospital system that made it possible to create a new technical medical system based on the American model.

In the end, the example of the canton of Vaud highlights a successful transformation of hospital medicine on the scale of a hospital system. This transformation was not without conflict, but the search for negotiated solutions between the various agents (doctors, philanthropists, insurance companies, the cantonal administration, politicians) and under the aegis of the state made it possible to set up an institutional framework that ensured the widespread development of the hospital system. This consensus-based growth, however, has come at a cost. Measured in terms of per capita health expenditure, the Swiss health system is one of the most expensive in the world. In 1970, it amounted to 326 US dollars PPP, similar to the US (327 US dollar PPP) and far ahead of major European countries such as Germany (252), France (192) and the UK (124).[2] Despite the adoption of a new hospital policy in the 1990s, based on the networking of hospitals and the introduction of management principles from the private sector, the Swiss health system is still one with the highest costs in the world.[3]

[1] GHRV archives, minutes of a meeting, 9 November 1966.

[2] OECD, Expenditure on healthcare per capita in PPPs, https://stats.oecd.org/# (accessed 17 February 2022).

[3] Donzé, *Bâtir*..., op. cit., chapter 6.

References

Archives

Archives of the Canton of Vaud (ACV), Lausanne
K VIII Department of Home Affairs
K IX Department of Public Works
K XIII Department of Public Instruction and Worship
S 54 Higher Education and Worship Service
S 73 Public Health Service
Private papers
Orthopaedic Hospice Papers
César Roux Papers
Charles Krafft Papers
Verdan Papers
Regional hospitals, annual reports

Archives of the Canton of Fribourg (ACF), Fribourg
Department of Public Health

Archives of Private and Regional Hospitals
Cecil Clinic (Lausanne), Blind People's Asylum Foundation (Lausanne), Children's Hospice (Lausanne), Orthopaedic Hospice (Lausanne), Cully Hospital, Montreux Hospital, Morges Hospital, Nyon Hospital, Rolle Hospital, Vevey-Samaritain Hospital, Vevey-Providence Hospital, Yverdon Hospital.

Archives of the Federation of Hospitals in Canton Vaud (AFHCV), Prilly

Archives of La Source Nursing School (ALS), Lausanne

Archives of the University of Lausanne

P.-Y. Donzé, *The Formation of the Swiss Hospital System (1840–1960)*,
https://doi.org/10.1007/978-981-19-3911-2

Cantonal and University Library, Lausanne

Charles Krafft Papers
César Roux Papers
Annual reports of regional hospitals

Schweizerische Wirtschaftsarchiv, Basel
M. Schaerer AG Papers

Printed Sources

Official Publications
Bulletin of the Grand Council meetings (BGC, *Bulletin des séances du Grand Conseil*), 1850–1960.
Feuille officielle suisse du commerce, 1883–1960.
Official Directory of the Canton of Vaud (ODCV, *Annuaire officiel du canton de Vaud*), 1816–1960.
Recueil des Lois, Décrets, Arrêtés et autres Actes du Gouvernement du Canton de Vaud, 1803–1960.
Report of the State Council (RSC, *Compte-rendu du Conseil d'Etat*), 1829–1960.

Periodicals
Annuaire statistique de la Suisse, 1900–1960.
Bulletin de la Fédération des Sociétés de secours mutuels de la Suisse romande, 1893–1950.
Bulletin de la Société médicale de la Suisse romande, 1866–1880.
Bulletin de la Société vaudoise de Secours mutuels, 1917–1958.
Bulletin de la Société vaudoise des ingénieurs et des architectes, 1875–1899.
Bulletin professionnel des médecins suisses, 1920–1960.
Bulletin technique de la Suisse romande, 1900–1960.
Catalogue des étudiants de l'Université de Lausanne, 1891–1922.
Centre anticancéreux romand, Rapports annuels, 1924–1958.
Helvetia chirurgica acta, 1945–1960.
Indicateur vaudois: Livre d'adresse de Lausanne et du canton de Vaud, various years.
Journal de la Société vaudoise d'utilité publique, 1832–1913.
La Construction moderne, 1934.
L'Efficient: Bulletin du Club d'Efficience de la Suisse romande, 1943–1960.
Kompass: Répertoire général de l'économie suisse, 1947.
Revue médicale de la Suisse romande, 1881–1960.
VESKA-Zeitschrift—Revue VESKA, 1937–1960.

Books and Articles
50e anniversaire de la Fédération des sociétés de secours mutuels de la Suisse romande: 1893–1943, Lausanne, 1943.
125e anniversaire de l'hôpital de Morges, Lausanne, Imprimeries réunies, 1994.
1867–1967, Hôpital d'Aigle: Cent années hospitalières, Aigle, Hôpital, 1967.

1869–1969, 100 ans au service de la communauté, Hôpital de Morges, La Chaux-de-Fonds, Courvoisier, 1969.
A votre santé: Histoire des institutions de soins à Sainte-Croix, Sainte-Croix, Les Cahiers du Balcon du Jura, 2000.
Académie suisse des sciences médicales, *50 Jahre Jubiläum: Schweizerische Akademie der medizinischen Wissenschaften*, Basel, ASSM, 1993.
ADEHR. Association des directeurs des établissements hospitaliers de Suisse romande. 20e anniversaire, Saignelégier, ADEHR, 1993.
André Golaz, 11 mai 1989, Morges, Hôpital, 1989.
Asile des aveugles. Lausanne. Centre d'accueil, d'instruction et d'adaptation pour aveugles et faibles de vue, 1843–1985, Renens, 1985.
Bardel Octave, *1846–1946: 100e anniversaire, Société vaudoise de secours mutuels, Notice historique*, Vevey, 1946.
Bolli Laurent, *Chronique de l'Asile des aveugles de Lausanne, 1843–1943*, Lausanne, Concorde, 1944.
Bonard Emile, *Histoire de l'Hôpital de Saint-Loup, 1852–1984*, Saint-Loup, Association des Amis de l'Hôpital de zone de Saint-Loup-Orbe, undated.
Bridgman Robert-Frédéric, «Problèmes de gestion hospitalière du point de vue administratif», *Revue économique et sociale*, 1965, pp. 75–80.
Centenaire de la Société vaudoise de médecine, 1829–1929, Lausanne, Concorde, 1929.
Centième anniversaire de l'hôpital orthopédique de la Suisse romande, Lausanne, Hospice orthopédique, 1976.
Ceppi Pierre et Jacques Adalbert, *Centenaire de l'hôpital de Sainte-Croix, 1875–1975*, Sainte-Croix, undated.
Chavanne D. A., *Notice sur l'hospice cantonal du canton de Vaud*, 1838.
Clinique La Source, 100 ans, 1891–1991, Lausanne, La Source, 1991.
Cornaz C., *La mutualité dans le canton de Vaud*, Lausanne, A. Fatio, 1880.
Decker Pierre, «Le problème de l'anesthésie en Suisse», *Helvetia chirurgica acta*, 1948, pp. 423–439.
Decker Pierre and Hessler W., «Les sulfamidés en chirurgie», *Helvetia Medica Acta*, vol. 11, 1944, pp. 337–401.
Dénéréaz L., «La cuisine électrique de l'Hôpital su Samaritain, à Vevey», *Bulletin technique de la Suisse romande*, 1933, pp. 34–36.
Dernière leçon de M. le Dr Pierre Decker, Professeur ordinaire de clinique chirurgicale à la Faculté de médecine, Lausanne, Université, 1957.
Dubs Jakob, *La chirurgie de guerre dans l'armée suisse: précis pour officiers et aspirants du service de santé*, Zurich, Morgarten, 1939.
Dufour René, «Essor de l'ophtalmologie à Lausanne au 19e siècle», *Advances in Ophtalmology*, 1978, n°36, pp. 12–20.
Dupont Emile, «Le service de chirurgie de l'Hôpital cantonal», *RMSR*, 1876, pp. 253–257 and 294–302.
Fell-Doriot Jeanne, *75 ans Fédération des sociétés de secours mutuels de la Suisse romande*, 1969.
Francken William, «Le rôle du Pavillon régional et les premières armes du Pavillon de la Côte», *RMSR*, 1924, pp. 469–470.
Germond H., «Notice sur les infirmeries locales dans la Suisse romande, présentée à la Société d'utilité publique du canton de Vaud, dans sa séance du 23 août 1870, à Avenches», *Journal de la Société vaudoise d'utilité publique*, 1870, pp. 251–262.

Gilliand Pierre, *Vieillissement démographique et planification hospitalière: Etude fondée sur les données de la Suisse et du canton de Vaud*, Lausanne, Département de l'Intérieur, 1969.
Golaz André, *Hôpital de zone—Réalisation et organisation*, Rennes, ENSP, 1968.
Gruner Erich (ed.), *L'Assemblée fédérale suisse, 1848–1920. Biographies*, Bern, Francke, 1966
Hahn Charles, *Chirurgien du cœur: L'une des conquêtes médicales du siècle par un grand patron de Suisse romande*, Lausanne, 24 Heures, 1987.
Infirmerie Comtesse, Romainmôtier, centenaire 1893–1993, Romainmôtier, Fondation Comtesse, 1993.
Infirmerie de Moudon—Notice historique, Mondon, L'Eveil, 1895.
Kinkelin Hermannn, *Les Sociétés de secours mutuels en Suisse en 1880*, Berne, 1887.
Kollros Jean-Charles, *100 ans, Hôpital de Montreux*, Montreux, Corbaz, 1977.
Kraege Charles, *Histoire de l'hospitalisation à Aigle de 1360 à 1991*, Aigle, 1992.
Krafft Charles, *La Source et Saint-Loup*, Lausanne, Imp. J. Couchoud, 1918.
L'infirmerie de Nyon, 1877–1927, Nyon, Imprimerie du Courrier de la Côte, 1927.
«La santé publique», *L'architecture aujourd'hui*, n°15, novembre 1947.
La construction des hôpitaux modernes et leurs installations: Ouvrage destiné à l'usage des médecins, architectes, ingénieurs, techniciens, personnel d'administration, étudiants et practiciens, Berne, Maison Schaerer SA, 1930.
Les établissements pour malades en Suisse de 1936 à 1942, Berne, Bureau fédéral de la Statistique, 1945.
Les sociétés de secours mutuels en Suisse en l'année 1903, Berne, Département fédéral de l'Industrie, 1907.
Liste des travaux du Centre anticancéreux romand, 1925–1944, Lausanne, La Concorde.
Louis Michaud, 1880–1956, Bâle, Benno Schwab & Cie, 1957.
de Mestral Combremont J., *Vies données… vies retrouvées. Les diaconesses de Saint-Loup*, Lausanne, Payot, 1932.
Naef Andreas, *De la tuberculose à la greffe du cœur: 1940–1990. Parcours d'un chirurgien*, Genève, Médecine & Hygiène, 1995.
Nicod Louis, «Historique médical de l'Hôpital orthopédique de la Suisse romande», *Revue médicale de la Suisse romande*, 1963, n°83, pp. 291–317.
Pasch T. and Frei F., «50 ans de la Société Suisse d'Anesthésiologie et de Réanimation (SSAR)», *Bulletin des médecins suisses*, 2002, pp. 2766–2770.
Piotet Gustave, *La médecine au service du malade*, Neuchâtel, La Baconnière, 1979.
Planification hospitalière 1966, Lausanne, Département de l'Intérieur, 1966.
Policlinique médicale universitaire, 100 ans, 1887–1987, Lausanne, PMU, 1987.
de Quervain Fritz, «Zur Operationstischfrage», *Zentralblatt für Chirurgie*, 1906, pp. 321–323.
Reynier Jean-Pierre de, «L'Hôpital de l'Enfance de 1861 à 1979», *Revue médicale de la Suisse romande*, 1980, pp. 557–565.
Roch M., «Médecine américaine et médecine suisse», *Revue médicale de la Suisse romande*, 1951, pp. 65–71.
Rollier Auguste, *Quarante ans d'héliothérapie*, Lausanne, Librairie de l'Université, 1944.
Saegesser Frédéric, «L'avenir de la chirurgie, tel que je le vois», *Société suisse de chirurgie, 1963–1988*, Bâle, Schwabe & Co AG, 1990, pp. 73–81.
Segond Victor, *La bienfaisance dans le canton de Vaud*, Nyon, Rauschet & Co, 1895.

Société suisse de chirurgie, 1913–1963, Basel, Schwabe, 1963.
Société suisse de chirurgie, 1963–1988, Basel, Schwabe, 1990.
Société vaudoise des Secours mutuels, *Notice historique sur la Société vaudoise des secours mutuels, 1846–1896*, Vevey, Imp. Säuberlin et Pfeiffer, 1896.
«Statistique des hôpitaux et hospices de la Suisse au 31.12.1909», *Journal de Statistique Suisse*, 1910, pp. 283–318.
Verdan Claude, «50e anniversaire de la fondation de la Clinique et permanence médicale de Longeraie, 1946–1996. Historique», *Revue médicale de la Suisse romande*, 1996, pp. 145–148.
Verdan Claude, *Histoire de la Société suisse de chirurgie plastique reconstructive et esthétique à l'occasion de son vingtième anniversaire, 1965–1985*, Lausanne, 1985.
Verdan Claude, *Mémoires d'un chirurgien*, Lausanne, Fondation Claude Verdan, 5 volumes, 1999–2001.
Vetter William and Vouga Jean-Pierre, «Le nouveau groupe opératoire de l'hôpital cantonal de Lausanne (Clinique de Chirurgie)», *Schweizerische Bauzeitung*, 8 May 1948.
Vincent J., *Aux écoutes de la souffrance: Histoire de l'Institution des diaconesses de Saint-Loup publiée, à l'occasion de son centenaire, par le Conseil général, 1842–1942*, Lausanne, La Concorde, 1942.

Academic Literature

Barras Vincent, «Le médecin de 1880 à la fin du XXe siècle», in Cabellat Louis (dir.), *Histoire du médecin*, Paris, Flammarion, 1999, pp. 269–307.
Barras Vincent and Lacharme Cécile, «L'Hospice cantonal», in *Vaud sous l'Acte de Médiation, 1803–1813: la naissance d'un canton confédéré*, Lausanne, Bibliothèque historique vaudoise, 2002, pp. 176–181.
Barras Vincent and Vouilloz Burnier Marie-France, *De l'hospice au réseau santé: Santé publique et systèmes hospitaliers valaisans, XIXe–XXe siècles*, Sierre, Monographic, 2004.
Berg Marc and Timmermans Stefan, *The Gold Standard: The Challenge of Evidence-Based Medicine and Standardization in Health Care*, Philadelphie, Temple University Press, 2003, 280 p.
Biaudet Jean-Charles, «L'écharpe, le marteau et le tourniquet: Mathias Mayor, un chirurgien vaudois du début du XIXe siècle», in Guy Saudan (ed.), *L'Eveil médical vaudoise, 1750–1850. Tissot, Venel, Mayor*, Lausanne, Université, 1987, pp. 105–175.
Bijker Wiebe, *Of Bicycles, Bakelites and Bulbs: Toward a Theory of Sociotechnical Change*, Cambridge, MIT Press, 1995.
Bijker Wiebe, Hughes Thomas and Pinch Trevor (eds.), *The Social Construction of Technological Systems: New Directions in the Sociology and History of Technology*, Cambridge, MIT Press, 1999.
Blanc Olivier, *Démographie et développement: Le canton de Vaud au XIXème siècle*, Lausanne, Office de statistique de l'Etat de Vaud, 1974.
Blume Stuart S., *Insight and Industry: On the Dynamics of Technological Change in Medicine*, Cambridge, MIT Press, 1992.
Borboën Marina, *Etude des livres opératoires de l'Hôpital cantonal de Lausanne de 1891 à 1930: Contexte et évolution de l'anesthésiologie*, Université de Lausanne, thèse de doctorat en médecine, 1996.

Bourgeois Daniel, *Business helvétique et Troisième Reich: Milieux d'affaires, politique étrangère, antisémitisme*, Lausanne, Ed. Page Deux, 1998.
Bridgman Perkins Barbara, «Shaping Institution-Based Specialism: Early Twentieth-Century Economic Organisation of Medicine», *Social History of Medicine*, 1997, pp. 419–435.
Caron François, *Les deux révolutions industrielles du 20e siècle*, Paris, Albin Michel, 1997.
Castroviejo Pedro M. Pérez, «La formación del sistema hospitalario vasco: administración y gestión económica, 1800–1936», *Transportes, Servicios y Telecomunicaciones*, 2002, pp. 73–97.
Centlivres Robert and Fleury Jean-Jacques, *De l'Eglise d'Etat à l'Eglise nationale (1839–1863)*, Lausanne, Eglise nationale vaudoise, 1963.
Chandler Alfred D., *The Visible Hand: The Managerial Revolution in American Business*, Cambridge: Belknap Press, 1977.
Cherry Steven, «Accountability, Entitlement, and Control Issues and Voluntary Hospital Funding c1860–1939», *Social History of Medicine*, 1996, pp. 215–233.
Cherry Steven, «Before the National Health Service: Financing the Voluntary Hospitals, 1900–1939», *Economic History Review*, 1997, pp. 305–326.
Cherry Steven, «Hospital Saturday, Workplace Collections and Issues in late Nineteenth-Century Hospital Funding», *Medical History*, 2000, pp. 461–488.
Christ Thierry, «Du zèle piétiste à l'activisme républicain: Démocratisation de la gestion et du contrôle de l'hôpital à Neuchâtel au 19e siècle», *Revue historique neuchâteloise*, 1999, pp. 19–31.
Clavel Anne-Marie and Prod'hom Louis-Samuel, *Historique de la mutation de l'Hôpital cantonal de Lausanne en Centre hospitalier universitaire vaudois de 1959 à 1990*, s.l., 1993.
Cohen Yves and Pestre Dominique, «Histoire des techniques» (dir.), in *Annales: Histoire, Sciences sociales*, 1998, pp. 721–943.
Cooter Roger, «The Meaning of Fractures: Orthopaedics and the Reform of British Hospitals in the Inter-War Period», *Medical History*, 1987, pp. 306–322.
Cooter Roger, *Surgery and Society in Peace and War: Orthopaedics and the Organisation of Modern Medicine, 1880–1948*, London, Macmillan, 1993, 416 p.
Cooter Roger, «War and Modern Medicine», in Bynum W. F. et Porter Roy, *Companion Encyclopedia of the History of Medicine*, New York, Routledge, 1993, vol. 2, pp. 1536–1573.
Cooter Rogger, Harrison Mark, Sturdy Steve (eds.), *War, Medicine and Modernity*, Thrup, Sutton Publishing, 1998.
Dirlewanger Dominique and Fussinger Catherine, «Les nécrologies des médecins romands: une autopsie du corps médical», *Revue historique vaudoise*, 1995, pp. 187–246.
Domin Jean-Paul, *Une histoire économique de l'hôpital (XIXe–XXe siècles)*, Paris: Comité d'histoire de la sécurité sociale, 2 vols, 2008 and 2013
Dommann Monika, *Durchsicht, Einsicht, Vorsicht: Eine Geschichte der Röntgenstrahlen, 1896–1963*, Zurich, Chronos, 2003.
Donzé Pierre-Yves, *Bâtir, gérer, soigner: Histoire des établissements hospitaliers de Suisse romande*, Genève, Georg, 2003.
Donzé Pierre-Yves and Fernández Pérez Paloma (eds), *The Business of Health: New Approaches to the Evolution of Health Systems in the World*, New York: Routledge, 2022.

Dreyfuss Véronique, *Le Bloc hospitalier du CHUV: Essai de géographie urbaine*, Lausanne, L'Aire, 1979.
Droux Joëlle, *L'attraction céleste: La construction de la profession d'infirmière en Suisse Romande (19e-20e siècles)*, Unpublished PhD thesis, University of Geneva, 2000.
Droux Joëlle, «Pédiatres et pédiatrie à Genève: l'enfance de l'art (1880–1950)», in Susannet Suter (ed.), *Âges et visages de la pédiatrie: La genèse du Département de pédiatrie, Genève*, Genève, Georg / HUG, 2001, pp. 43–60.
Ehrenström Philippe, «Affirmation et structuration de la profession médicale, Genève, 1880–1914», *Revue suisse d'histoire*, 1992, pp. 220–226.
Fairman Julie, «Economically Practical and Critically Necessary? The Development of Intensive Care at Chestnut Hill Hospital», *Bulletin of the History of Medicine*, 2000, pp. 80–106.
Faure Olivier, *Genèse de l'hôpital moderne: les hospices civils de Lyon de 1802 à 1845*, Lyon, Presses universitaires de Lyon, 1982.
Faure Olivier, «20 ans d'histoire de la santé», *Revue historique vaudoise*, 1995, pp. 315–327.
Faure Olivier, «La médicalisation vue par les historiens», in Aïach Pierre and Delanoë Daniel, *L'ère de la médicalisation: Ecce homo sanitas*, Paris, Economica, 1998, pp. 53-68.
Fee Elizabeth, «The Social History of the Hospital: From Charity Care to the Management of Medicine: A Review Essay», *Radical History Review*, 1984, pp. 472–481.
Fernández Pérez Paloma, *The Emergence of Modern Hospital Management and Organisation in the World 1880s–1930s*, Bradford: Emerald, 2021.
Fleury Antoine and Joye Frédéric, *Les débuts de la politique de la recherche en Suisse: Histoire de la création du Fonds national de la recherche scientifique*, Genève, Droz, 2002.
Ford Chapin Christy, *Ensuring America's Health: The Public Creation of the Corporate Health Care System*, Cambridge, Cambridge University Press, 2015.
Foucault Michel, *Naissance de la clinique*, Paris, PUF, 1963.
Foucault Michel, «L'incorporation de l'hôpital dans la technologie moderne», in *Dits et écrits*, Paris, Gallimard, 1998, vol. 3, pp. 508–521.
Francillon Denise, «La Source: Enjeux et perspectives d'une école-hôpital», *Mémoire vive*, 1992, pp. 33–42.
Francillon Denise (ed.), *Valérie de Gasparin, une conservatrice révolutionnaire*, Lausanne/Le Mont-sur-Lausanne, Ecole de La Source/Ed. Ouverture, 1994.
Francillon Denise, «Du métier de garde-malade à la profession d'infirmière: de la dépendance à la professionnalisation», *Revue historique vaudoise*, 1995, pp. 293–313.
Fussinger Catherine and Tevaearai Deodaat, *Lieux de folie, monuments de raison: Architecture et psychiatrie en Suisse romande, 1830–1930*, Lausanne, Presses polytechniques et universitaires romandes, 1998.
Garden Maurice, *Histoire économique d'une entreprise de santé: le budget des Hospices civils de Lyon, 1800–1976*, Lyon, PUL, 1980.
Gasser Paul, *Charles Krafft (1863–1921), ein Pionier der Appendektomie und der Krankenpfkege in Europa*, Basel, Schwabe & Co, 1977.
Gille Bertrand (ed.), *Histoire des techniques*, Paris, Gallimard, 1978.

Goebel Thomas, «American Medicine and the "Organisational Synthesis": Chicago Physicians and the Business of Medicine, 1900–1920», *Bulletin of the History of Medicine*, 1994, pp. 639–663.

Gorsky Martin and Sheard Sally (eds.), *Financing Medicine: The British Experience Since 1750*, New York: Routledge, 2006.

Grandshaw Lindsay, «"Fame and Fortune by Means of Bricks and Mortar": The Medical Profession and Specialist Hospitals in Britain», in Roy Porter and Lindsay Grandshaw (eds.), *Hospitals in History*, New York, Routledge, 1989, pp. 199–220.

Hamilton David, «The Nineteenth-Century Surgical Revolution—Antisepsis or Better Nutrition?», *Bulletin of the History of Medicine*, 1982, pp. 30–40.

Harrison Mark, Jones Margaret and Sweet Helen (eds.), *From Western Medicine to Global Medicine: The Hospital Beyond the West*, New Delhi: Orient Blackswan, 2009.

Hayter Charles R., «The Clinic as Laboratory: The Case of Radiation Therapy, 1896–1920», *Bulletin of the History of Medicine*, 1998, pp. 663–688.

Heller Geneviève, *Charlotte Olivier: La lutte contre la tuberculose dans le canton de Vaud*, Lausanne, Ed. d'en bas, 1992.

Heller Geneviève, «Les lieux de la maladie: quelques repères historiques», in Hagmann Hermann-Michel and Fragnière Jean-Pierre (eds.), *Maintien à domicile: Le temps de l'affirmation*, Lausanne, Réalités sociales, 1997, pp. 15–25.

Howell Joel, *Technology in the Hospital: Transforming Patient Care in the Early Twentieth Century*, Baltimore, Johns Hopkins University Press, 1995.

Hughes Thomas P., *Networks of Power: Eectrification in Western Society, 1880–1930*, Baltimore, Johns Hopkins University Press, 1983.

Imbert Jean (ed.), *Histoire des hôpitaux en France*, Toulouse, Privat, 1982.

Imbert Jean, «L'évolution de l'architecture hospitalière: piété, salubrité, bien-être», *Bulletin de la Société française d'histoire des hôpitaux*, 1984, n°49, pp. 25–38.

Jones Colin and Porter Roy (eds.), *Reassessing Foucault: Power, Medicine and the Body*, New York, Routledge, 1994.

Kaba Mariama, *Une histoire de l'orthopédie: L'Hôpital orthopédique de la Suisse romande dans le contexte international (18e–21e siècle)*, Lausanne, BHMS, 2018.

Keel Othmar, *L'avènement de la médecine clinique moderne en Europe, 1750–1815*, Genève, Georg, 2001.

Keel Othmar and Hudon Philippe, «L'essor de la pratique clinique dans les armées européennes (1750–1800)», in *Gesnerus*, 1997, pp. 37–58.

Killian Hans, *Meister der Chirurgie und die Chirurgenschulen im gesamten deutschen Sprachraum*, Stuttgart, Georg Thieme Verlag, 1980.

Kunitz Stephen, «Efficiency and Reform in the Financing and Organisation of American Medicine in the Progressive Era», *Bulletin of the History of Medicine*, 1981, pp. 497–515.

Labisch Alfons and Spree Reinhardt, «Neuere Entwicklungen und aktuelle Trends in der Sozialgeschichte der Medizin in Deutschland—Rückschau und Ausblick», *Vierteljahrschrift für Sozial- und Wirtschaftsgeschichte*, 1997, pp. 171–210 and 305–321.

Labisch Alfons and Spree Reinhardt (eds.), *Krankenhaus-Report 19. Jahrhundert: Krankenhausträger, Krankenhausfinanzierung, Krankenhauspatienten*, Francfort, Campus Verlag, 2001.

Lasserre André, *Finances publiques et développement: Le canton de Vaud, 1831–1913*, Lausanne, Bibliothèque historique vaudoise, 1980.

Latour Bruno and Woolgar Steve, *Laboratory Life: The Social Construction of Scientific Facts*, London, Sage, 1979.

Lawrence Christopher, «Democratic, Divine and Heroic: The History and Historiography of Surgery», in *Medical Theory, Surgical Practice: Studies in the History of Surgery*, London/New York, Routledge, 1992, pp. 1–47.

Lehmann-Jomini Catherine, *La genèse de l'Infirmerie de Lavaux: 1878–1942: Cas particulier dans le développement des hôpitaux régionaux vaudois*, unpublished master thesis, University of Lausanne, 1978.

Leimgruber Matthieu, *Taylorisme et management en Suisse romande (1917–1950)*, Lausanne, Antipodes, 2001.

Léonard Jacques, *Les médecins de l'Ouest au XIXe siècle*, Paris, Champion.

Loetz Francisca, *Von Kranken zum Patienten. „Medikalisierung" und medizinische Vergesellschaftung am Beispiel Badens 1750–1850*, Stuttgart, Franz Steiner Verlag, 1993.

Löwy Ilana (ed.), *Medicine and Change: Historical and Sociological Studies of Medical Innovation*, London, INSRM/ John Libbey, 1993.

Lynaugh Joan, *The Community Hospitals of Kansas City, Missouri, 1870–1915*, New York/London, Garland, 1989.

Marchand Bruno (ed.), *Jean-Pierre Vouga, architecte de l'Etat*, Payot, Lausanne, 2000.

Mayer Roger, «Il y a 75 ans naissait le second service de médecine de l'Hôpital cantonal de Genève», *Revue médicale de la Suisse romande*, 1991, pp. 901–928.

Meuwly Olivier, *La politique vaudoise au 20e siècle: De l'Etat radical à l'émiettement du pouvoir*, Lausanne, PPUR, 2003.

Muheim David, *Le mutualisme contre l'assurance sociale: La Fédération des Sociétés de secours mutuels de la Suisse romande et les premiers projets d'assurance maladie (1893–1912)*, unpublished master of thesis, University of Lausanne, 1998.

Murken Axel Hinrich, «Das deutsche Baracken- und Pavillon-Krankenhaus von 1866 bis 1906», in *Studien zur Krankenhausgeschichte im 19: Jahrhundert im Hinblick auf die Entwicklung in Deutschland*, Göttingen, Vandenhoeck & Ruprecht, 1976, pp. 72–104.

Mützenberg Gabriel, *Une femme de style: Valérie de Gasparin*, Le Mont-sur-Lausanne, Ed. Ouverture, 1995.

Olivier Eugène, *Médecine et santé dans le Pays de Vaud. 2e partie: Au XVIIIe siècle: 1675–1798* , Lausanne, Payot, 1962.

Pickstone John, *Medicine and Industrial Society: A History of Hospital Development in Manchester and Its Region, 1752–1946*, Manchester, Manchester University Press, 1985.

Pickstone John, *Ways of Knowing: A New History of Science, Technology and Medicine*, Manchester, Manchester University Press, 2000.

Porter Roy, «The Gift Relation: Philanthropy and Provincial Hospitals in 18th Century England», in Granshaw Lindsay et Porter Roy (eds.), *Hospitals in History*, New York, 1989, pp. 149–178.

Porter Roy and Wear Andrew (eds.), *Problems and Methods in the History of Medicine*, London, Croom Helm, 1987.

Premuda Loris, «La naissance des spécialités», in *Histoire de la pensée médicale en Occident*, vol. 3, Paris, Seuil, 1999, pp. 253–269.

Prod'hom Louis-Samuel, Clavel Anne-Marie and Hamel J.P., «L'hôpital universitaire: hier-aujourd'hui-demain», *Revue médicale de la Suisse romande*, 1991, pp. 45–58.

Reverby Susan, «Stealing the Golden Eggs: Ernest Amory Codman and the Science and Management of Medicine», *Bulletin of the History of Medicine*, 1981, pp. 156–171.

De Riedmatten Soun, Rosetti Daniel and Fussinger Catherine, «La création de l'assurance maladie, un danger pour le corps médical? (1893–1911)», *Revue historique* vaudoise, 1995, pp. 247–292.

Rosen George, «Changing Attitudes of the Medical Profession to Specialization», *Bulletin of the History of Medicine*, 1942, pp. 343–354.

Rosenberg Charles, «Inward Vision and Outward Glance: The Shaping of the American Hospital, 1880–1914», in *Bulletin of the History of Medicine*, 1979, pp. 346–391.

Rosner David, *A Once Charitable Enterprise: Hospitals and Health Care in Brooklyn and New York, 1885–1915*, Cambridge, Cambridge University Press, 1982.

Saudan Guy (ed.), *L'éveil médical vaudois, 1750–1850, Tissot—Venel—Mayor*, Lausanne, Université, 1987.

Saudan Guy, «Dispensaire et policlinique à Lausanne: 100 ans de médecine et société», *Revue médicale de la Suisse romande*, 1989, pp. 267–277.

Schlich Thomas, *Surgery, Science and Industry: A Revolution in Fracture Care, 1950s–1990s*, Basingstoke, Palgrave Macmillan, 2002.

Shumsky Neil Larry, «The Municipal Clinic of San Francisco: A Study in Medical Structure», *Bulletin of the History of Medicine*, 1978, pp. 542–559.

Secrétan Claude, *L'hôpital de Cery, 1873–1973*, Lausanne, Payot, 1973.

Spree Reinhardt, «Krankenhasuentwicklung und Sozialpolitik in Deutschland während des 19. Jahrhunderts», *Historische Zeitschrift*, 1995, pp. 75–105.

Stanton Jennifer, «Making Sense of Technologies in Medicine», *Social History of Medicine*, 1999, pp. 437–448.

Stanton Jennifer (ed.), *Innovations in Health and Medicine: Diffusion and Resistance in the Twentieth Century*, New York, Routledge, 2002.

Starr Paul, *The Social Transformation of American Medicine: The Rise of a Sovereign Profession and the Making of a Vast Industry*, New York, Basic Books, 1982.

Sturdy Steve, «The Political Economy of Scientific Medicine: Science, Education and the Transformation of Medical Practice in Sheffield, 1890–1922», *Medical History*, 1992, pp. 125–159.

Terrier Georges, «Le Dr Fritz de Quervain à la Chaux-de-Fonds (1894–1910)», *Revue médicale de la Suisse romande*, 1998, pp. 193–201.

Tissot Laurent, *Politique, société et enseignement supérieur dans le canton de Vaud: L'Université de Lausanne, 1890–1916*, Lausanne, Payot, 1996.

Tröhler Ulrich, *Der Nobelpreisträger Theodor Kocher, 1841–1917. Auf dem Weg zur physiologischen Chirurgie*, Bâle, Birkhauser, 1984.

Ueyama Takahiro, «Capital, Profession and Medical Technology: The Electro-Therapeutic Institutes and the Royal College of Physicians, 1888–1922», *Medical History*, 1997, pp. 150–181.

Vilar-Rodríguez Margarita and Pons-Pons Jerònia, "The Historical Creation of the Hospital System in Spain: Private Hospital Sector Strategies in Relation to the Development of the Public System", in Martin Gorsky, Margarita Vilar-Rodríguez and Jerònia Pons-Pons (eds), *The Political Economy of the Hospital in History*, Huddersfield: University of Huddersfield Press, 2020, pp. 17–59.

Vogel Morris J., «The Transformation of American Hospital, 1850–1920», in Reverby S. and Rosner D. (eds.), *Health Care in America: Essays in Social History*, Philadelphia, 1979, pp. 105–116.
Vogel Morris J., «Managing Medicine: Creating a Profession of Hospital Administration in the United States, 1895–1915», in Granshaw Lindsay and Porter Roy (eds.), *Hospitals in History*, New-York, 1989, pp. 243–260.
Waddington Keir, *Charity and the London Hospitals, 1850–1898*, Woodbrifge, The Boydell Press, 2000.
Weisz George, «The Emergence of Medical Specialization in the Nineteenth Century», *Bulletin of the History of Medicine*, 2003, pp. 536–575.
Wisard François, *L'université vaudoise d'une guerre à l'autre: Politique, finances, refuge*, Lausanne, Payot, 1998.

FSC
www.fsc.org
MIX
Papier | Fördert gute Waldnutzung
FSC® C083411

Kolibri 360 GmbH
Ferdinand-Jühlke-Straße 7
99095 Erfurt, Deutschland
produktsicherheit@kolibri360.de